Atrial Fibrillation and Heart Failure

Editors

ANDREW A. GRACE
SANJIV M. NARAYAN
MARK D. O'NEILL

HEART FAILURE CLINICS

www.heartfailure.theclinics.com

Consulting Editors
MANDEEP R. MEHRA
JAVED BUTLER

Founding Editor
JAGAT NARULA

October 2013 • Volume 9 • Number 4

ELSEVIER

1600 John F. Kennedy Boulevard • Suite 1800 • Philadelphia, Pennsylvania, 19103-2899

http://www.theclinics.com

HEART FAILURE CLINICS Volume 9, Number 4
October 2013 ISSN 1551-7136, ISBN-13: 978-0-323-22720-9

Editor: Barbara Cohen-Kligerman
Developmental Editor: Susan Showalter

Heart Failure Clinics (ISSN 1551-7136) is published quarterly by Elsevier Inc., 360 Park Avenue South, New York, NY 10010-1710. Months of publication are January, April, July, and October. Business and editorial offices: 1600 John F. Kennedy Boulevard, Suite 1800, Philadelphia, PA 19103-2899. Periodicals postage paid at New York, NY, and additional mailing offices. Subscription prices are USD 235.00 per year for US individuals, USD 386.00 per year for US institutions, USD 80.00 per year for US students and residents, USD 280.00 per year for Canadian individuals, USD 442.00 per year for Canadian institutions, USD 300.00 per year for international individuals, USD 442.00 per year for international institutions, and USD 100.00 per year for Canadian and foreign students/residents. To receive student and resident rate, orders must be accompanied by name of affiliated institution, date of term, and the *signature* of program/residency coordinator on institution letterhead. Orders will be billed at individual rate until proof of status is received. Foreign air speed delivery is included in all *Clinics* subscription prices. All prices are subject to change without notice. **POSTMASTER:** Send address changes to *Heart Failure Clinics*, Elsevier Health Sciences Division, Subscription Customer Service, 3251 Riverport Lane, Maryland Heights, MO 63043. **Customer Service: 1-800-654-2452 (US and Canada). From outside of the US and Canada, call 314-447-8871. Fax: 314-447-8029. For print support, e-mail: JournalsCustomerService-usa@elsevier.com. For online support, e-mail: JournalsOnlineSupport-usa@elsevier.com.**

Reprints. For copies of 100 or more of articles in this publication, please contact the Commercial Reprints Department, Elsevier Inc., 360 Park Avenue South, New York, NY 10010-1710. Tel.: 212-633-3874; Fax: 212-633-3820; E-mail: reprints@elsevier.com.

Heart Failure Clinics is covered in *MEDLINE/PubMed (Index Medicus)*.

Printed in the United States of America.

Contributors

CONSULTING EDITORS

MANDEEP R. MEHRA, MD
Professor of Medicine, Harvard Medical School; Co-Director, BWH Cardiovascular; and Executive Director, Center for Advanced Heart Disease, Brigham and Women's Hospital, Boston, Massachusetts

JAVED BUTLER, MD, MPH
Professor of Medicine; Director, Heart Failure Research, Emory University, Atlanta, Georgia

EDITORS

ANDREW A. GRACE, MB, PhD, FRCP
Department of Biochemistry, University of Cambridge; Papworth Hospital, Cambridge, United Kingdom

SANJIV M. NARAYAN, MD, PhD, FRCP, FHRS
Professor of Medicine, Director of Electrophysiology, San Diego VA Healthcare System, University of California, San Diego, San Diego, California

MARK D. O'NEILL, DPhil, FRCP, FHRS
Consultant Cardiologist and Reader in Clinical Cardiac Electrophysiology, Divisions of Imaging Sciences and Biomedical Engineering and Cardiovascular Medicine, Medical Engineering Centre, St. Thomas' Hospital, London, United Kingdom

AUTHORS

ISSAM H. ABU-TAHA, PhD
Faculty of Medicine, Institute of Pharmacology, University Duisburg-Essen, Essen, Germany

AYOTUNDE BAMIMORE, MB, ChB
Electrophysiology Fellow/Clinical Instructor, Division of Cardiology, University of North Carolina, Chapel Hill, Chapel Hill, North Carolina

S. SERGE BAROLD, MD, FACC, FAHA, FHRS
Clinical Professor of Medicine Emeritus, University of Rochester School of Medicine and Dentistry, Rochester, New York

JOHN G.F. CLELAND, MD, FRCP, FACC, FESC
Department of Cardiology, Castle Hill Hospital, Hull York Medical School, University of Hull, Kingston-upon-Hull, United Kingdom

EUGENE C. DEPASQUALE, MD
Clinical Instructor, Ahmanson-UCLA Cardiomyopathy Center, David Geffen School of Medicine, Los Angeles, California

BENJAMIN DICKEN, MBBS, MRCP
Department of Cardiology, Castle Hill Hospital, Hull York Medical School, University of Hull, Kingston-upon-Hull, United Kingdom

DOBROMIR DOBREV, MD
Faculty of Medicine, Institute of Pharmacology, University Duisburg-Essen, Essen; Division of Experimental Cardiology, Medical Faculty Mannheim, Heidelberg University; DZHK (German Centre for Cardiovascular Research) partner site Mannheim/Heidelberg, Mannheim, Germany

GREGG C. FONAROW, MD
Eliot Corday Professor of Cardiovascular
Medicine and Science, Co-Chief of Clinical
Cardiology, UCLA Division of Cardiology,
Director, Ahmanson-UCLA Cardiomyopathy
Center, David Geffen School of Medicine,
Los Angeles, California

DARREL P. FRANCIS, FRCP, MD
International Centre for Circulatory Health,
National Heart and Lung Institute, Imperial
College London, London, United Kingdom

ANDREAS GOETTE, MD
Department of Cardiology and Intensive Care
Medicine, St. Vincenz Hospital Paderborn
GmbH, EUTRAF Working Group, University
Hospital Magdeburg, Paderborn, Germany

ANDREW A. GRACE, MB, PhD, FRCP
Department of Biochemistry, University of
Cambridge; Papworth Hospital, Cambridge,
United Kingdom

PATRICK M. HECK, BM BCh
Department of Cardiology, Papworth Hospital,
Papworth Everard, Cambridge, United Kingdom

JORDI HEIJMAN, PhD
Faculty of Medicine, Institute of Pharmacology,
University Duisburg-Essen, Essen, Germany

BENGT HERWEG, MD, FACC, FHRS
Associate Professor of Medicine, Director,
Electrophysiology and Arrhythmia Services,
Department of Cardiovascular Disease,
University of South Florida Morsani College of
Medicine, Tampa, Florida

FREIDOON KESHAVARZI, MD, MRCP
Department of Cardiology, Castle Hill Hospital,
Hull York Medical School, University of Hull,
Kingston-upon-Hull, United Kingdom

SENTHIL KIRUBAKARAN, MRCP, MD
Cardiothoracic Department, Guy's and St
Thomas' NHS Trust, London, United Kingdom

PETER M. KISTLER, MBBS, PhD
Associate Professor, Department of
Cardiology, Baker IDI, Melbourne; Department
of Cardiovascular Medicine, Alfred Heart
Centre, Alfred Hospital, Baker IDI Heart and
Diabetes Institute, University of Melbourne,
Victoria, Australia

**STEPHEN R. LARGE, MA, MS, FRCS,
FRCP, MBA**
Papworth Hospital, Cambridge,
United Kingdom

JUSTIN M.S. LEE, BM BCh
Department of Cardiology, Papworth
Hospital, Papworth Everard, Cambridge,
United Kingdom

GREGORY Y.H. LIP, MD
Professor of Cardiovascular Medicine,
University of Birmingham Centre
for Cardiovascular Sciences, City
Hospital, Birmingham, West Midlands,
United Kingdom

**PAUL MOUNSEY, BSc, BM BCh, PhD,
MRCP, FACC**
Chief of Electrophysiology and Professor of
Medicine, Division of Cardiology, University of
North Carolina, Chapel Hill, Chapel Hill,
North Carolina

SANJIV M. NARAYAN, MD, PhD
Professor of Medicine, Director of
Electrophysiology, San Diego VA Healthcare
System, University of California, San Diego,
San Diego, California

SAMER A.M. NASHEF, MB ChB, FRCS, PhD
Papworth Hospital, Cambridge,
United Kingdom

MARK D. O'NEILL, DPhil, FRCP, FHRS
Consultant Cardiologist and Reader in
Clinical Cardiac Electrophysiology,
Divisions of Imaging Sciences and
Biomedical Engineering and Cardiovascular
Medicine, Medical Engineering Centre,
St. Thomas' Hospital, London,
United Kingdom

PIERPAOLO PELLICORI, MD
Department of Cardiology, Castle Hill Hospital,
Hull York Medical School, University of Hull,
Kingston-upon-Hull, United Kingdom

MICHIEL RIENSTRA, MD, PhD
Department of Cardiology, University Medical
Center Groningen, University of Groningen,
Groningen, The Netherlands

EDUARD SHANTSILA, PhD
Research Fellow, University of Birmingham Centre for Cardiovascular Sciences, City Hospital, Birmingham, West Midlands, United Kingdom

JAGMEET P. SINGH, MD, PhD, DPhil
Cardiac Arrhythmia Service, Massachusetts General Hospital, Associate Professor of Medicine, Harvard Medical School, Boston, Massachusetts

NITESH SOOD, MD
Division of Cardiology, Lahey Clinic, Tufts University, Burlington, Massachusetts

JONATHAN S. STEINBERG, MD, FACC, FHRS
Director, Arrhythmia Institute, Valley Health System, Ridgewood, New Jersey; Professor of Medicine, Columbia University College of Physicians and Surgeons, New York, New York

ISABELLE C. VAN GELDER, MD, PhD
Department of Cardiology, University Medical Center Groningen, University of Groningen, Groningen, The Netherlands

ESZTER M. VEGH, MD
Cardiac Arrhythmia Service, Massachusetts General Hospital, Harvard Medical School, Boston, Massachusetts

NIELS VOIGT, MD
Faculty of Medicine, Institute of Pharmacology, University Duisburg-Essen, Essen; Division of Experimental Cardiology, Medical Faculty Mannheim, Heidelberg University, Mannheim, Germany

ZACHARY I. WHINNETT, BMedSci, BMBS, MRCP, PhD
International Centre for Circulatory Health, National Heart and Lung Institute, Imperial College London, London, United Kingdom

Contents

The prevalence of both chronic heart failure and atrial fibrillation is increasing as a result of systemic multimorbid risk and improved therapy of acute heart disease. Current treatment options are unsatisfactory especially regarding antiarrhythmic drugs. We propose that a systems biology approach to increase understanding of cardiac arrhythmias offers the best immediate way forward. Such an approach would be based on an accumulation of large clinical datasets, and application of next-generation sequencing in conjunction with selected experimental and computer-based models. Such an approach would in turn facilitate the development and targeted application of currently available and novel therapeutic approaches.

In patients with atrial fibrillation (AF) undergoing cardiac resynchronization therapy (CRT) for heart failure, continuous monitoring of the percentage of biventricular (BiV%) pacing has shown that the greatest improvement and reduction in mortality occur with a BiV pacing greater than 98%. Continuous monitoring of BiV pacing has improved the CRT management of patients with AF. Continuous monitoring has generated important new questions about anticoagulant therapy, which require randomized trials. Anticoagulant therapy should probably be considered in patients who have a high risk of thromboembolism according to standard scoring systems.

In the last few years, there has been a major shift in the treatment of atrial fibrillation (AF) in the setting of hear failure (HF), from rhythm to ventricular rate control in most patients with both conditions. In this article, the authors focus on ventricular rate control and discuss the indications; the optimal ventricular rate-control target, including detailed results of the Rate Control Efficacy in Permanent Atrial Fibrillation: a Comparison Between Lenient versus Strict Rate Control II (RACE II) study; and the pharmacologic and nonpharmacologic options to control the ventricular rate during AF in the setting of HF.

Atrial fibrillation (AF) and heart failure (HF) are common cardiovascular pathologies with severe prognostic implications that show bidirectional interactions. Rate and rhythm control are the main therapeutic strategies for patients with AF and HF. There is a paucity of safe and effective antiarrhythmic drugs for rhythm control of AF in HF, with amiodarone and (in the United States) dofetilide as the only imperfect options. The basic mechanisms of AF are discussed and the evidence and limitations of AF rhythm control options for patients with HF are reviewed. In addition, novel potential antiarrhythmic strategies for rhythm control of AF are highlighted.

Atrial fibrillation (AF) is a common arrhythmia that occurs as the result of various pathophysiologic processes. Heart failure increases the likelihood of AF. Several aspects of the morphologic and electrophysiologic alterations promoting AF in heart failure (congestive heart failure [CHF]) have been studied in animal models and patients with CHF. Under these conditions, ectopic activity originating from the pulmonary veins or other sites is more likely to occur and trigger longer episodes of AF. This article summarizes the impact of angiotensin-converting enzyme inhibitors, angiotensin II receptor blockers and statins, so-called upstream therapy, in patients who have CHF with AF.

Heart failure and atrial fibrillation are major problems of modern cardiology with important clinical, prognostic, and socioeconomic implications. The risks are high morbidity, impaired quality of life, poor outcome, and increased risk of stroke. Oral anticoagulation with vitamin K antagonists or novel licensed medicines should be considered unless contraindicated. Possible benefits of sinus rhythm maintenance are not entirely clear and need to be explored further. Relatively scarce data are available on stroke prevention in atrial fibrillation in heart failure with preserved ejection fraction; this requires further research.

The prevalence of atrial fibrillation (AF) and heart failure increases with advancing age. It is estimated that the annual incidence of AF in the general heart failure population is approximately 5%, whereas as many as 40% of patients with advanced heart failure have AF. The goals of therapy in patients with heart failure and AF are symptom control and prevention of arterial thromboembolism. The adverse hemodynamic events of AF may lead to symptom deterioration and reduced exercise capacity. This review addresses the impact of AF on heart failure outcomes as they pertain to prognosis and management.

Atrial fibrillation (AF) is an important and often-underrecognized cause of cardiovascular morbidity and mortality. It is an arrhythmia that is commonly seen in the older patient; the median age of patients with AF in early studies was 75 years. Heart failure (HF) is also more frequently seen in the older patient with an approximate doubling of HF prevalence with each decade of life. There is clear interaction between

AF and HF, with evidence that HF can lead to AF and AF exacerbates HF. This review focuses on the specific aspect of AF management in elderly patients with HF.

Case Selection for Cardiac Resynchronization in Atrial Fibrillation

John G.F. Cleland, Freidoon Keshavarzi, Pierpaolo Pellicori, and Benjamin Dicken

Remarkably little evidence exists that cardiac resynchronization therapy (CRT) is effective in patients who have atrial fibrillation (AF) but who otherwise seem suitable for this treatment. The landmark trials of CRT generally excluded patients with AF because atrioventricular (AV) resynchronization was considered a possibly important mechanism by which CRT might deliver its benefits. The only landmark trial that included many patients with AF confirmed marked benefit among patients in sinus rhythm but no benefit among those with AF. Evidence is lacking that biventricular rather than AV resynchronization is an important mechanism for delivering the benefits of CRT.

Cardiac Resynchronization Therapy Mechanisms in Atrial Fibrillation

Zachary I. Whinnett and Darrel P. Francis

This article examines how to assess the reliability of potential techniques for performing optimization of biventricular pacemakers in patients with atrial fibrillation. It explores the magnitude of improvement that is likely to be obtained with the optimization of biventricular pacing in this clinical setting and discusses the lessons that can be learned with regard to the mechanisms of action of biventricular pacing in the general heart failure population.

The Role of Ablation of the Atrioventricular Junction in Patients with Heart Failure and Atrial Fibrillation

Eszter M. Vegh, Nitesh Sood, and Jagmeet P. Singh

Ablation of the atrioventricular junction (AVJ) is a technically easy procedure that is safe and has a high success rate as an intervention for effective ventricular rate control in patients in symptomatic atrial fibrillation. AVJ ablation has been reported to improve quality of life, left ventricular ejection fraction, and exercise duration in these patients and minimize the incidence of inappropriate shocks. Because right ventricular pacing after AVJ ablation may result in decrease in left ventricular function and worsening of heart failure symptoms, there is increasing evidence to support the effectiveness of cardiac resynchronization therapy in atrial fibrillation populations.

Ablation of Atrial Tachycardia and Atrial Flutter in Heart Failure

Ayotunde Bamimore and Paul Mounsey

Atrial tachycardia and atrial flutter are common tachyarrhythmias in the heart failure population. They commonly lead to, exacerbate, and increase the morbidity and mortality associated with heart failure and, thereby, warrant urgent and early definitive therapy in the form of catheter ablation. Catheter ablation requires careful patient stabilization and extensive preprocedural planning, particularly with regards to anesthesia, strategy, catheter choice, mapping system, and fluid balance, to increase efficacy and limit adverse effects. Heart failure may limit the success of catheter ablation with higher reported recurrence rates, and in selected patients, a hybrid epicardial-endocardial ablation can be considered.

Atrial fibrillation in the presence of heart failure is an independent predictor of mortality and is associated with increased hospitalizations and worsening New York Heart Association functional class. Despite these associations, large-scale trials have not shown a benefit in rhythm restoration. However, further analysis of these trials showed that patients who remained in sinus rhythm did have improved survival rates. Studies to examine the efficacy of catheter ablation of atrial fibrillation were therefore conducted and reported efficacy rates ranging from 50% to 92% at maintaining sinus rhythm with associated improvements in left ventricular ejection fraction, quality of life, and New York Heart Association functional class.

Surgery to correct a structural heart valve problem can restore sinus rhythm in approximately one-fifth of patients with atrial fibrillation (AF), and the addition of a maze procedure will increase this proportion. Evidence shows that the maze procedure may restore atrial function in some patients and may have beneficial effects on functional symptoms and prognosis. The role of the maze procedure as an isolated treatment for lone AF in the context of heart failure with no structurally correctable cause is unknown. Future progress will determine the appropriate indications for treatment and the risks and benefits of any intervention.

HEART FAILURE CLINICS

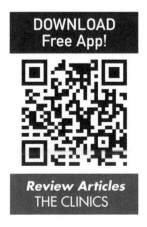

NOW AVAILABLE FOR YOUR iPhone and iPad

Foreword
Atrial Fibrillation and Heart Failure: It Takes Two to Tango

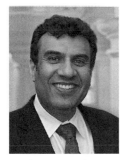
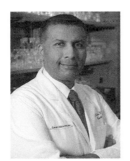

Mandeep R. Mehra, MD   Javed Butler, MD, MPH
Consulting Editors

Even as we celebrate control of preclinical risk markers such as hypertension, endorse campaigns to reduce adverse cardiovascular consequences of tobacco, and gain comfort in strategies to target episodes of crises such as sudden death and acute coronary syndromes, the growing combined burden of atrial fibrillation and heart failure remains a gnawing sore. It is estimated that unless tackled meticulously by 2050, the epidemics of atrial fibrillation and heart failure will gulp down the cardiovascular economic resources and create a frightening combined morbidity.

Atrial fibrillation can cause heart failure by reducing atrial contribution to cardiac output and decreasing diastolic filling time (including influencing myocardial coronary blood flow). This may be of particular importance among patients with heart failure and preserved ejection fraction. If the rapid heart rates are left unchecked, tachycardia-induced cardiomyopathy can result. Heart failure can raise intra-atrial filling pressures, stimulate stretch-induced fibrosis, and promote aberrant cellular signaling that can perpetuate atrial fibrillation even further, rendering it difficult to treat. The neurohormonal milieu activated in heart failure has been shown to induce these very structural cellular and tissue changes in the atria that set up the nidus for a complex interplay between these two syndromes.

Thus, it is not at all surprising that the onset of atrial fibrillation in the journey of heart failure syndromes signals an adverse prognosis and decreases the quality of life for our patients. Therapy targeted as an anti-arrhythmic can often destabilize the heart failure syndrome by promoting pro-arrhythmia and negative myocardial effects. Similarly, the presence of heart failure reduces the effectiveness of such therapy and the ability to optimally titrate treatment to control the arrhythmia. Complex therapeutics and smaller gains have propelled the scientific community to seek mechanical treatment options using ablative techniques with variable success.

Heart Failure Clin 9 (2013) xiii–xiv
http://dx.doi.org/10.1016/j.hfc.2013.08.001
1551-7136/13/$ – see front matter © 2013 Elsevier Inc. All rights reserved.

Also, considering the increased risk of stroke in those patients, recent research has also focused on developing novel drugs and devices that are more effective or have a better safety profile for stroke prevention in atrial fibrillation.

In this timely issue of *Heart Failure Clinics*, the combined editorial force of Drs Andrew A. Grace, Sanjiv M. Narayan, and Mark D. O'Neill bring to our readers an extraordinary compilation of articles that outline the current and future challenges in this arena. We invite you to review their thoughtful coverage of this issue in a "one-stop shop" of the state of art in this evolving important field.

Mandeep R. Mehra, MD
Center for Advanced Heart Disease
Brigham and Women's Hospital
75 Francis Street
A Building, 3rd Floor, Room AB324
Boston, MA 02115, USA

Javed Butler, MD, MPH
Emory Clinical Cardiovascular Research Institute
1462 Clifton Road NE, Suite 504
Atlanta, GA 30322, USA

E-mail addresses:
MMEHRA@partners.org (M.R. Mehra)
javed.butler@emory.edu (J. Butler)

Preface
Atrial Fibrillation and Heart Failure

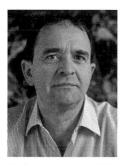

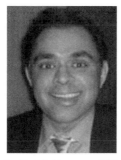

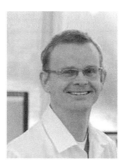

Andrew A. Grace, MB, PhD, FRCP

Sanjiv M. Narayan, MD, PhD, FRCP, FHRS

Mark D. O'Neill, DPhil, FRCP, FHRS

Editors

Atrial fibrillation and heart failure each have major medical impact. The substantial scale of their independent influence on morbidity, mortality, and public health has however only been appreciated recently. This realization has already had population benefit with improved early detection and prophylaxis against stroke and progressive pump failure.

Their frequent coexistence, while long recognized, adds new layers to management decisions and the situations that can then arise are addressed in this volume. Our target audience are the subscribers to the *Heart Failure Clinics* series and the objective has been to enhance patient care. The authors of individual articles, while mostly having as their primary interest cardiac arrhythmia, actually represent a broad diversity of interests and talents and present contrasting but complementary perspectives.

The prevalence of atrial fibrillation and heart failure will continue to rise and treatment options are set to expand. Accordingly, the complexity of the decisions for this group is set to increase. It is hoped that the perspectives in this issue will assist the broader community in making the smartest, most effective choices to achieve the very best in patient care.

Andrew A. Grace, MB, PhD, FRCP
Department of Biochemistry
University of Cambridge
Hopkins Building, Tennis Court Road
CB2 1QW, UK
Papworth Hospital
Cambridge CB23 3RE, UK

Sanjiv M. Narayan, MD, PhD, FRCP, FHRS
San Diego VA Healthcare System
University of California, San Diego
3350 La Jolla Village Drive
San Diego, CA 92161, USA

Mark D. O'Neill, DPhil, FRCP, FHRS
Divisions of Imaging Sciences & Biomedical
Engineering & Cardiovascular Medicine
Medical Engineering Centre
3rd Floor, Lambeth Wing
St. Thomas' Hospital
London SE1 7EH, UK

E-mail addresses:
aag1000@cam.ac.uk (A.A. Grace)
snarayan@ucsd.edu (S.M. Narayan)
mark.oneill@kcl.ac.uk (M.D. O'Neill)

http://dx.doi.org/10.1016/j.hfc.2013.08.002

Common Threads in Atrial Fibrillation and Heart Failure

Andrew A. Grace, MB, PhD, FRCP[a,b],*,
Sanjiv M. Narayan, MD, PhD[c]

KEYWORDS

- Chronic heart failure • Atrial fibrillation • Systems biology • Genetics • Genomics • Remodeling

KEY POINTS

- The prevalence of both chronic heart failure and atrial fibrillation is increasing as a result of systemic *multimorbid* risk and improved therapy of acute heart disease.
- Atrial and ventricular tissues are exposed to the same toxicities but the time-dependent responses of different chambers in individuals while apparently idiosyncratic are likely to have an intrinsic/genetic determination.
- Current treatment options are unsatisfactory, especially regarding the availability of effective and safe antiarrhythmic drugs.
- The proposal is that a *systems biology* approach to increase understanding of cardiac arrhythmias offers the best immediate way forward. Such an approach would be based on an accumulation of large clinical datasets, and application of next-generation sequencing in conjunction with selected experimental and computer-based models. Such an approach would in turn facilitate the development and targeted application of currently available and novel therapeutic approaches.

INTRODUCTION

Chronic heart failure (CHF) and atrial fibrillation (AF) are inextricably linked and usually the phenotypic outcome of an exposure to common risks.[1–4] Accordingly, a principal thread is that they each represent chamber-specific expressions of a more global disease of cardiac muscle. The relative contribution of atrial versus ventricular manifestations in an individual is then founded on a combination of intrinsic genetic and acquired/epigenetic influences.[5–8]

When primary clinical expression of disease affects the ventricles, symptoms are likely to be those of pump failure.[9–11] Alternatively, if the primary expression is atrial, then rhythm disturbance will probably be the first thing that brings an individual to the physician's attention.[1,12] Of course it has been recognized for some time that the first presentation in 30% to 35% of patients with CHF may also include explicit clinical evidence of AF.[13,14] Nevertheless, whatever the primary clinical evidence, we propose that this will be only the most obvious expression of disease and

The British Heart Foundation, the Medical Research Council, the Wellcome Trust, and the Biotechnology and Biological Research Council, UK supports A.A. Grace. S.M. Narayan is supported by grants from the National Institutes of Health (R01 HL83359, K24 HL103800).

Commercial and Funding Relationships: A.A. Grace is Founder and equity holder in Electus Medical Inc, Consultant to Medtronic Inc and Xention Ltd. S.M. Narayan is equity holder in Topera Medical Inc, and reports having received honoraria from Medtronic, St. Jude Medical, and Biotronik.

[a] Department of Biochemistry, University of Cambridge, Hopkins Building, Tennis Court Road, Cambridge CB2 1QW, UK; [b] Papworth Hospital, Cambridge CB23 3RE, UK; [c] San Diego VA Healthcare System, University of California, San Diego, 3350 La Jolla Village Drive, San Diego, CA 92161, USA

* Corresponding author. Department of Biochemistry, University of Cambridge, Hopkins Building, Tennis Court Road, Cambridge CB2 1QW, UK.

E-mail address: aag1000@cam.ac.uk

Heart Failure Clin 9 (2013) 373–383
http://dx.doi.org/10.1016/j.hfc.2013.07.011
1551-7136/13/$ – see front matter © 2013 Elsevier Inc. All rights reserved.

in fact contractile and electrical reserve will likely be compromised across all compartments essentially from the outset. Of course when electrical failure (fibrillation) is the first expression of ventricular disease (which most likely will arise at some point in the natural history in fully 50% of patients with CHF), then survival is unlikely unless prompt defibrillation is applied.[10]

After initial presentation, the clinical picture evolves over time based on differential and/or specific chamber remodeling that varies widely among individuals.[15–18] Of course, once patients present with symptoms, drugs will be prescribed that again interface with underlying disease processes to modify progression and the consequences for atrial versus ventricular clinical expression.[1] Disease progress will also be based on the presence and continuing activity of risk factors.[5,19,20]

In this article, we introduce this issue by concentrating on those clinically relevant overlapping mechanisms of disease common to both AF and CHF. The mechanisms more apposite to CHF alone have been covered previously in other contributions in this series and elsewhere.[16]

COEXISTENCE AND RISING PREVALENCE

Approximately 40% of individuals presenting with either CHF or AF will develop clinical evidence of the other condition during further periods of observation.[13] The prevalence of the 2 conditions is rising,[21] but although the incidence of AF continues to rise, CHF incidence may be starting to plateau.[10,21]

Heart failure as a primary diagnosis tends to present in the older population and affects in broad terms 10% of men and 8% of women older than 60 years,[10] with the prevalence of CHF likely to rise to more than 750,000 in the United States over the next 4 decades.[21] AF has a prevalence again in the United States that is currently estimated in the range of 2.7 to 6.1 million, and is anticipated to rise inexorably, with estimates reaching 16 million by 2050.[22] This upward trend is also consistently seen in Europe and elsewhere.[23,24] In the prospective Framingham Heart Study, 1470 participants developed either new AF or new CHF, with 383 (26%) developing both.[13] What is clear is that the more advanced the clinical CHF, the greater is its association with AF (**Fig. 1**).[25] The overall prevalence of AF in CHF is in the range of 13% to 27%.[1,12]

The nature of the relationship between AF and CHF, however, is complex and case specific.[1,4,12] On occasion there will be a common setting for both, such as the individual with dilated cardiomyopathy who presents with AF.[12] In other cases, CHF, for example due to an ST elevation myocardial infarction, may lead secondarily to AF. From the practical clinical standpoint, it is prudent to assume that all patients will have the potential to develop the other condition given time.[1]

COINCIDENT RISK FACTORS

The common etiologic thread linking the coincidence of AF and CHF is that each arises in response to an accumulated exposure of cardiac muscle to a common set of "cardiovascular" risk factors.[5,8,26] These comorbid risks tend to increase with age, thereby explaining the age-related increase in prevalence of each phenotype.[19,27] The simple proposition is that "acquired" conditions,

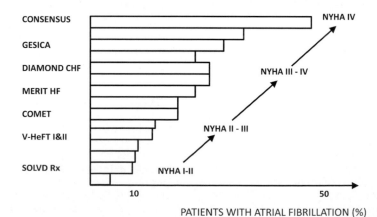

Fig. 1. Atrial fibrillation in patients with symptomatic heart failure: prevalence of atrial fibrillation related to New York Heart Association symptomatic classification in various clinical studies. These relationships highlight the relationship but raise issues of causality and mechanism. (*Adapted from* Savelieva I, John Camm A. Atrial fibrillation and heart failure: natural history and pharmacologic treatment. Europace 2004;5(Suppl 1):S5–19; with permission.)

including hypertension, diabetes, and chronic renal disease, interact with an underlying genetic susceptibility of the individual cardiac chambers, leading to disease expression.[8] The general background risk is therefore set by the increasingly prevalent chronic disease state of *multimorbidity* exposing vulnerable individuals to the development of a disease complex affecting all the cardiac chambers, albeit to a variable clinically explicit extent.[20]

Genetic Variants

Some well-described *monogenic* variants can result in both AF and CHF.[8,12] These include familial cardiomyopathies,[12] laminopathies[28] and some ion channel variants (eg, mutations in the *cardiac sodium channel gene, SCN5A*), that can result in both a cardiomyopathic phenotype and AF.[29,30] Although these combinations are relatively rare, they provide insights into "common" CHF by demonstrating the sheer impact of genetic variants on disease expression.[8,19,31]

There are a number of well-described genetic determinants of AF.[7,8,19,30] In this context, the familial occurrence of AF is clear and having an affected parent leads to a doubling of risks in offspring.[8] Ion channel genes are strongly implicated in some families with AF, and patients with ion channel diseases have an increased risk of AF.[8,19] Although there have been practical difficulties in the genetic elucidation of AF, a number of susceptibility alleles have been identified.[7,8,19] Genetic sequence variants at chromosomal location 4q25, representing a noncoding region with the nearest candidate gene being *Pitx2c*, have been strongly associated with AF.[7,32] The relative importance of the interaction between such variants and CHF phenotypes remains the subject of intense study.

Conversely, genetic influences on "common" CHF have been somewhat elusive.[33] Candidate gene studies have identified polymorphic variants that modify risk and are associated with disease progression.[33] Many of these variants encode receptors or the postreceptor cell-signaling machinery of the sympathetic and renin-angiotensin pathways.[33]

It seems highly likely that the capacity to develop either ventricular pump disease or AF in the face of a range of insults will be essentially person specific and determined by the carriage of genetic modifiers.[8,19,31,33] We would therefore anticipate that next-generation sequencing applied to large, well-phenotyped populations will provide genetic/genomic insights of practical value to personalized disease management.[19,31]

Coronary Heart Disease

The direct association of coronary disease with AF is modest,[8] with much of the association being indirect following, for example, myocardial infarction.[12] Coronary disease is, however, the main cause of CHF through both direct and rather more indirect routes.[10] Indeed, substantially improved management of acute coronary disease is a major driver of the current prevalence of CHF,[9,10] with individuals receiving effective immediate coronary intervention likely for all practical purposes to remain at risk of subsequent cardiac muscle attrition and possible CHF.[10] In the wake of an acute coronary event, other manifestations of heart disease dependent on intrinsic susceptibility to, respectively, AF, pump failure, and ventricular fibrillation are all possible.[19]

Obesity and Other Metabolic Factors

Metabolic disease represents a clear and present threat to worldwide public health.[34] Accordingly, whereas hypertension remains a prominent risk factor for CHF and AF, obesity is now also a clearly proven important risk for the development of both.[35,36] In a large community-based sample, obese subjects had an approximately doubling of the risk of CHF.[35] Similarly, for AF, the Framingham Heart Study estimated that obesity was associated with a 50% increase in the risk of AF,[36] further supported from Olmsted County where obesity accounted for 60% of the enhanced age-adjusted and sex-adjusted increase in AF incidence.[22] Furthermore, the Women's Health Study documented both a linear association between body mass index (BMI) and AF, and also that short-term changes in BMI were associated with AF risk.[37] Although some of the influences of obesity may be hemodynamic, such as through impaired ventricular relaxation or atrial stretch, more direct metabolic effects also seem likely (see later in this article).[19]

CONVENTIONAL INTERPRETATIONS OF MECHANISM

Widely diverse presentations and patterns of disease development are well-recognized features of both AF and CHF.[1,4,12] Unsurprisingly, the range of behaviors, emerging clinical scenarios, and complexity expands considerably when both conditions coexist.[1] These characteristics of heterogeneity have served to limit recruitment to clinical studies and thus slowed the acquisition of robust practically useful clinical trial–based data.[1,8]

Initial presentations of combined AF and CHF, although usually occurring against a background of a systemic predisposition, can have a more cardiac-specific trigger, such as acute myocardial infarction or myocarditis.[4,12] In patients presenting with rapidly conducted AF, if the rate remains uncontrolled, then an undefined proportion may go on to develop CHF through the well-recognized clinical progression that defines tachycardiopathy.[12] Conversely, in those with severe pump failure, AF may well supervene, although similarly this is not always the case.[13] These variations in the clinical course support an intrinsic susceptibility in the different chambers.[15,19,26]

Impact of Rate, Rhythm, and Stretch

The intuitive view is that AF can damage the ventricles through junctional transmission of rapid irregular impulses,[12] with the reaction appearing idiosyncratic with no obvious threshold/cutoff in terms of rates/durations.[4,12] Conversely, if the ventricles are failing, then they, in their turn, can negatively influence the atria through their failure to empty and reduced diastolic filling times (Fig. 2).[12,38] The evidence to support these various views comes from a range of clinical observations and experimental models.[12,15,16,39,40] This bidirectional clinical interaction will be further influenced through systemic effects arising as a result of the circulation being compromised in the face of rapid rates and/or impaired hemodynamics.

Atrial damage in response to a loss of normal ventricular function is generally thought to arise fundamentally through the actions of atrial "stretch."[1,12,26,39,40] The most prevalent idea is that stretch-activated channels, usually membrane bound, play a key role with downstream alterations

in calcium signaling, action potential shortening, and an increased dispersion of refractoriness.[1,26,40] In addition, at the physically observable level, atrial chamber dilatation increases the endocardial surface area (critical mass) that may further facilitate both the initiation and perpetuation of fibrillation.[41] In rabbit hearts, gadolinium and tarantula toxin extract have been shown to inhibit some of these processes.[42] In sheep atria, stretch increased both the rate of AF and facilitated the conduction of rapid activity from the pulmonary veins to the left atrial body,[43] with reversal of stretch being potentially antiarrhythmic.[44]

Systemic Influences

The interest in metabolic determinants of arrhythmias is increasing.[19,45,46] The common cumulative exposure of atria and ventricles to metabolic risks activate highly promiscuous biologic pathways.[17,19] Indeed, inflammatory pathways invoked in vascular and ventricular disease have significant importance for AF.[47,48] Oxidative stress has been strongly implicated as a mechanism for human AF,[47,49,50] with transcriptomes/metabolomes showing coordinated downregulation of enzymes controlling fatty acid oxidation.[16,45] In addition, the propensity to canine AF directly correlates to cellular bioenergetic status[26] and mice with cardiac-specific Rac1GTPase overexpression and AF have activated nicotinamide adenine dinucleotide phosphate (NADPH) oxidase.[51] Furthermore, it has now been shown that DNA from degraded mitochondria promotes inflammation, leading to myocellular damage and CHF, with likely implications for the pathogenesis

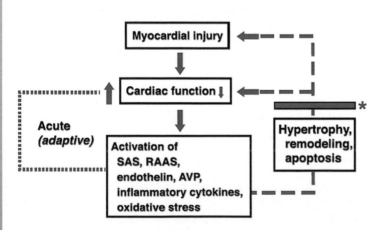

Fig. 2. Interplay between cardiac function and neurohumoral and cytokine systems. Myocardial injury, which may have any of a number of causes, might depress cardiac function, which in turn may cause activation of the sympathoadrenal system (SAS) and the renin-angiotensin-aldosterone system (RAAS) and the elaboration of endothelin, arginine vasopressin (AVP), and cytokines, such as tumor necrosis factor-α. In acute heart failure (left), these are adaptive and tend to maintain arterial pressure and cardiac function. In chronic heart failure (right), they cause maladaptive hypertrophic remodeling and apoptosis, which cause further atrial and ventricular injury and impairment of cardiac function with electrophysiological consequences. The horizontal line on the right shows that chronic maladaptive influences can be inhibited by angiotensin-converting enzyme inhibitors, β-adrenergic blockers, angiotensin II type 1 receptor blockers, and/or aldosterone antagonists. *, one proposed area of intervention to block remodeling. (From Braunwald E. Heart failure. JACC Heart Fail 2013;1:1–20; with permission.)

of AF (**Fig. 3**).[52,53] Additionally, mitochondria have been proposed as an appropriate target for drug intervention in CHF.[54] In sum, the body of biologic evidence supporting the importance of metabolism linking epidemiologic observations through mechanisms to clinical outcomes is now substantial.[19,36,46]

Structural and Electrical Remodeling

At a multicellular tissue level, physiologic substrates for pump failure and arrhythmogenesis evolve over time.[15,16,39] Several components of electrical remodeling are analogous between atria and ventricles: for instance, the calcium overload that characterizes ventricular phenotypes has also been described in the atria.[15,55] Although it was originally thought that functional substrates for AF were defined simply by shortened action potentials and hence abbreviated refractoriness,[39,56] it has since been recognized that structural changes ensue with scarring and fibrosis.[57] Temporal evolution of these derangements is collectively termed "remodeling," during which the relative contributions of functional and anatomic aspects of the substrate to AF change.[15,26] Remodeling shows wide interindividual variation governed by many factors (eg, genetic, individual behavior, epigenetic, and the responses to administered treatment).[19,26,40] Rapid rates undoubtedly promote remodeling in both atria and ventricles, and indeed have been used to generate animals prone to both CHF and AF.[16,40]

Although clinicians clearly recognize remodeling in their patients, the underlying biology remains poorly understood.[15,58] Some patients progress from relatively infrequent runs of self-terminating AF to more persistent patterns over relatively short time frames, whereas in others, clinical evidence of arrhythmia may even regress.[59] Similarly, as presented previously, the ventricle in some patients may be compromised quickly, whereas others may sustain exposure to rapid rates with no obvious sequelae for long periods.[1,12]

Atrial Structural and Functional Remodeling

Structural abnormalities of the atria may be linked even more tightly with atrial fibrillation than previously recognized.[4,16,40,57,60] One recent notable histologic study in humans indicated, for example, that the extent of atrial fibrosis was not directly associated with age, as previously highlighted,[61–63] but instead with the presence and severity of AF.[64] During AF in failing hearts, there is a heterogeneous distribution of fibrosis at the posterior left atrial wall that likely influences dynamic pattern of AF activation and signal complexity.[65] However, although a clear relationship has been identified between the presence of late gadolinium enhancement in the atrium and responses to AF therapy,[66] the relationship between structural remodeling of the atrium and left ventricular function has yet to be established.[66] Intriguingly, transcriptomic studies indicate a

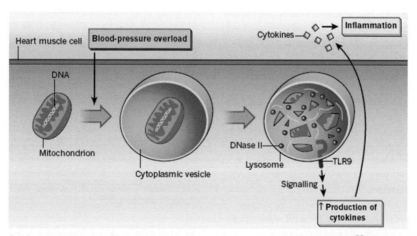

Fig. 3. Mitochodrial DNA induces inflammation and heart failure: Oka and colleagues[52] carried out experiments in mice that suggest a possible mechanism contributing to heart failure. Various processes that put stress on the heart, such as blood-pressure overload, may damage mitochondria in heart muscle cells. These mitochondria are engulfed into cytoplasmic vesicles and transported to lysosomes (intracellular organelles in which mitochondrial components are digested by various enzymes, such as DNase II, which degrades DNA). If mitochondrial DNA accumulates, then the protein TLR9 is activated. Signals from TLR9 induce the production of cytokine proteins, which are then secreted from the cell and act on the same and other heart cells to induce inflammation and contribute over time to adverse organ remodeling. (*From* Konstantinidis K, Kitsis RN. Cardiovascular biology: escaped DNA inflames the heart. Nature 2012;485(7397):179–80; with permission.)

ventricularization of atrial gene expression during AF.[26,67]

Fibrillation Mechanisms

Common themes are emerging that link preclinical and clinical observations, and are helping to rationalize our understanding of the initiation and perpetuation of fibrillation.[68,69] In preclinical models, there is considerable evidence that fibrillation in both atrial and ventricular compartments are sustained by stable localized sources[68,70,71] formed, in turn, by the interaction of action potential duration alternans and conduction velocity slowing to create localized electrical spiral waves (reentry) or regions of triggered focal activity.[68,70,72]

The clinical relevance of the initiation and perpetuation of fibrillation has attracted considerable attention.[39,68] Two principal hypotheses have been advanced to explain the "substrates" (mechanisms that sustain) of human AF.[19,39] The multiple wavelet hypothesis is based on mapping in dogs and humans and proposes that multiple non-localized interacting circuits meander around the atria.[73] The alternative localized source hypothesis proposes that rapidly conducted impulses (eg, from focal delayed afterdepolarization-mediated sources or electrical spiral waves [rotors]) result in complex fibrillatory activity.[68,74–76]

With the increasing application and positive results of ablation therapy, the perceived importance of localized sources for atrial fibrillation has gained ground.[76,77] There is general acceptance that triggers, such as ectopic beats from the pulmonary veins, can initiate AF, whereas steep restitution and exaggerated dispersion of refractoriness observed around those pulmonary veins[62,78–82] and patterns of left atrial ion channel expression facilitate wave break and the initiation of reentry.[18,19,26] Recent clinical work now describes atrial rotors seemingly directly amenable to ablation, with the most recent observations suggesting a central role in forming the "substrates" that sustain AF after it has been triggered in a wide range of patients, including those with paroxysmal atrial fibrillation.[83,84]

NATURAL HISTORY OF THE HEART FAILURE/ATRIAL FIBRILLATION RELATIONSHIP
Structural Clinical Phenotypes

The proportion of patients presenting with heart failure with preserved ejection fraction (HFpEF) is increasing in proportion to those with heart failure with reduced ejection fraction (HFrEF),[85] and is of particular relevance due to an association of HFpEF with AF.[6,11,14,21,86] The presence and severity of diastolic dysfunction is independently predictive of AF,[6,86] with those patients having distinct associated cellular phenotypes supporting separation and possible association with AF.[87] The loss of effective atrial contractile function is possibly more important to those with HFpEF rather than those with HFrEF. In addition, left atrial functional impairment that limits exercise capacity may have an impact on prognosis.[88]

Influence of Atrial Fibrillation on Heart Failure Outcomes

The prognostic significance of AF on CHF is becoming clearer, and new-onset AF may provide a grave indicator in patients with CHF.[1,12,89] This risk may be intrinsic or may arise following initiation of antiarrhythmic therapy.[89,90] In a recent study in which AF was present in a third of CHF cases, use of antiarrhythmic medications was associated with adverse hospital outcomes, longer hospital stay, and higher risks of in-hospital death.[91] This has also been reported in patients without CHF in a substudy of the Atrial Fibrillation Follow-Up Investigation of Rhythm Management (AFFIRM) trial.[92] Notably, in a propensity-matched study, AF actually had no intrinsic association with mortality, although it was associated with an increased risk of CHF hospitalization.[93]

Drug Interactions with Substrate

One major practical issue in the management of patients with AF and CHF is that the responses of the ventricular myocardium to antiarrhythmic drugs that act through ion channel blockade is modified.[16,89,90,94] Indeed, transcriptional shifts in the expression of genes encoding cardiac ion channels may increase susceptibility to adverse drug reactions.[16,89] Most specifically, downregulation of potassium channel gene expression with action potential prolongation might increase susceptibility to, for example, the addition of potassium channel blockers, such as D-sotalol.[16,95] A further interaction that is not fully explained is the negative impact of dronedarone on prognosis in patients with significant impairment of ventricular pump function.[96,97]

SYSTEMATIC APPROACHES TO COMPLEX CARDIAC DISEASE

To integrate and make sense of the enormous amount of accumulating biologic and clinical information relevant to the conditions discussed here, a *systems biology* approach to disease analysis seems appropriate.[19,98] Although semantics remain contentious for our practical purposes,

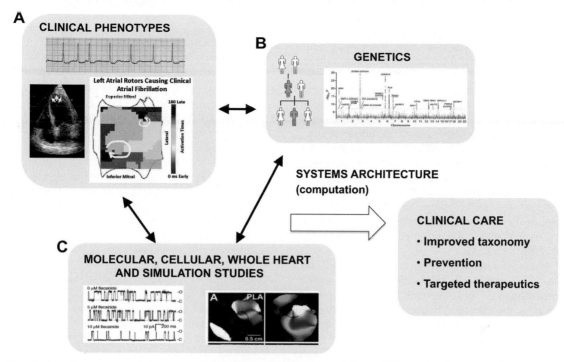

Fig. 4. A systems approach to an analysis of atrial fibrillation and heart failure: the final objective is a new taxonomy of disease susceptibility of clinical utility that integrates multiparameter data. Accordingly, clinical (*A*) and genetic (*B*) inputs are used in conjunction with appropriately designed mechanistic studies (*C*) in clinical and model systems. Iterative computer-based modeling provides an architectural framework leading to improved taxonomy, allowing for tailoring of medical treatment (precision medicine). *Arrows* show defined patient-specific abnormalities in cardiac function (in this case, apical hypertrophy).

we can define a *systems* approach as an analytic framework characterized by integrated descriptions of multiple biologic processes based on systematic measurement (**Fig. 4**).[19] Such a strategy requires as a starting point large high-quality data sets describing the phenotypes and natural history of disease. Once appropriate populations of patients are identified, then genetic and genomic analysis can ideally be complemented by the use of experimental systems to model functional consequences. For overlapping phenotypes, in this case AF and CHF, this is a substantial problem, with the situation for CHF further complicated by limitations to the quantification of the phenotype. Technical advances in relevant genomic technologies and the acquisition of target populations are particularly valuable, although the absence of genetically manipulable model systems relevant to CHF provide some limitations.[10,00]

We do, however, think it likely that, over time, relationships between atrial and ventricular biology, even in such complex settings, will become tractable.[19,98] This may be most amenable initially through unpicking electrophysiological phenotypes in which the prospects for quantification seem higher.[19,99] In view of the sheer volume of information obtained from such systems approaches, computational models to elaborate underlying network architecture will almost certainly be of value.[99] There are already examples of the use of computerized models to analyze the generation of fibrillation within the context of CHF.[69,99–101] The important goal when developing disease models is to allow the responses to therapeutic interventions to be assessed.[19]

SUMMARY

Atrial fibrillation and heart failure have much in common and tend to occur in the same vulnerable populations.[1,9,10,12] Affected individuals are often older and frequently have underlying systemic *multimorbidity*.[20] Although the initial manifestation of atrial disease is through arrhythmia, there are also significant issues with contractile performance.[88] The first manifestation of ventricular disease is most usually contractile, but those chambers also remain electrically sensitive with a risk of fibrillation and sudden cardiac death.[10]

The complex clinical settings caused by the interaction of 2 independently highly heterogeneous disorders explain why there have been few practically useful prospective clinical evaluations addressing the combined clinical scenario.[92,102,103] We are, however, optimistic that significant advances will be made, although necessarily in a stepwise fashion. We strongly advocate that attention is paid to further characterization of the myocardial substrates for disease. We believe such an approach will lead to opportunities for a greater understanding of the underlying biology, greater opportunities for accurate risk stratification, and the possibility of rescue via pharmacologic therapy, tissue ablation or regenerative therapy, or by appropriate devices.[76,84,104,105]

We see a systems approach to this highly complex, yet increasingly tractable, problem, using a combination of well-selected translational model systems, the managed collection of large amounts of data and computerized modeling, as offering the best hope in achieving medium-term to long-term advances.[19] In the interim, we will also need a community-wide effort to more vigorous multifaceted approaches to prevention, which will be reliant also on the identification of novel risk factors plus early disease detection.[5] The fact that populations of patients with both AF and CHF continue to increase should motivate funding agencies to make targeted research in this area a priority.

REFERENCES

1. Anter E, Jessup M, Callans DJ. Atrial fibrillation and heart failure: treatment considerations for a dual epidemic. Circulation 2009;119(18): 2516–25.

2. Carson PE, Johnson GR, Dunkman WB, et al. The influence of atrial fibrillation on prognosis in mild to moderate heart failure. The V-HeFT Studies. The V-HeFT VA Cooperative Studies Group. Circulation 1993;87(Suppl 6):VI102–10.

3. Stevenson WG, Stevenson LW. Atrial fibrillation in heart failure. N Engl J Med 1999;341(12): 910–1.

4. Ben Morrison T, Jared Bunch T, Gersh BJ. Pathophysiology of concomitant atrial fibrillation and heart failure: implications for management. Nat Clin Pract Cardiovasc Med 2009;6(1):46–56.

5. Benjamin EJ, Chen PS, Bild DE, et al. Prevention of atrial fibrillation: report from a National Heart, Lung, and Blood Institute workshop. Circulation 2009; 119(4):606–18.

6. Tsang TS, Gersh BJ, Appleton CP, et al. Left ventricular diastolic dysfunction as a predictor of the first diagnosed nonvalvular atrial fibrillation in 840 elderly men and women. J Am Coll Cardiol 2002; 40(9):1636–44.

7. Ellinor PT, Lunetta KL, Albert CM, et al. Meta-analysis identifies six new susceptibility loci for atrial fibrillation. Nat Genet 2012;44(6):670–5.

8. Magnani JW, Rienstra M, Lin H, et al. Atrial fibrillation: current knowledge and future directions in epidemiology and genomics. Circulation 2011; 124(18):1982–93.

9. Yancy CW, Jessup M, Bozkurt B, et al. 2013 ACCF/AHA guideline for the management of heart failure: a report of the American College of Cardiology Foundation/American Heart Association Task Force on practice guidelines. J Am Coll Cardiol 2013. [Epub ahead of print].

10. Braunwald E. Heart failure. JACC Heart Fail 2013; 1:1–20.

11. Lee DS, Gona P, Vasan RS, et al. Relation of disease pathogenesis and risk factors to heart failure with preserved or reduced ejection fraction: insights from the Framingham Heart Study of the National Heart, Lung, and Blood Institute. Circulation 2009;119(24):3070–7.

12. Darby AE, Dimarco JP. Management of atrial fibrillation in patients with structural heart disease. Circulation 2012;125(7):945–57.

13. Wang TJ, Larson MG, Levy D, et al. Temporal relations of atrial fibrillation and congestive heart failure and their joint influence on mortality: the Framingham Heart Study. Circulation 2003; 107(23):2920–5.

14. Olsson LG, Swedberg K, Ducharme A, et al. Atrial fibrillation and risk of clinical events in chronic heart failure with and without left ventricular systolic dysfunction: results from the Candesartan in Heart Failure–Assessment of Reduction in Mortality and morbidity (CHARM) program. J Am Coll Cardiol 2006;47(10):1997–2004.

15. Nattel S, Maguy A, Le Bouter S, et al. Arrhythmogenic ion-channel remodeling in the heart: heart failure, myocardial infarction, and atrial fibrillation. Physiol Rev 2007;87(2):425–56.

16. Aiba T, Tomaselli GF. Electrical remodeling in the failing heart. Curr Opin Cardiol 2010;25(1):29–36.

17. Barth AS, Kumordzie A, Frangakis C, et al. Reciprocal transcriptional regulation of metabolic and signaling pathways correlates with disease severity in heart failure. Circ Cardiovasc Genet 2011;4(5): 475–83.

18. Michael G, Xiao L, Qi XY, et al. Remodelling of cardiac repolarization: how homeostatic responses can lead to arrhythmogenesis. Cardiovasc Res 2009;81(3):491–9.

19. Grace AA, Roden DM. Systems biology and cardiac arrhythmias. Lancet 2012;380(9852): 1498–508.

20. Tinetti ME, Fried TR, Boyd CM. Designing health care for the most common chronic condition—multimorbidity. JAMA 2012;307(23):2493–4.

21. Go AS, Mozaffarian D, Roger VL, et al. Heart disease and stroke statistics—2013 update: a report from the American Heart Association. Circulation 2013;127(1):e6–245.

22. Miyasaka Y, Barnes ME, Gersh BJ, et al. Secular trends in incidence of atrial fibrillation in Olmsted County, Minnesota, 1980 to 2000, and implications on the projections for future prevalence. Circulation 2006;114(2):119–25.

23. Miyasaka Y, Barnes ME, Gersh BJ, et al. Incidence and mortality risk of congestive heart failure in atrial fibrillation patients: a community-based study over two decades. Eur Heart J 2006;27(8):936–41.

24. Stefansdottir H, Aspelund T, Gudnason V, et al. Trends in the incidence and prevalence of atrial fibrillation in Iceland and future projections. Europace 2011;13(8):1110–7.

25. Savelieva I, John Camm A. Atrial fibrillation and heart failure: natural history and pharmacological treatment. Europace 2004;5(Suppl 1):S5–19.

26. Wakili R, Voigt N, Kaab S, et al. Recent advances in the molecular pathophysiology of atrial fibrillation. J Clin Invest 2011;121(8):2955–68.

27. Lopez-Otin C, Blasco MA, Partridge L, et al. The hallmarks of aging. Cell 2013;153(6):1194–217.

28. Fatkin D, MacRae C, Sasaki T, et al. Missense mutations in the rod domain of the lamin A/C gene as causes of dilated cardiomyopathy and conduction-system disease. N Engl J Med 1999;341(23):1715–24.

29. Olson TM, Michels VV, Ballew JD, et al. Sodium channel mutations and susceptibility to heart failure and atrial fibrillation. JAMA 2005;293(4):447–54.

30. Darbar D, Kannankeril PJ, Donahue BS, et al. Cardiac sodium channel (SCN5A) variants associated with atrial fibrillation. Circulation 2008;117(15):1927–35.

31. Kathiresan S, Srivastava D. Genetics of human cardiovascular disease. Cell 2012;148:1242–57.

32. Gudbjartsson DF, Arnar DO, Helgadottir A, et al. Variants conferring risk of atrial fibrillation on chromosome 4q25. Nature 2007;448(7151):353–7.

33. Cappola TP, Dorn GW 2nd. Clinical considerations of heritable factors in common heart failure. Circ Cardiovasc Genet 2011;4(6):701–9.

34. O'Rahilly S. Human genetics illuminates the paths to metabolic disease. Nature 2009;462(7271):307–14.

35. Kenchaiah S, Evans JC, Levy D, et al. Obesity and the risk of heart failure. N Engl J Med 2002;347(5):305–13.

36. Wang TJ, Parise H, Levy D, et al. Obesity and the risk of new-onset atrial fibrillation. JAMA 2004;292(20):2471–7.

37. Tedrow UB, Conen D, Ridker PM, et al. The long- and short-term impact of elevated body mass index on the risk of new atrial fibrillation: the WHS (Women's Health Study). J Am Coll Cardiol 2010;55(21):2319–27.

38. Rosenberg MA, Gottdiener JS, Heckbert SR, et al. Echocardiographic diastolic parameters and risk of atrial fibrillation: the Cardiovascular Health Study. Eur Heart J 2012;33(7):904–12.

39. Nattel S. New ideas about atrial fibrillation 50 years on. Nature 2002;415(6868):219–26.

40. Schotten U, Verheule S, Kirchhof P, et al. Pathophysiological mechanisms of atrial fibrillation: a translational appraisal. Physiol Rev 2011;91(1):265–325.

41. Byrd GD, Prasad SM, Ripplinger CM, et al. Importance of geometry and refractory period in sustaining atrial fibrillation: testing the critical mass hypothesis. Circulation 2005;112(Suppl 9):I7–13.

42. Bode F, Sachs F, Franz MR. Tarantula peptide inhibits atrial fibrillation. Nature 2001;409(6816):35–6.

43. Kalifa J, Jalife J, Zaitsev AV, et al. Intra-atrial pressure increases rate and organization of waves emanating from the superior pulmonary veins during atrial fibrillation. Circulation 2003;108(6):668–71.

44. John B, Stiles MK, Kuklik P, et al. Reverse remodeling of the atria after treatment of chronic stretch in humans: implications for the atrial fibrillation substrate. J Am Coll Cardiol 2010;55(12):1217–26.

45. Mayr M, Yusuf S, Weir G, et al. Combined metabolomic and proteomic analysis of human atrial fibrillation. J Am Coll Cardiol 2008;51(5):585–94.

46. Barth AS, Tomaselli GF. Cardiac metabolism and arrhythmias. Circ Arrhythm Electrophysiol 2009;2(3):327–35.

47. Reilly SN, Jayaram R, Nahar K, et al. Atrial sources of reactive oxygen species vary with the duration and substrate of atrial fibrillation: implications for the antiarrhythmic effect of statins. Circulation 2011;124(10):1107–17.

48. Friedrichs K, Klinke A, Baldus S. Inflammatory pathways underlying atrial fibrillation. Trends Mol Med 2011;17(10):556–63.

49. Li J, Solus J, Chen Q, et al. Role of inflammation and oxidative stress in atrial fibrillation. Heart Rhythm 2010;7(4):438–44.

50. Mihm MJ, Yu F, Carnes CA, et al. Impaired myofibrillar energetics and oxidative injury during human atrial fibrillation. Circulation 2001;104(2):174–80.

51. Adam O, Frost G, Custodis F, et al. Role of Rac1 GTPase activation in atrial fibrillation. J Am Coll Cardiol 2007;50(4):359–67.

52. Oka T, Hikoso S, Yamaguchi O, et al. Mitochondrial DNA that escapes from autophagy causes inflammation and heart failure. Nature 2012;485(7397):251–5.

53. Konstantinidis K, Kitsis RN. Cardiovascular biology: escaped DNA inflames the heart. Nature 2012;485(7397):179–80.

54. Bayeva M, Gheorghiade M, Ardehali H. Mitochon-dria as a therapeutic target in heart failure. J Am Coll Cardiol 2013;61(6):599–610.

55. El-Armouche A, Boknik P, Eschenhagen T, et al. Molecular determinants of altered Ca2+ handling in human chronic atrial fibrillation. Circulation 2006;114(7):670–80.

56. Wijffels MC, Kirchhof CJ, Dorland R, et al. Atrial fibrillation begets atrial fibrillation. A study in awake chronically instrumented goats. Circulation 1995; 92(7):1954–68.

57. Ausma J, Wijffels M, Thone F, et al. Structural changes of atrial myocardium due to sustained atrial fibrillation in the goat. Circulation 1997; 96(9):3157–63.

58. Du J, Xie J, Zhang Z, et al. TRPM7-mediated Ca2+ signals confer fibrogenesis in human atrial fibrilla-tion. Circ Res 2010;106(5):992–1003.

59. Jahangir A, Lee V, Friedman PA, et al. Long-term progression and outcomes with aging in patients with lone atrial fibrillation: a 30-year follow-up study. Circulation 2007;115(24):3050–6.

60. Spach MS. Mounting evidence that fibrosis gener-ates a major mechanism for atrial fibrillation. Circ Res 2007;101(8):743–5.

61. Kistler PM, Sanders P, Fynn SP, et al. Electrophys-iologic and electroanatomic changes in the human atrium associated with age. J Am Coll Cardiol 2004;44(1):109–16.

62. Stiles MK, John B, Wong CX, et al. Paroxysmal lone atrial fibrillation is associated with an abnormal atrial substrate: characterizing the "second factor." J Am Coll Cardiol 2009;53(14):1182–91.

63. Roberts-Thomson KC, Stevenson IH, Kistler PM, et al. Anatomically determined functional conduc-tion delay in the posterior left atrium relationship to structural heart disease. J Am Coll Cardiol 2008;51(8):856–62.

64. Platonov PG, Mitrofanova LB, Orshanskaya V, et al. Structural abnormalities in atrial walls are associ-ated with presence and persistency of atrial fibrilla-tion but not with age. J Am Coll Cardiol 2011; 58(21):2225–32.

65. Tanaka K, Zlochiver S, Vikstrom KL, et al. Spatial distribution of fibrosis governs fibrillation wave dy-namics in the posterior left atrium during heart fail-ure. Circ Res 2007;101(8):839–47.

66. Higuchi K, Akkaya M, Akoum N, et al. Cardiac MRI assessment of atrial fibrosis in atrial fibrillation: im-plications for diagnosis and therapy. Heart 2013. [Epub ahead of print].

67. Barth AS, Merk S, Arnoldi E, et al. Reprogramming of the human atrial transcriptome in permanent atrial fibrillation: expression of a ventricular-like genomic signature. Circ Res 2005;96(9):1022–9.

68. Pandit SV, Jalife J. Rotors and the dynamics of car-diac fibrillation. Circ Res 2013;112(5):849–62.

69. Rappel WJ, Narayan SM. Theoretical consider-ations for mapping activation in human cardiac fibrillation. Chaos 2013;23(2):023113.

70. Davidenko JM, Pertsov AV, Salomonsz R, et al. Stationary and drifting spiral waves of excitation in isolated cardiac muscle. Nature 1992; 355(6358):349–51.

71. Mandapati R, Skanes A, Chen J, et al. Stable microreentrant sources as a mechanism of atrial fibrillation in the isolated sheep heart. Circulation 2000;101(2):194–9.

72. Klos M, Calvo D, Yamazaki M, et al. Atrial septopul-monary bundle of the posterior left atrium provides a substrate for atrial fibrillation initiation in a model of vagally mediated pulmonary vein tachycardia of the structurally normal heart. Circ Arrhythm Electro-physiol 2008;1(3):175–83.

73. Moe GK, Rheinboldt WC, Abildskov JA. A computer model of atrial fibrillation. Am Heart J 1964;67:200–20.

74. Mines GR. On dynamic equilibrium in the heart. J Physiol 1913;46(4–5):349–83.

75. Lewis T. Oliver-Sharpey Lectures on the nature of flutter and fibrillation of the auricle. Br Med J 1921;1(3146):551–5.

76. Narayan SM, Krummen DE, Shivkumar K, et al. Treatment of atrial fibrillation by the ablation of localized sources: CONFIRM (Conventional Abla-tion for Atrial Fibrillation With or Without Focal Im-pulse and Rotor Modulation) trial. J Am Coll Cardiol 2012;60:628–36.

77. Haissaguerre M, Jais P, Shah DC, et al. Sponta-neous initiation of atrial fibrillation by ectopic beats originating in the pulmonary veins. N Engl J Med 1998;339(10):659–66.

78. Narayan SM, Bayer JD, Lalani G, et al. Action potential dynamics explain arrhythmic vulnerability in human heart failure: a clinical and modeling study implicating abnormal calcium handling. J Am Coll Cardiol 2008;52(22):1782–92.

79. Rostock T, Steven D, Lutomsky B, et al. Atrial fibrillation begets atrial fibrillation in the pulmo-nary veins on the impact of atrial fibrillation on the electrophysiological properties of the pulmo-nary veins in humans. J Am Coll Cardiol 2008; 51(22):2153–60.

80. Narayan SM, Franz MR, Clopton P, et al. Repolari-zation alternans reveals vulnerability to human atrial fibrillation. Circulation 2011;123(25):2922–30.

81. Markides V, Schilling RJ, Ho SY, et al. Characteriza-tion of left atrial activation in the intact human heart. Circulation 2003;107(5):733–9.

82. Lalani GG, Schricker A, Gibson M, et al. Atrial conduction slows immediately before the onset of human atrial fibrillation: a bi-atrial contact map-ping study of transitions to atrial fibrillation. J Am Coll Cardiol 2012;59(6):595–606.

83. Shivkumar K, Ellenbogen KA, Hummel JD, et al. Acute termination of human atrial fibrillation by identification and catheter ablation of localized rotors and sources: first multicenter experience of focal impulse and rotor modulation (FIRM) ablation. J Cardiovasc Electrophysiol 2012;23(12): 1277–85.

84. Narayan SM, Krummen DE, Clopton P, et al. Direct or coincidental elimination of stable rotors or focal sources may explain successful atrial fibrillation ablation: on-treatment analysis of the CONFIRM trial (Conventional Ablation for AF With or Without Focal Impulse and Rotor Modulation). J Am Coll Cardiol 2013;62(2):138–47.

85. Owan TE, Hodge DO, Herges RM, et al. Trends in prevalence and outcome of heart failure with preserved ejection fraction. N Engl J Med 2006; 355(3):251–9.

86. Bhatia RS, Tu JV, Lee DS, et al. Outcome of heart failure with preserved ejection fraction in a population-based study. N Engl J Med 2006; 355(3):260–9.

87. van Heerebeek L, Borbely A, Niessen HW, et al. Myocardial structure and function differ in systolic and diastolic heart failure. Circulation 2006; 113(16):1966–73.

88. Kusunose K, Motoki H, Popovic ZB, et al. Independent association of left atrial function with exercise capacity in patients with preserved ejection fraction. Heart 2012;98(17):1311–7.

89. Grace AA, Camm AJ. Quinidine. N Engl J Med 1998;338(1):35–45.

90. Kannankeril P, Roden DM, Darbar D. Drug-induced long QT syndrome. Pharmacol Rev 2010;62(4): 760–81.

91. Mountantonakis SE, Grau-Sepulveda MV, Bhatt DL, et al. Presence of atrial fibrillation is independently associated with adverse outcomes in patients hospitalized with heart failure: an analysis of get with the guidelines–heart failure. Circ Heart Fail 2012; 5(2):191–201.

92. Saksena S, Slee A, Waldo AL, et al. Cardiovascular outcomes in the AFFIRM trial (Atrial Fibrillation Follow-Up Investigation of Rhythm Management). An assessment of individual antiarrhythmic drug therapies compared with rate control with propensity score–matched analyses. J Am Coll Cardiol 2011;58(19):1975–85.

93. Ahmed MI, White M, Ekundayo OJ, et al. A history of atrial fibrillation and outcomes in chronic advanced systolic heart failure: a propensity-matched study. Eur Heart J 2009;30(16):2029–37.

94. Dobrev D, Carlsson L, Nattel S. Novel molecular targets for atrial fibrillation therapy. Nat Rev Drug Discov 2012;11(4):275–91.

95. Waldo AL, Camm AJ, deRuyter H, et al. Effect of d-sotalol on mortality in patients with left ventricular dysfunction after recent and remote myocardial infarction. The SWORD Investigators. Survival With Oral d-Sotalol. Lancet 1996;348(9019):7–12.

96. Kober L, Torp-Pedersen C, McMurray JJ, et al. Increased mortality after dronedarone therapy for severe heart failure. N Engl J Med 2008;358(25): 2678–87.

97. Connolly SJ, Camm AJ, Halperin JL, et al. Dronedarone in high-risk permanent atrial fibrillation. N Engl J Med 2011;365(24):2268–76.

98. Rudy Y, Ackerman MJ, Bers DM, et al. Systems approach to understanding electromechanical activity in the human heart: a National Heart, Lung, and Blood Institute workshop summary. Circulation 2008;118(11):1202–11.

99. Trayanova NA. Whole-heart modeling: applications to cardiac electrophysiology and electromechanics. Circ Res 2011;108(1):113–28.

100. Thul R, Coombes S, Roderick HL, et al. Subcellular calcium dynamics in a whole-cell model of an atrial myocyte. Proc Natl Acad Sci U S A 2012;109(6):2150–5.

101. Comtois P, Nattel S. Impact of tissue geometry on simulated cholinergic atrial fibrillation: a modeling study. Chaos 2011;21(1):013108.

102. Roy D, Talajic M, Nattel S, et al. Rhythm control versus rate control for atrial fibrillation and heart failure. N Engl J Med 2008;358(25):2667–77.

103. Talajic M, Khairy P, Levesque S, et al. Maintenance of sinus rhythm and survival in patients with heart failure and atrial fibrillation. J Am Coll Cardiol 2010;55(17):1796–802.

104. Saumarez RC, Chojnowska L, Derksen R, et al. Sudden death in noncoronary heart disease is associated with delayed paced ventricular activation. Circulation 2003;107(20):2595–600.

105. Saumarez RC, Pytkowski M, Sterlinski M, et al. Paced ventricular electrogram fractionation predicts sudden cardiac death in hypertrophic cardiomyopathy. Eur Heart J 2008;29(13):1653–61.

Continuous Monitoring of Atrial Fibrillation in Heart Failure

Bengt Herweg, MD, FHRS[a],*, S. Serge Barold, MD, FHRS[b],
Jonathan S. Steinberg, MD, FHRS[c,d]

KEYWORDS

- Atrial fibrillation • Heart failure • Cardiac resynchronization • Dual-chamber pacemaker
- Continuous cardiac monitoring • Stroke • Thromboembolism

KEY POINTS

- Knowledge of atrial fibrillation (AF) in heart failure has increased dramatically because of the widespread use of continuous monitoring provided by implanted cardiac rhythm devices.
- Continuous monitoring has improved cardiac resynchronization therapy (CRT) management of patients with AF.
- Data from continuous monitoring have generated new questions about anticoagulant therapy in patients with only asymptomatic AF and in those with very short atrial high-rate episodes.
- Anticoagulant therapy should be considered in patients who have a high risk of thromboembolism according to standard scoring systems.

Atrial fibrillation (AF) is found in up to 30% to 40% of patients with heart failure, depending on the underlying cause and severity of heart failure. Each complicates the course of the other. Paroxysmal AF is self-terminating, usually within 48 hours. Although AF paroxysms may continue for up to 7 days, the 48-hour time point is clinically important; after this period, the likelihood of spontaneous conversion is low and anticoagulation must be considered. Persistent AF is present when an AF episode either lasts longer than 7 days or requires termination by cardioversion, either with drugs or by direct current cardioversion. AF increases the risk of thromboembolic complications (particularly stroke) and may lead to worsening of symptoms. Heart failure can be both a consequence of AF (eg, tachycardiomyopathy or decompensation in acute-onset AF) and a cause of the arrhythmia as a result of increased atrial pressure, volume overload, or excessive neurohumoral stimulation. Patients with paroxysmal AF have a similar risk of thromboembolism to those with sustained AF. This risk can be significantly lowered by oral anticoagulation. Heart failure and AF share risk factors such as hypertension, valve disease, coronary artery disease, and diabetes mellitus. Both heart failure and AF independently increase the mortality risk, and, when both conditions occur together, the mortality risk is even higher.

Disclosures: Dr Herweg reports receiving fellowship support from Medtronic, and minor consulting fees from St. Jude Medical and Biosense-Webster. Dr Barold has no disclosures. Dr Steinberg reports receiving consulting fees from Medtronic, Boston-Scientific, Philips, St. Jude Medical, Janssen, Biosense-Webster and Sanofi. He is also receiving research grant support from Jansen, Medtronic and Biosense-Webster.

[a] Department of Cardiovascular Disease, University of South Florida Morsani College of Medicine, South Tampa Campus (5th Floor), Two Tampa General Circle, Tampa, FL 33606, USA; [b] 5806 Mariner's Watch Drive, Tampa, FL 33615, USA; [c] Arrhythmia Institute, Valley Health System, 223 North Van Dien Avenue, Ridgewood, NJ 07450, USA; [d] Department of Medicine, Columbia University College of Physicians & Surgeons, 630 W 168 Street, New York, NY 10032, USA
* Corresponding author. Department of Cardiovascular Disease, University of South Florida Morsani College of Medicine, South Tampa Campus (5th Floor), Two Tampa General Circle, Tampa, FL 33606.
E-mail address: bherweg@health.usf.edu

Detection of AF can be achieved by a 12-lead electrocardiogram (ECG, Holter [24 hour or 7 day), noninvasive and invasive event monitoring, and from data stored in a pacemaker, implantable cardioverter defibrillator (ICD), or a device for cardiac resynchronization therapy (CRT) by virtue of continuous monitoring via the atrial channel. Resting 12-lead ECGs and ambulatory monitoring (in the absence of an implanted device) provide only a snapshot of the ECG, with resulting limited information that underestimates the true prevalence of AF (**Fig. 1**). Asymptomatic AF may be as much as 6 to 8 times more common than symptomatic AF and seems to be a precursor of symptomatic AF.[1,2] In the last few years, research interest has grown in the clinical relevance of AF at an even earlier stage, before its clinical detection. Earlier detection of AF in the asymptomatic phase (as with cardiac rhythm devices) might allow the timely introduction of therapies to protect the patient, not only from the consequences of AF but also from progression from an easily treated condition into one that becomes refractory to therapy.

Contemporary pacemakers and CRT devices are equipped with reliable and extensive diagnostic and memory features yielding full disclosure of the number, duration, and overall burden of atrial tachyarrhythmias. These advanced diagnostic features have shown the high frequency of symptomatic and asymptomatic atrial arrhythmias in patients with heart failure and an implanted cardiac rhythm device. Device interrogation also provides estimates of the percentage of biventricular (BiV%) pacing in patients receiving CRT, a measurement of the utmost importance in achieving a satisfactory clinical response. Other important data from implanted devices include the ventricular rate (VR) during atrial tachyarrhythmias and stored electrograms that permit the precise diagnosis of the atrial tachyarrhythmia (eg, AF vs atrial flutter vs atrial tachycardia [AT]) and characterize the initiation/termination of arrhythmias. Many arrhythmias may not be true AF but rather ATs or atrial flutters with rates that exceed the programmable recording threshold. These arrhythmias are therefore referred to as atrial high-rate episodes (AHRE) and their therapy differs from that of AF. Manual overreading of all recorded episodes is good practice, because a device may not arrive at the correct diagnosis. Problematic situations include far-field R wave oversensing and other extraneous signals, such as external electromagnetic signals, which a device interprets and records as AF. Because of intermittent atrial undersensing, a single prolonged episode may be recorded as multiple shorter episodes, so that the overall arrhythmia burden may be more reliable than number of episodes. Many workers refer to all atrial tachyarrhythmias simply as AF, because AF constitutes most atrial arrhythmias in patients with cardiac rhythm devices.[2–6]

AF BURDEN

Over the last decade, the term burden has become frequently used when discussing AF. AF burden generally means the percentage of time that a patient is in AF calculated from the total time in AF divided by the total monitored time. AF burden using this definition can be adequately assessed only by some method of continuous monitoring for prolonged periods. Such assessments involve continuously applied monitors, implanted monitors, or interrogation of cardiac rhythm devices. The AF burden calculated from the ECG recordings in terms of total time in AF during a specific period is sometimes called the ECG AF burden. This burden can be further subdivided into total time in AF, the number of AF (re)occurrences in a specific period, or duration of the AF-free period until the recurrence of AF, or a combination of these. AF burden may provide a more clinically useful assessment of AF than the time to the first recurrence of AF. In addition, cardiac rhythm device–based AF recordings have become a useful guide to assess interventional procedures, the need for anticoagulation, and to understand the importance of asymptomatic AF. AF recurrence should not always be considered as treatment

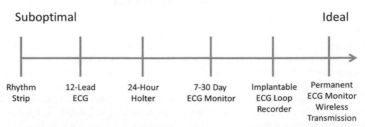

Fig. 1. The spectrum of ambulatory monitoring modalities. As one moves from left to right, the duration of monitoring increases, which in turn increases the diagnostic yield.

failure. A reduction of AF burden may constitute a therapeutic success because of less frequent, briefer, or less symptomatic episodes. However, in highly symptomatic patients, any AF recurrence may be unacceptable.

There is growing clinical interest in symptomatic and asymptomatic device-recorded AHRE as possible precursors of thromboembolic complications in patients with a pacemaker or ICD.[2–10] Timely diagnosis of both paroxysmal AF or atrial flutter has important implications for anticoagulant therapy for stroke prevention.[11–18]

INCIDENCE AND PROGNOSIS OF AF DURING CRT

Device-based continuous monitoring of AF in CRT patients has improved the diagnosis and therapy for AF in this group of patients. The bulk of our knowledge regarding the role of CRT in patients with permanent AF is based on nonrandomized, observational data. Marijon and colleagues[4] analyzed the incidence of AF in CRT patients in a prospective study and found that 34 of 173 (27.5%) patients developed paroxysmal AF during a follow-up of 9.9 ± 3.6 months. About half of the patients with AF had a past history of AF. Boriani and colleagues[19] evaluated 1404 CRT patients for a median follow-up of 18 months. All were in sinus rhythm at the time of entry into the study. AF was documented in 443 of 1404 patients (32%). The duration of AF ranged from more than 10 minutes to weeks. AF developed in 222 CRT patients without a previous history of AF (22%) and 221 CRT patients with a previous history of AF (16%). The observations of Leclercq and colleagues[5] involving 120 CRT patients followed for a mean of 183 ± 23 days showed an AF incidence of 21%. A previous history of AF was present in 29% of patients, and those with new-onset AF after CRT constituted 17% of all the patients. Thus, the incidence of AF in patients with heart failure treated with CRT ranges from 30% to 35% for paroxysmal AF and around 20% to 25% for permanent AF. This finding should not be surprising given the association of AF with the severity of heart failure. This association carries a worse prognosis than heart failure with sinus rhythm.

SIGNIFICANCE OF THE VR

A VR in AF controlled at rest may not be controlled during exercise. Furthermore, pronounced RR interval variability in AF may decrease the number of resynchronized beats. In the AF group (443 patients), Boriani and colleagues[19] calculated the average VR of each patient at 115 ± 15 bpm. An uncontrolled VR occurred in 150 of 443 (34%) of the patients. In the patients with new-onset AF, 93 of 222 (42%) were found to have uncontrolled VR, whereas in those with a known history of AF, 43 of 221 (26%) showed uncontrolled VR ($P = .001$). An uncontrolled VR, which occurred in one-third of CRT patients, was associated with a worse clinical outcome of combined heart failure hospitalization or death ($P = .046$).

The traditional recommendation in AF to control the resting VR at 80 bpm increasing to only 110 bpm with exertion is an effort that is difficult to achieve in heart failure. This arbitrary goal was recently challenged by the results of the Rate Control Efficacy in Permanent Atrial Fibrillation II (RACE II) trial, which showed that lenient rate control was not inferior to strict rate control in terms of cardiovascular morbidity and mortality. However, rate control between groups did not differ that much and the composite endpoint was very heterogenous. Furthermore, the trial did not evaluate the safety of a lenient strategy in patients with heart failure.[20] Consequently, it would be unwise to extrapolate the data from the RACE II trial to the management of patients with heart failure.

PROGNOSIS OF AF DURING CRT

Boriani and colleagues[19] found that age ($P = .046$) and uncontrolled VR ($P = .028$) in CRT patients with AF were the only independent predictors of clinical outcome assessed by the combined end point of heart failure hospitalizations or death. In a study involving 1193 CRT patients (initially all in sinus rhythm), Santini and colleagues[3] found AF in 361 patients (30%) over a mean follow-up of 13 months (the study overlapped that of Boriani and colleagues).[19] AF (especially persistent AF) correlated with the composite end point of death and heart failure hospitalization ($P = .005$). Prognostic data were also obtained in a recent subanalysis of MADIT-CRT (Multicenter Automatic Defibrillator Implantation Trial–Cardiac Resynchronization Therapy).[21] The cumulative probability of both the combined end point of heart failure or all-cause mortality was higher among patients who developed atrial tachyarrhythmia during the first year.

ABLATION OF THE ATRIOVENTRICULAR JUNCTION TO OPTIMIZE CRT

It seems reasonable to start with pharmacologic therapy to optimize rate control in AF patients requiring CRT. When after careful evaluation by device interrogation, Holter monitoring, and exercise testing, the amount of true BiV pacing is suboptimal, atrioventricular junctional (AVJ) ablation should be considered. The impressive results after AVJ ablation suggest that the procedure should be performed in most patients with permanent AF as well as in those with frequent and prolonged episodes of paroxysmal AF.[22–28] However, a few claim good results with rate control rather than ablation.[29] There are no reports of increased mortality associated with AVJ ablation. The procedure carries the theoretic risk of device failure and death in pacemaker-dependent patients and eliminates fusion with spontaneously conducted beats during sinus rhythm. A randomized clinical trial to test the value of routine AVJ ablation is desirable.

IMPORTANCE OF THE BIV%: MORE IS ALWAYS BETTER

In the study of Boriani and colleagues,[19] the BiV% in the AF group was 95% versus 98% in the entire patient population. When patients with AF were in sinus rhythm, the BiV% was 98% versus 71% during AF, P<.01. Suboptimal CRT was defined as BiV% less than 95%, which was predicted by the occurrence of persistent or permanent AF (P<.001), and uncontrolled VR (P = .002). BiV% was inversely correlated to the VR in AF, decreasing by 7% for each 10-bpm increase in VR.

Koplan and colleagues[30] conducted a retrospective analysis in 1800 of CRT patients to evaluate the significance of BiV% and its relationship to a combined clinical end point of death and heart failure hospitalization. Patients who showed a

BiV% greater than 92% had a 44% reduction in clinical end points compared with patients with BiV% 0% to 92% (P<.0001). Patients with BiV % 98% to 99% had similar outcomes as the patients with BiV% 93% to 97% and also similar outcomes as patients paced 100% of the time. Patients with a history of atrial arrhythmias were more likely to pace 92% or lower (P<.001).

The importance of a high BiV% has recently been confirmed in a large cohort of 36,935 patients who participated in the US LATITUDE (LATITUDE, Patient Management System, Boston-Scientific, Natick, MA, USA) patient management system, in which the patients were followed in a remote monitoring network.[31] The mortality was inversely associated with BiV% in the presence of both normal sinus and atrial paced rhythm and with AF (Fig. 2). The greatest reduction in mortality was observed with BiV% greater than 98%. Patients with BiV% greater than 99.6% experienced a 24% reduction in mortality (P<.001), whereas those with BiV% less than 94.8% had a 19% increase in mortality. The optimal BiV% cut-point was 98.7%.

The delivery of a stimulus does not guarantee effective CRT. The BiV% based on device interrogation data overestimates the percentage of truly resynchronized beats, because it does not account for fusion and pseudofusion between intrinsic (not paced) and paced beats. Kamath and colleagues[32] used 12-lead Holter monitoring to assess the incidence of ineffective capture in 19 patients with AF undergoing CRT (Fig. 3). The study clearly showed that although device interrogation showed

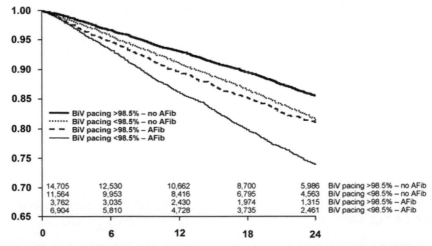

Fig. 2. In a large cohort of 36,935 patients followed up in a remote monitoring network (LATITUDE patient management system) a high BiV% achieved, specifically greater than 98.5%, was associated with a reduction in mortality. As expected, patients with AF had a worse outcome than those without AF. However, this was lessened if the high BiV% could be achieved in the AF population, usually after an AVJ ablation. (*From* Hayes DL, Boehmer JP, Day JD, et al. Cardiac resynchronization therapy and the relationship of percent biventricular pacing to symptoms and survival. Heart Rhythm 2011;8:1473; with permission.)

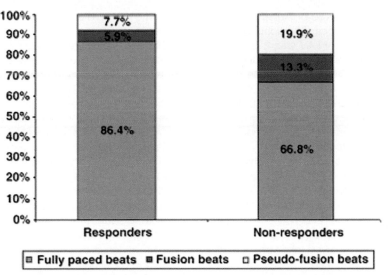

Fig. 3. 24-Hour Holter data for CRT responders and nonresponders with permanent AF. CRT responders had a higher percentage of fully paced beats than nonresponders. Nonresponders to CRT had a significantly higher percentage of ineffective pacing, because of a combination of fusion and pseudofusion beats. (*From* Kamath GS, Cotiga D, Koneru JN, et al. The utility of 12-lead Holter monitoring in patients with permanent atrial fibrillation for the identification of nonresponders after cardiac resynchronization therapy. J Am Coll Cardiol 2009;53:1050–5; with permission.)

more than 90% BiV pacing, only 9 patients (47%) received effective BiV pacing. It is imperative to examine rhythm strips and ECGs of nonresponders to verify that the beats are truly resynchronized. Certain device algorithms aimed at maximizing BiV pacing in patients with AF with a relatively fast VR may also lead to a false sense of reassurance about the BiV% pacing.

ANALYSIS OF THE RAFT STUDY IN PATIENTS WITH PERMANENT AF: SUBOPTIMAL DOSE OF CARDIAC RESYNCHRONIZATION?

The RAFT (Resynchronization for Ambulatory Heart Failure Trial) AF study constitutes the largest randomized report examining the role of CRT in patients with permanent AF.[33] Patients with permanent AF were randomized to CRT-ICD (n = 114) or ICD (n = 115). Cardiovascular death was similar between treatment arms (hazard ratio, 0.97; 95% confidence interval [CI], 0.55–1.71; *P* = .91); however, there was a trend for fewer heart failure hospitalizations with CRT-ICD (hazard ratio, 0.58; 95% CI, 0.38–1.01; *P* = .052). The findings were disappointing, contrary to prevailing belief that patients with AF improve with CRT, albeit less than in patients in sinus rhythm. To be eligible for the study, patients were required to have a resting heart rate of 60 beats per minute or lower and 90 beats per minute or lower after a 6-minute walk test. Only 1 patient underwent an AVJ ablation. There

was no statistically significant difference of reaching a composite end point of all-cause mortality or heart failure hospitalization for those receiving BiV pacing less than 90% versus 90% or more or less than 95% versus 95% or more (only one-third of patients received BiV pacing ≥95%). Furthermore, the CRT-ICD arm had the conducted AF response algorithm (Medtronic, Minneapolis, MN, USA) enabled. This feature regularizes the pacing rate by adjusting the pacemaker escape interval after each ventricular beat. In this way, the delivery of BiV pacing was enhanced at a rate that closely matches the relatively fast spontaneous VR. Therefore, as a result of fusion and pseudofusion, the percentage of truly resynchronized beats was likely overestimated. The investigators of the RAFT study indicated that the standard medical rate control of permanent AF may have been insufficient to allow effective delivery of CRT therapy.

IMPACT OF STRUCTURAL CHANGES ON THE DEVELOPMENT OF ATRIAL TACHYARRHYTHMIAS DURING CARDIAC RESYNCHRONIZATION

The change in the left atrial volume (LAV) and incidence of atrial tachyarrhythmias was evaluated in a substudy of the MADIT-CRT trial.[21] In the total population of 1820 patients, there were 139 patients with atrial tachyarrhythmia (AF 47%). A low LAV reduction was defined as less than 20% and a high LAV reduction as 20% or higher. Based on the 1-year follow-up echocardiographic data, the mean percent reduction of LAV was 3-fold higher in patients treated with a CRT-D (D = ICD) device compared with the ICD-only group. The median reduction in LAV was 29% (20%–30%) in the CRT-D group versus 10% (5%–14%) in the ICD-only group (P<.001). As expected, reduction in LAV was highly correlated with reduction in the left ventricular end-systolic volume.

The cumulative probability of atrial tachyarrhythmias (at 2.5 years) in MADIT-CRT was lowest among high LAV responders to CRT-D (3%) and significantly higher among both low LAV responders to CRT-D (9%) and ICD-only patients (7%; P = .03 for the difference among the 3 groups). Multivariate analysis showed that high LAV responders experienced a 53% reduction in the risk of subsequent atrial tachyarrhythmia compared with low LAV responders in the CRT-D group and patients in the ICD-only group (P = .01).

REMOTE MONITORING

Implantable CRT devices are capable of automatic daily transmission of device data consisting of full interrogation and monitoring to a remote service center. Internet-based remote device interrogation systems provide clinicians with frequent (such as daily) and complete access to stored data. Easy access to these stored data permits clinicians to make diagnostic and therapeutic decisions sooner, thus avoiding potential long-term sequelae as a result of untreated clinical disorders. Such follow-up systems can automatically send reports and special alerts on a daily basis, thereby allowing physicians to respond more proactively to paroxysmal or asymptomatic AF. AF is more likely to be detected early with daily remote monitoring compared with traditional follow-up visits.[11–15,34]

MONITORING FOR AF BY CONVENTIONAL PACEMAKERS

Almost 10 years ago, in a landmark study of 110 patients with previous AF and a dual-chamber pacemaker, Israel and colleagues[35] reported recurrent AF in 88% of patients by review of stored electrograms and in 46% of patients by ECG recordings during follow-up (19 ± 11 months). AF lasted >48 hours in 50 patients, 19 of whom (38%) were completely asymptomatic and in sinus rhythm at subsequent follow-up. These observations clearly indicated clinical usefulness of pacemaker diagnostics. Continuous arrhythmia monitoring by cardiac rhythm devices has become the gold standard for AF diagnosis using continuous monitoring.

Devices vary in their capability to detect and record AHREs and are manufacturer specific. However, devices generally provide a reliable way to quantify AF burden. Devices do not simply average atrial cycles, and they vary in their rate detection and recordings. Therefore, evaluation of AHREs requires interpretation of the stored atrial rate data based on knowledge of how a particular device processes the data.

AHREs are not synonymous with AF, because they are dependent on the rate cut-off and duration of the high rate. As a rule, AHREs should be evaluated with the corresponding stored atrial electrograms. However, manual adjudication may not be necessary in some pacemaker-based recordings, provided the accuracy of AF detection without electrograms has been proven. Not all mode switches are necessarily caused by AF and should not be a surrogate for AF. Mode switches are less precise than full data disclosure with electrograms. Atrial oversensing can cause overestimation of AF episodes, whereas undersensing of AF may cause underestimation.

In 2003, Glotzer and colleagues[1] analyzed AHREs from MOST (Mode Selection Trial) and documented that AHREs greater than 5 minutes in duration and rate greater than 220 bpm were detected in 51% of patients during a mean of 27 months after implantation of a dual-chamber pacemaker for sinus node dysfunction. Patients with at least 1 episode of AHRE were 2.5 times more likely to die, 2.8 times more likely to die or have a nonfatal stroke, and nearly 6 times as likely to develop AF as patients without any AHRE. However, this was a retrospective analysis, including only 312 patients, and more than one-third of those with AHRE already had a clinical diagnosis of AF. In TRENDS (The Relationship Between Daily Atrial Tachyarrhythmia Burden From Implantable Device Diagnostics and Stroke Risks Study), it was shown that patients with a daily burden of AT of more than 5.5 hours had a 2.4-fold increase in the risk of thromboembolism, compared with patients with no AT.[2] In these trials, subclinical AF also increased the risk of clinical AF 5-fold to 6-fold, which suggests that subclinical AF could be regarded as a precursor to clinical AF. Whether the number of subclinical AF episodes, the AF burden (percentage of time spent in AF divided by total time), or the duration of the longest AF episode may be the best predictor for subsequent stroke, is still under debate.

Capucci and colleagues[36] reported the thromboembolic complications on a long-term follow-up (median 22 months) of 725 patients with permanent

Medtronic DDDR pacemakers for bradycardia and suffering from AF. Previous embolism, ischemic cardiomyopathy, hypertension, diabetes mellitus, and, in general, the presence of stroke risk factors resulted in the association of higher risk of embolism. Patients with device-detected AF recurrences longer than 1 day had a risk of embolism 3.1 times increased compared with patients without or with shorter AF recurrences, showing that AF recurrences longer than 1 day are independently associated with arterial embolism (P<.0001).

ASSERT (Asymptomatic Atrial Fibrillation and Stroke Evaluation in Pacemaker Patients and the AF Reduction Atrial Pacing Trial) enrolled 2580 patients, 65 years of age or older, with

hypertension and no history of AF or related tachyarrhythmias in whom a pacemaker or defibrillator had recently been implanted (2451 pacemakers and 129 ICDs [St. Jude Medical, Saint Paul, MN, USA]), all capable of storing high-atrial-rate electrograms. The patients were monitored for 3 months to detect subclinical atrial tachyarrhythmias (episodes of atrial rate >190 bpm for >6 minutes) and then followed for a mean of 2.5 years for the primary outcome of ischemic stroke or systemic embolism (**Fig. 4**).[37–39] Kaufman and colleagues[38] reported the adjudicated AHREs derived from the programmed AT/AF algorithms. Of these AHREs, 82.7% were true AT/AF episodes, and 17.3%

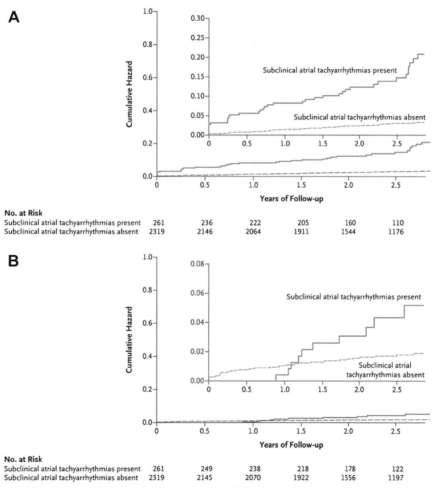

Fig. 4. The risk of clinical atrial tachyarrhythmias and of ischemic stroke or systemic embolism, according to the presence or absence of subclinical atrial tachyarrhythmia's (ASSERT trial). (*A*) The risk of electrocardiographically documented clinical atrial tachyarrhythmias after the 3-month visit, according to whether subclinical atrial tachyarrhythmias were or were not detected between enrollment and the 3-month visit. (*B*) The risk of ischemic stroke or systemic embolism after the 3-month visit, according to whether subclinical atrial tachyarrhythmias were or were not detected between enrollment and the 3-month visit. The insets show the same data on an enlarged y-axis. (*From* Healey JS, Connolly SJ, Gold MR, et al, ASSERT Investigators. Subclinical atrial fibrillation and the risk of stroke. N Engl J Med 2012;366:126; with permission.)

were inappropriate AT/AF episodes, highlighting the importance of individual electrogram review. The positive-predictive value for detecting true AT/AF improved with increased episode duration.

Subclinical (asymptomatic) atrial tachyarrhythmias were detected in 10% of the patients (n = 261) within 3 months after device implantation, and at least once in 34.7% of the patients during the follow-up of 2.5 years. Subclinical AF episodes were almost 8 times as common as clinical AF (P<.001). Subclinical atrial tachyarrhythmias often preceded the development of clinical AF. Clinical AF developed in only 15.7% of the patients with subclinical AF, suggesting that there is a time lag between subclinical events and clinical detection. Subclinical atrial tachyarrhythmias were associated with an increased risk of clinical AF (P<.001) and of ischemic stroke or systemic embolism (P = .007). The population attributable risk of stroke or systemic embolism associated with subclinical atrial tachyarrhythmias was 13%. The risk was virtually unchanged after adjustment for baseline risk factors for stroke (P = .008). During the follow-up period, 11 of the 261 patients (4.2%) in whom subclinical atrial tachyarrhythmias had been detected before 3 months had an ischemic stroke or systemic embolism (a rate of 1.69% per year), compared with 40 of the 2319 in whom subclinical atrial tachyarrhythmias had not been detected (1.7%, a rate of 0.69% per year, P = .007).

The ASSERT study did not show a strong temporal relationship between AHRE and thromboembolic events. The median interval between the most recent previous AHRE and the thromboembolic complication was 47 days, and only 27% of patients with AHRE who suffered a thromboembolic complication were in AF at the time of that event. This finding is in keeping with the published report from the TRENDS trial, which found that in patients with AHRE and a thromboembolic event, only 30% were in AF at the time of the event, and in the remaining patients, the most recent AHRE was an average of 168 ± 199 days earlier.[2]

MONITORING BY CARDIAC RESYNCHRONIZATION DEVICES

Shanmugam and colleagues[18] studied 560 patients with heart failure (median left ventricular ejection fraction 27%) with a CRT device (past history of paroxysmal AF in 178 patients). AHRE burden was defined as the duration of mode switch in a 24-hour period with atrial rates of more than 180 bpm. The investigators did not adjudicate the individual AHRE, but defined them as significant if they were documented for at least 1% of any day (14 minutes). Thromboembolic complications developed in 2% of patients (n=11) and were 9 times more likely to develop among patients who had at least 3.8 hours of AHRE detected during any day. Sarkar and colleagues[40] retrospectively evaluated 519 CRT patients with paroxysmal AF (n = 519, 33% of all the CRT patients) and documented a greater risk of hospitalization for heart failure (P<.001) in patients with AF compared with patients with no AF. The risk increased further (P<.001) if there was 1 day of poor rate control during persistent AF or a high burden of paroxysmal AF in the last 30 days. Thus, a high burden of paroxysmal AF (>6 hours) with good or poor rate control is a risk factor for heart failure hospitalization in the next 30 days. The amount of AF, and the changes in rate control status during AF, may provide an opportunity to proactively reduce hospitalizations.

SUMMARY

In the last decade, our knowledge of AF in heart failure has increased dramatically, in large part because of the widespread use of continuous monitoring, mostly provided by implanted cardiac rhythm devices. Continuous monitoring has improved CRT management of patients with AF. New knowledge acquired from continuous monitoring has generated important questions, especially in patients with only asymptomatic AF and in those with very short AHREs. The answers to these questions require randomized trials.

- Several studies support a link between AHRE detected by implantable cardiac rhythm devices and the occurrence of stroke or systemic embolism. The minimum duration of subclinical or asymptomatic AF associated with a higher risk of thromboembolism remains debatable (ranging from 6 minutes in the ASSERT trial to 5.5 hours in the TRENDS study).
- Considering that there is frequently a long interval between AHRE and thromboembolic events, a causative relationship is questionable. It is more likely that AHRE are one of many features of the complex pathophysiologic mechanism that leads to cardioembolic events.
- The prevalence of subclinical atrial tachyarrhythmias may be higher in patients with pacemakers than in other high-risk patient groups. Sinus node dysfunction is associated with an increased risk of AF. Furthermore, patients with AV nodal disease may be more likely to be asymptomatic when atrial

tachyarrhythmias occur because of reduced AV conduction.

- Monitoring of the VR with ambulatory devices or implantable cardiac rhythm devices in patients with heart failure should be used to determine whether excessive VRs are present, targeting a resting VR of less than 80 bpm and peak activity rates of less than 110 to 120 bpm. The results of the RACE II trial that lenient rate control is not inferior to strict rate control should not be extrapolated to patients with heart failure.
- Although there is a strong association between AHRE and stroke, authorities believe that more data in the form of randomized studies are needed before routine oral anticoagulation can be recommended. Anticoagulant therapy should probably be considered in high-risk patients with asymptomatic AF from the CHADS2 score (or CHA2DS$_2$-VASc score) of 2 or greater (heart failure = 1) considering also the bleeding risk (HASBLED score, European Society of Cardiology).[41] In the ASSERT trial the absolute rate of stroke increased with increasing CHADS$_2$ score, reaching a rate of 3.78% per year in patients with subclinical atrial tachyarrhythmias and a CHADS2 score of greater than 2.
- The incidence of AF in patients with heart failure treated with CRT ranges from 30% to 35% for paroxysmal AF and around 20% to 25% for permanent AF. In CRT patients, AF is associated with an increase in heart failure hospitalizations and death. The greatest mortality reduction in CRT patients with AF was observed with BiV% greater than 98%. One should always aim for a BiV% of 100%. Small gains in BiV% are important. AVJ ablation will become more widely used, because it permits CRT delivery close to 100% of the time with regularization of the RR intervals, elimination of fusion and pseudofusion beats, and discontinuation of some AV nodal blocking drugs.

REFERENCES

1. Glotzer TV, Hellkamp AS, Zimmerman J, et al, MOST Investigators. Atrial high rate episodes detected by pacemaker diagnostics predict death and stroke: report of the Atrial Diagnostics Ancillary Study of the MOde Selection Trial (MOST). Circulation 2003; 107(12):1614–9.
2. Glotzer TV, Daoud EG, Wyse DG, et al. The relationship between daily atrial tachyarrhythmia burden from implantable device diagnostics and stroke risk: the TRENDS study. Circ Arrhythm Electrophysiol 2009;2:474–80.
3. Santini M, Gasparini M, Landolina M, et al, Cardiological centers participating in ClinicalService Project. Device-detected atrial tachyarrhythmias predict adverse outcome in real-world patients with implantable biventricular defibrillators. J Am Coll Cardiol 2011;57: 167–72.
4. Marijon E, Jacob S, Mouton E, et al, Mona Lisa Study Group. Frequency of atrial tachyarrhythmias in patients treated by cardiac resynchronization (from the Prospective, Multicenter Mona Lisa Study). Am J Cardiol 2010;106:688–93.
5. Leclercq C, Padeletti L, Cihák R, et al, CHAMP Study Investigators. Incidence of paroxysmal atrial tachycardias in patients treated with cardiac resynchronization therapy and continuously monitored by device diagnostics. Europace 2010;12:71–7.
6. Yannopoulos D, Lurie KG, Sakaguchi S, et al. Reduced atrial tachyarrhythmia susceptibility after upgrade of conventional pulse generator to cardiac resynchronization therapy in patients with heart failure. J Am Coll Cardiol 2007;50:1246–51.
7. Maisel WH, Stevenson LW. Atrial fibrillation in heart failure: epidemiology, pathophysiology, and rationale for therapy. Am J Cardiol 2003;91:2D–8D.
8. Tolosana JM, Hernandez Madrid A, Brugada J, et al, SPARE Investigators. Comparison of benefits and mortality in cardiac resynchronization therapy in patients with atrial fibrillation versus patients in sinus rhythm (Results of the Spanish Atrial Fibrillation and Resynchronization [SPARE] Study). Am J Cardiol 2008;102:444–9.
9. Molhoek SG, Bax JJ, Bleeker GB, et al. Comparison of response to cardiac resynchronization therapy in patients with sinus rhythm versus chronic atrial fibrillation. Am J Cardiol 2004;94:1506–9.
10. Linde C, Leclercq C, Rex S, et al. Long-term benefits of biventricular pacing in congestive heart failure: results from the MUltisite STimulation in cardiomyopathy (MUSTIC) study. J Am Coll Cardiol 2002;40: 111–8.
11. De Ruvo E, Gargaro A, Sciarra L, et al. Early detection of adverse events with daily remote monitoring versus quarterly standard follow-up program in patients with CRT-D. Pacing Clin Electrophysiol 2011; 34:208–16.
12. Burri H, Quesada A, Ricci RP, et al. The MOnitoring Resynchronization dEvices and CARdiac patiEnts (MORE-CARE) study: rationale and design. Am Heart J 2010;160:42–8.
13. Ricci RP, Morichelli L, Gargaro A, et al. Home monitoring in patients with implantable cardiac devices: is there a potential reduction of stroke risk? Results from a computer model tested through Monte Carlo simulations. J Cardiovasc Electrophysiol 2009;20: 1244–51.

14. Borleffs CJ, Ypenburg C, van Bommel RJ, et al. Clinical importance of new onset atrial fibrillation after cardiac resynchronization therapy. Heart Rhythm 2009;6:305–10.

15. Crossley GH, Aonuma K, Haffajee C, et al, Concerto-AT Study Investigators. Atrial fibrillation therapy in patients with a CRT defibrillator with wireless telemetry. Pacing Clin Electrophysiol 2009;32:13–23.

16. Ip J, Waldo AL, Lip GY, et al, IMPACT Investigators. Multicenter randomized study of anticoagulation guided by remote rhythm monitoring in patients with implantable cardioverter-defibrillator and CRT-D devices: rationale, design, and clinical characteristics of the initially enrolled cohort. The IMPACT study. Am Heart J 2009;58:364–70.

17. Khoo CW, Krishnamoorthy S, Lim HS, et al. Atrial fibrillation, arrhythmia burden and thrombogenesis. Int J Cardiol 2012;157:318–23.

18. Shanmugam N, Boerdlein A, Proff J, et al. Detection of atrial high-rate events by continuous home monitoring: clinical significance in the heart failure-cardiac resynchronization therapy population. Europace 2012;14:230–7.

19. Boriani G, Gasparini M, Landolina M, et al, on behalf of the Clinical Service Cardiac Centres. Incidence and clinical relevance of uncontrolled ventricular rate during atrial fibrillation in heart failure patients treated with cardiac resynchronization therapy. Eur J Heart Fail 2011;13(8):868–76.

20. Van Gelder IC, Groenveld HF, Crijns HJ, RACE II Investigators. Lenient versus strict rate control in patients with atrial fibrillation. N Engl J Med 2010;362:1363–73.

21. Brenyo A, Link MS, Barsheshet A, et al. Cardiac resynchronization therapy reduces left atrial volume and the risk of atrial tachyarrhythmias in MADIT-CRT (Multicenter Automatic Defibrillator Implantation Trial with Cardiac Resynchronization Therapy). J Am Coll Cardiol 2011;58:1682–9.

22. Gasparini M, Auricchio A, Regoli F, et al. Four-year efficacy of cardiac resynchronization therapy on exercise tolerance and disease progression: the importance of performing atrioventricular junction ablation in patients with atrial fibrillation. J Am Coll Cardiol 2006;48:734–43.

23. Gasparini M, Auricchio A, Metra M, et al, Multicentre Longitudinal Observational Study (MILOS) Group. Long-term survival in patients undergoing cardiac resynchronization therapy: the importance of performing atrio-ventricular junction ablation in patients with permanent atrial fibrillation. Eur Heart J 2008;29:1644–52.

24. Ferreira AM, Adragão P, Cavaco DM, et al. Benefit of cardiac resynchronization therapy in atrial fibrillation patients vs. patients in sinus rhythm: the role of atrio-ventricular junction ablation. Europace 2008;10:809–15.

25. Dong K, Shen WK, Powell BD, et al. Atrioventricular nodal ablation predicts survival benefit in patients with atrial fibrillation receiving cardiac resynchronization therapy. Heart Rhythm 2010;7:1240–5.

26. Bradley DJ, Shen WK. Atrioventricular junction ablation combined with either right ventricular pacing or cardiac resynchronization therapy for atrial fibrillation: the need for large-scale randomized trials. Heart Rhythm 2007;4:224–32.

27. Foley PW, Leyva F. Long-term survival in patients undergoing cardiac resynchronization therapy: the importance of atrio-ventricular junction ablation in patients with permanent atrial fibrillation. Eur Heart J 2008;29:2182.

28. Kaszala K, Ellenbogen KA. Role of cardiac resynchronization therapy and atrioventricular junction ablation in patients with permanent atrial fibrillation. Eur Heart J 2011;32:2344–6.

29. Himmel F, Reppel M, Mortensen K, et al. A strategy to achieve CRT response in permanent atrial fibrillation without obligatory atrioventricular node ablation. Pacing Clin Electrophysiol 2012;35:943–7.

30. Koplan BA, Kaplan AJ, Weiner S, et al. Heart failure decompensation and all-cause mortality in relation to percent biventricular pacing in patients with heart failure: is a goal of 100% biventricular pacing necessary? J Am Coll Cardiol 2009;53:355–60.

31. Hayes DL, Boehmer JP, Day JD, et al. Cardiac resynchronization therapy and the relationship of percent biventricular pacing to symptoms and survival. Heart Rhythm 2011;8:1469–75.

32. Kamath GS, Cotiga D, Koneru JN, et al. The utility of 12-lead Holter monitoring in patients with permanent atrial fibrillation for the identification of nonresponders after cardiac resynchronization therapy. J Am Coll Cardiol 2009;53:1050–5.

33. Healey JS, Hohnloser SH, Exner DV, et al, RAFT Investigators. Cardiac resynchronization therapy in patients with permanent atrial fibrillation: results from the Resynchronization for Ambulatory Heart Failure Trial (RAFT). Circ Heart Fail 2012;5(5):566–70.

34. Caldwell JC, Contractor H, Petkar S, et al. Atrial fibrillation is under-recognized in chronic heart failure: insights from a heart failure cohort treated with cardiac resynchronization therapy. Europace 2009;11:1295–300.

35. Israel CW, Gronefeld G, Ehrlich JR, et al. Long-term risk of recurrent atrial fibrillation as documented by an implantable monitoring device: implications for optimal patient care. J Am Coll Cardiol 2004;43:47–52.

36. Capucci A, Santini M, Padeletti L, et al, Italian AT500 Registry Investigators. Monitored atrial fibrillation duration predicts arterial embolic events in patients suffering from bradycardia and atrial fibrillation

implanted with antitachycardia pacemakers. J Am Coll Cardiol 2005;46:1913–20.

37. Hohnloser SH, Capucci A, Fain E, et al. ASymptomatic atrial fibrillation and Stroke Evaluation in pacemaker patients and the atrial fibrillation reduction atrial pacing Trial (ASSERT). Am Heart J 2006;152:442–7.

38. Kaufman ES, Israel CW, Nair GM, et al, ASSERT Steering Committee and Investigators. Positive predictive value of device-detected atrial high-rate episodes at different rates and durations: an analysis from ASSERT. Heart Rhythm 2012;9:1241–6.

39. Healey JS, Connolly SJ, Gold MR, et al, ASSERT Investigators. Subclinical atrial fibrillation and the risk of stroke. N Engl J Med 2012;366:120–9.

40. Sarkar S, Koehler J, Crossley GH, et al. Burden of atrial fibrillation and poor rate control detected by continuous monitoring and the risk for heart failure hospitalization. Am Heart J 2012;164:616–24.

41. Camm AJ, Kirchhof P, Lip GY, et al. Guidelines for the management of atrial fibrillation: the task force for the management of atrial fibrillation of the European Society of Cardiology (ESC). Eur Heart J 2010;31(19):2369–429.

Ventricular Rate Control of Atrial Fibrillation in Heart Failure

Michiel Rienstra, MD, PhD, Isabelle C. Van Gelder, MD, PhD*

KEYWORDS

- Atrial fibrillation • Heart failure • Ventricular rate • Treatment • Rate control

KEY POINTS

- Ventricular rate control in patients with atrial fibrillation (AF) and chronic heart failure (HF) is recommended as the first-line therapy in the acute phase.
- The decision for long-term ventricular rate control should be based on patient symptoms and the cause of HF.
- If the ventricular rate control is adopted, a target of less than 110 beats per minute is appropriate for most patients.
- Stricter rate control may be indicated in patients with persisting AF-related symptoms under lenient rate control or in the setting of HF with ongoing ischemia, severe diastolic dysfunction, hypertrophic cardiomyopathy, hypotension, or signs of pulmonary congestion, although the beneficial effects of stricter rate control have not yet been proven.
- Ventricular rate control is generally easy to achieve, although frequent dose adjustments, combinations of drugs, and medication changes may be needed.

INTRODUCTION

Atrial fibrillation (AF) and heart failure (HF) often coexist.[1,2] The prevalence of AF in patients with chronic HF in cardiology practices in Europe is 42%.[3] The incidence and the prevalence of AF increase with the severity of HF.[4] From several small studies, it is known that AF begets HF and HF begets AF in the first place because both have shared risk factors, like hypertension and ischemia.[5,6] The loss of atrioventricular synchrony (loss of atrial kick), the rapid ventricular rate, the irregular ventricular response (R-R irregularity), and the development of tachycardiomyopathy during AF may adversely affect ventricular function and overall hemodynamic status.[7–13] The onset of AF is associated with a worsening of the New York Heart Association (NYHA) functional class for HF and a decline in peak exercise capacity, a lower cardiac index, and increased mitral and tricuspid regurgitation in patients with mild to moderate chronic HF.[14] The increased atrial pressure and volume, the activation of the renin-angiotensin-aldosterone system, and the activation of the sympathetic nervous system that occurs in chronic HF may result in atrial stretch and interstitial fibrosis.[10,15–17]

In the last few years, there has been a major shift in the treatment of AF in the setting of HF, from rhythm to ventricular rate control in most patients with both conditions. In the present article, the authors focus on ventricular rate control and discuss

No conflicts of interest.

Department of Cardiology, University Medical Center Groningen, University of Groningen, Groningen, Hanzeplein 1, PO Box 30.001, Groningen 9700 RB, The Netherlands

* Corresponding author. Department of Cardiology, Thoraxcenter, University Medical Center Groningen, University of Groningen, Hanzeplein 1, PO Box 30.001, Groningen 9700 RB, The Netherlands.

E-mail address: I.C.van.Gelder@umcg.nl

Heart Failure Clin 9 (2013) 397–406

http://dx.doi.org/10.1016/j.hfc.2013.07.004

the indications; the optimal ventricular rate-control target, including ventricular results in the Rate Control Efficacy in Permanent Atrial Fibrillation: a comparison Between Lenient versus Strict Rate Control II (RACE II) study[18]; and the pharmacologic and nonpharmacologic options to control the ventricular rate during AF in the setting of HF.

INDICATIONS FOR VENTRICULAR RATE CONTROL OF AF IN HF

The treatment of patients with AF and chronic HF may differ from patient to patient. Initial acute therapy includes adequate ventricular rate control and anticoagulation based on the thromboembolic risk.[19] Before choosing ventricular rate control as a long-term strategy, symptoms and potential further deterioration of HF need to be considered.[19] Previously, 6 randomized controlled trials (the Atrial Fibrillation Follow-up Investigation of Rhythm Management [AFFIRM], the Rate Control versus Electrical Cardioversion for Persistent Atrial Fibrillation [RACE], the Pharmacologic Intervention in Atrial Fibrillation [PIAF], the Strategies of Treatment of Atrial Fibrillation [STAF], the How to Treat Chronic Atrial Fibrillation [HOT CAFE], and the Japanese Rhythm Management Trial for Atrial Fibrillation [J-RHYTHM]) showed that a ventricular rate-control strategy (see **Table 1** for the variety in ventricular rate-control criteria) is not inferior to rhythm control with regard to cardiovascular morbidity and mortality.[20–25] Although in most of these studies only a subset of patients had chronic HF, the large randomized Rhythm Control versus Rate Control for Atrial Fibrillation and Heart Failure trial confirmed that in 1376 patients with AF and chronic HF (AF-CHF), a routine strategy of rhythm control does not reduce the rate of death from cardiovascular causes, symptoms, functional status, quality of life, and left ventricular ejection fraction (LVEF), as compared with a ventricular rate-control strategy.[26–28]

Table 1
Heart rate criteria used in the rate versus rhythm control trials

Trial	Year	Primary Endpoint	Ventricular Rate Control Criteria
PIAF[22]	2000	Symptoms related to AF	Diltiazem 90 mg, 2–3 times per day, additional rate-control therapy at discretion of physician
AFFIRM[20]	2002	All-cause mortality	≤80 bpm and ≤110 bpm during moderate exercise; on Holter mean ventricular rate ≤100 bpm and not >110% of the maximum predicted heart rate
RACE[21]	2002	Composite of cardiovascular death, HF hospitalization, thromboembolic complications, bleeding, pacemaker implantation, and severe adverse effects or antiarrhythmic drugs	<100 bpm
STAF[23]	2003	Composite of all-cause mortality, stroke or transient ischemic attack, systemic embolism, and cardiopulmonary resuscitation	Not specified
HOT CAFE[24]	2004	All-cause mortality, thromboembolic complications and intracranial or other major hemorrhage	70–90 bpm, <140 bpm during moderate exercise
AF-CHF[26]	2008	Cardiovascular death	≤80 bpm and ≤110 bpm during 6-min walk test
J-RHYTHM[25]	2009	Composite of all-cause mortality, symptomatic cerebral infarction, systemic embolism, major bleeding, HF hospitalization, physical/psychological disability requiring alteration of assigned strategy	60–80 bpm

Abbreviations: AF, atrial fibrillation; HF, heart failure; bpm, beat per minute.
Adapted from Groenveld HF, Crijns HJ, Tijssen JG, et al. Rate control in atrial fibrillation, insight into the RACE II study. Neth Heart J 2013;21(4):200; with permission.

However, since in the randomized controlled trials patients with severe symptoms were not included, rhythm control is still indicated in those patients who are severely symptomatic. But in the majority of patients with minor or absence of symptoms of AF long-term ventricular rate control is recommended. Previously, several small patient studies reported that AF adversely affects ventricular function and overall hemodynamic status.[7–13] Conversely, adequate ventricular rate control may improve left ventricular function.[13,29] In the aforementioned randomized controlled trials and their substudies, no evidence for the development of tachycardiomyopathy with ventricular rate control was found. In addition, in patients with chronic HF, no further deterioration of left ventricular function was observed.[26,28,30,31] Accordingly, no superior efficacy of rhythm control was observed. Furthermore, the safety of a rhythm-control strategy is a concern because patients with HF may be prone to proarrhythmic side effects of the antiarrhythmic drugs used to maintain sinus rhythm.[19] This inclination may further limit the applicability of a rhythm-control strategy in patients with HF. A rate-control strategy is, thus, established as one of the evidence-based strategies for managing patients with AF in the setting of chronic HF.

However, because the randomized controlled trials typically enrolled patients without severe symptoms, rhythm control should be strongly considered in the subset of patients who are severely symptomatic. In patients with HF with severe diastolic dysfunction or restrictive physiology (eg, hypertrophic cardiomyopathy), the loss of atrial kick during AF may be of great hemodynamic importance and lead to symptoms, and a rhythm-control strategy may still be indicated.

OPTIMAL VENTRICULAR RATE-CONTROL TARGET OF AF IN HF

The optimal target for ventricular rate control in patients with AF and chronic HF is the subject of an ongoing debate. So far, there has been 1 randomized controlled trial designed to address this specific question: the RACE II study.[18] In this pivotal trial, 614 patients with permanent AF and a resting ventricular rate of more than 80 beats per minute (bpm) were included. Of the total, 60 patients (10%) had a prior HF hospitalization, 93 patients (15%) had an LVEF of 40% or less, and 214 patients (35%) had dyspnea and were in the NYHA functional class II or III. The primary outcome was a composite of death from cardiovascular causes, hospitalization for HF and stroke, systemic embolism, bleeding, and life-threatening arrhythmic events and was assessed during 2 to 3 years of follow-up. The lenient ventricular rate-control target was a resting ventricular rate of less than 110 bpm, and the strict ventricular rate-control targets were a resting ventricular rate less than 80 bpm and a ventricular rate during moderate exercise of less than 110 bpm. During the dose-adjustment phase, patients were administered one or more negative dromotropic drugs (ie, beta-blockers, nondihydropyridine calcium channel blockers, and digoxin), used alone or in combination and at various doses, until the ventricular rate targets were achieved. The mean resting ventricular rate at the end of the dose-adjustment phase was 93 ± 9 bpm in the lenient-control group, as compared with 76 ± 12 bpm in the strict-control group ($P<.001$). There was no difference in the occurrence of the composite primary end point (38 in the lenient-control group and 43 in the strict-control group) or in its individual components. Furthermore, a predefined substudy of the RACE II trial was performed to assess the effect of the stringency of ventricular rate control on quality of life and symptoms.[32] General health-related quality of life was assessed using the Medical Outcomes Study 36-Item Short-Form Health Survey; the severity of AF-related symptoms was assessed with the University of Toronto AF Severity Scale (AF severity scale); and the severity of fatigue was measured using the Multidimensional Fatigue Inventory-20. At baseline, 58% of patients experienced symptoms of AF, predominantly dyspnea, fatigue, and palpitations. There were no differences in symptoms of AF at either baseline or at the end of the study between the lenient- and strict-control groups. Furthermore, the stringency of the rate control did not improve quality of life, measured on any of the used questionnaires. Instead, changes in quality of life were related to age, symptoms, severity of underlying disease, and female sex.[32] RACE II, thus, demonstrated that stringency of ventricular rate control had no influence on symptoms, quality of life, cardiovascular morbidity, and mortality. The main concern of high ventricular rates accompanying AF is the development of tachycardiomyopathy.[7–13] An echocardiographic substudy of RACE II investigated left ventricular and atrial remodeling in patients with permanent AF treated with lenient or strict rate control.[33] In general, no important adverse atrial or ventricular remodeling during the 3-year follow-up was observed. In addition, lenient rate control did not cause significant adverse atrial and ventricular remodeling compared with strict rate control.[33]

It is important to note that only a minority of patients with AF and HF were included in RACE II, although, as in the main trial, no effect of ventricular rate-control stringency on cardiovascular morbidity and mortality was consistently seen in those patients with AF and HF.[61] At this point, data from RACE II are some of the sparse data that are available on ventricular rate control in patients with AF and HF. Grogan and colleagues[13] reported in 1992 that adequate rate control, using mainly digoxin and amiodarone, improved left ventricular function in 10 patients with presumed idiopathic dilated cardiomyopathy with impaired left ventricular function. However, no specific rate-control target was defined. Khand and colleagues[35] performed the first randomized, double-blinded, placebo-controlled study. In total, 47 patients with persistent AF and systolic chronic HF were included. In the first 4 months, digoxin was compared with the combination of digoxin and carvedilol. In the 6 months thereafter, digoxin was withdrawn in a double-blinded manner in the carvedilol-treated arm, thus allowing a comparison between digoxin and carvedilol. Compared with digoxin alone, combination therapy lowered the ventricular rate on 24-hour Holter monitoring and during submaximal exercise, and LVEF and symptoms improved. There were no significant differences found between digoxin alone and carvedilol alone. Again, no prespecified ventricular rate-control targets were applied. More recently, Silvet and colleagues[36] performed an open-label, crossover, interventional study including patients with AF and chronic systolic HF. Quality of life and exercise tolerance were assessed before and after attempting strict ventricular rate control. Patients were treated with increasing doses of metoprolol succinate to achieve a target resting ventricular rate of less than 70 bpm. On monthly visits, the dose of the medication was increased in 25-mg to 50-mg steps until the ventricular rate target was reached or until side effects occurred. Quality of life and exercise tolerance were measured after at least 2 weeks of stable medication dose. After a mean follow-up of 98 days, the resting ventricular rate decreased from 94 ± 14 bpm to 85 ± 12 bpm ($P = .005$). Only 2 patients achieved the goal of a resting ventricular rate of less than 70 bpm. Side effects prevented further up-titration of metoprolol in the remaining patients. Both the primary outcome, meters walked during a 6-minute walk test, and quality of life as measured by the Minnesota Living With Heart Failure Questionnaire did not change.

Long-term prognostic information was provided by several subanalyses of randomized controlled trials and the aforementioned RACE II study.[18,37–40] A substudy of the Second Prospective Randomised Study of Ibopamine on Mortality and Efficacy (PRIME II) aimed to study heart rate in patients with AF and chronic systolic HF.[37] In total,

77 patients with AF at inclusion and advanced systolic HF were studied and dichotomized according to the median heart rate of 80 bpm at inclusion (39 patients with low heart rate and 38 patients with high heart rate). Both patient groups were remarkably comparable; after a mean follow-up of 3.3 ± 0.9 years, mortality was comparable (62% vs 55%). If anything, lower heart rates were related to impaired prognosis. The Candesartan in Heart Failure: Assessment of Reduction in Mortality and Morbidity (CHARM) Program enrolled 7599 patients with a clinical diagnosis of chronic HF that were enrolled in CHARM-Alternative (n = 2028, LVEF <40% and not receiving an angiotensin-converting enzyme inhibitor because of previous intolerance), CHARM-Added (n = 2548, LVEF <40% receiving angiotensin-converting enzyme inhibitor treatment), and the CHARM-Preserved study (n = 3023, LVEF >40%). Among all 3 CHARM studies, 1148 patients with AF at randomization were included. There was no association between ventricular rate and cardiovascular morbidity and mortality found in patients with AF; this is in great contrast to patients with sinus rhythm.[41] In the Permanent Atrial Fibrillation Outcome Study Using Dronedarone on Top of Standard Therapy (PALLAS), which was prematurely stopped for safety reasons, the high rate of cardiovascular events occurring directly after the institution of dronedarone may be related to excessive rate control. The ventricular rate at 1 month in survivors in the dronedarone arm had decreased by 7.6 ± 14.5 bpm.[42] Based on the studies described earlier, there is no evidence supporting the deleterious effects of a lenient ventricular rate-control approach in patients with AF.

At present, the European Society of Cardiology's 2010 AF guidelines[43] state that it is reasonable to initiate treatment with a lenient rate-control protocol aimed at a resting heart rate of less than 110 bpm and to adopt a stricter rate-control strategy (a resting heart rate of less than 80 bpm and heart rate during moderate exercise of less than 110 bpm) when symptoms persist or tachycardiomyopathy occurs, despite lenient rate control. After achieving the strict heart rate target, a 24-hour Holter monitor is recommended to assess safety (Fig. 1). No specific ventricular rate-control targets for patients with HF are described. The 2011 AF guidelines of the American College of Cardiology (ACC)/American Heart Association (AHA)/Heart Rhythm Society recommend strict ventricular rate control for patients with AF in the setting of chronic HF, with a ventricular rate target of 60 to 80 bpm at rest and 90 to 115 bpm during moderate exercise.[19] The 2009 chronic HF guidelines recommend a more lenient

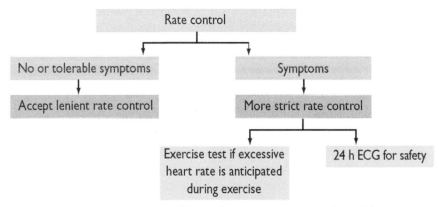

Fig. 1. Ventricular rate control approach according to the European Society of Cardiology's 2010 AF guidelines. (*Adapted from* Camm AJ, Kirchhof P, Lip GY, et al. Guidelines for the management of atrial fibrillation: the Task Force for the Management of Atrial Fibrillation of the European Society of Cardiology (ESC). Eur Heart J 2010;31:2369–429; with permission.)

approach, with a target ventricular rate of less than 80 to 90 bpm at rest and less than 110 to 130 during moderate exercise.[44]

Based on the available literature, there is no evidence supporting that different long-term ventricular rate-control targets should be recommended in patients with AF in the setting of chronic HF. In general, ventricular rates during AF of less than 110 bpm seem sufficient, although the persistence of symptoms or the presence of ongoing ischemia, signs of pulmonary congestion, severe diastolic dysfunction, and hypertrophic (obstructive) cardiomyopathy may warrant stricter targets; however, the beneficial effects of stricter rate control have not been proven.

PHARMACOLOGIC VENTRICULAR RATE CONTROL OF AF IN HF

Ventricular rate control is generally easy to achieve, although frequent dose adjustments, combinations of drugs, and medication changes may be needed.[18,36,45] In randomized controlled studies, pharmacologic ventricular rate control has been achieved in 70% to 80% of patients, dependent primarily on the rate-control target that was attempted.[18,45,46] As previously described, there is no evidence of any adverse influence on left ventricular function; serious adverse effects from rate-control drugs are uncommon. However, the rate-control strategy is not without adverse effects.[18,20,21] Negative dromotropic treatment that slows ventricular rates may lead to symptomatic bradycardia and eventually to otherwise unnecessary pacemaker implantation.

Ventricular rate control can be achieved by beta-blockers, nondihydropyridine calcium channel antagonists, digoxin, and amiodarone alone or in combination. Beta-blockers are the most effective rate-control agents[26] that reduce morbidity and mortality in HF patients and have a class IA recommendation[44] in the current chronic HF guidelines. This recommendation also holds for patients with AF and chronic HF, although the data are less convincing, as was shown in a recent meta-analysis including 8680 patients with chronic HF, of whom 1677 had AF from 4 selected randomized placebo-controlled beta-blocker trials.[47] In a systematic review by Segal and colleagues,[48] beta-blockers were proven safe and effective for control of heart rate in patients with AF and superior to placebo. Beta-blockers are effective for controlling ventricular rates in rest and during exercise[48] and provide better control of ventricular rates during exercise than digoxin.[49] Beta-blockers should be initiated cautiously in patients with AF and chronic systolic HF.[44] Patients taking beta-blockers may experience slow rates at rest or compromised exercise tolerance when the ventricular rate response is restrained excessively.[48]

Individual patient responses to a specific type of beta-blockers may depend on the presence of the beta-1-adrenoceptor Arg389Gly polymorphism; however, because data are sparse and sometimes conflicting, this has not yet found its way into clinical practice. The common single nucleotide polymorphism in the beta-1-adrenoceptor (Arg389Gly), a replacement of arginine with glycine at position 389, results in reduced cyclic adenosine monophosphate synthesis.[50,51] Around 40% of people of European ancestry are heterozygous and approximately 7% homozygous for the Gly389 genetic variant. Parvez and colleagues[52] reported that in the Vanderbilt AF registry, 543 patients with AF with the homozygous Arg389 genotype are more resistant to pharmacologic rate control (using different beta-blockers) than patients with AF with sinus rhythm, but only 11% of the patients in that study had HF. Two substudies of large randomized trials in patients with AF and chronic HF have been reported. The effect of this polymorphism on the ventricular rate response by beta-blockers was investigated in a pharmacogenetics substudy of the Cardiac Insufficiency Bisoprolol Study in Elderly study (CIBIS-ELD). This substudy included 528 patients (421 with sinus rhythm and 107 with AF) with chronic HF.[53] Patients were randomized to bisoprolol or carvedilol. Patients in sinus rhythm responded essentially identically to bisoprolol and carvedilol, independent of genotype. However, patients with AF who were homozygous for Arg389 had a 12-bpm lower response to carvedilol (but not bisoprolol) than carriers of at least one Gly389 allele. The immediate response to carvedilol did not differ between genotypes. Although intriguing, the absence of a ventricular rate response to carvedilol in Arg389-homozygous carriers contradicts a higher expected activity and prior reports of maintained responses to beta-blockers for this genotype. In a post hoc analysis of the Beta-Blocker Evaluation of Survival Trial (BEST), there was no difference observed in achieving the study-defined ventricular rate-control target in patients with AF and HF with the beta-1-adrenoceptor Arg389Gly polymorphism.[54]

Digoxin can be used for ventricular rate control in patients with AF and chronic systolic HF. A systematic review reported that digoxin slows the ventricular rate at rest, but not during exercise, in patients with AF.[48,49] The combination of a beta-blocker and digoxin improves ventricular rate control, reduces symptoms, and may improve ventricular function to a greater extent than either drug alone.[35] However, digoxin has a narrow therapeutic range; frequent drug interactions occur, so cautious use of low-dose digoxin is indicated in older patients, those with renal insufficiency, and those who are using other drugs that may raise digoxin concentrations. The most frequent adverse effects of digoxin are ventricular arrhythmias, atrioventricular block, and sinus pauses; all effects are dose dependent. Previously, concerns have been raised that digoxin use may be associated with mortality when used in patients with AF[55,56]; however, whether this is a true digoxin effect or is caused by bias by indication remains uncertain. It has been postulated that the excess mortality may result from high-dose digoxin because this was not observed in multiple other AF trials using lower-dose digoxin. At this point, recommendations for the use of low-dose digoxin have not been modified.

Amiodarone is also effective for ventricular rate control of AF in patients with chronic HF.[49] However, because of its potential noncardiac toxicity, amiodarone is considered a second-line drug for rate control after a beta-blocker and digoxin are proven ineffective. In the United States and some other countries, amiodarone is not approved for use as a ventricular rate-control drug, and its use is off label.[19] Acute ventricular rate control with amiodarone intravenously or at high oral doses is effective in lowering the ventricular rate in patients with AF with high ventricular rates and hemodynamic compromise, although strict hemodynamic monitoring is indicated.[57]

The nondihydropyridine calcium channel antagonists verapamil and diltiazem should be used cautiously or avoided in patients with HF caused by systolic dysfunction because of their negative inotropic effects, although these drugs seem to be useful in HF with preserved ejection fraction.[19]

NONPHARMACOLOGIC VENTRICULAR RATE CONTROL OF AF AND HF

Permanent complete atrioventricular node ablation provides highly effective ventricular rate control and improves symptoms in selected patients.[58–61] In general, patients most likely to benefit from this therapy are those who are severely symptomatic and with uncontrollable ventricular rates with antiarrhythmic or negative dromotropic drugs.[19,61] This approach has several limitations varying from the loss of atrioventricular synchrony if patients have intermittent sinus rhythm and an atrial lead is not present, lifelong pacemaker dependency, and the potential risk of development or deterioration of HF caused by right ventricular pacing-induced left ventricular dyssynchrony, affecting left ventricular structure and function.[62–68] The ACC/AHA/European Society of Cardiology's guidelines state that nonpharmacologic therapy should be considered when pharmacologic measures fails.[19] In patients with AF and chronic HF, lifelong right ventricular pacing is a great concern and biventricular pacing is an option. In several acute hemodynamic studies compared with right ventricular pacing, left ventricular pacing improves systolic function and diastolic filling and decreases mitral regurgitation.[69,70] Two randomized studies compared different pacing modes in patients undergoing atrioventricular node ablation for permanent AF. The Optimal Pacing Site study found that left ventricular and biventricular pacing provided modest or no additional favorable effect compared with right ventricular pacing.[71] The left ventricular–based cardiac stimulation study, Post

AtrioVentricular Nodal Ablation Evaluation, showed that biventricular pacing significantly improved the 6-minute walk test and LVEF compared with right ventricular pacing after 6 months of follow-up, with the greatest beneficial effects in those with impaired systolic function or with symptomatic HF.[72] Therefore, the guidelines[19] state that for those with impaired left ventricular function not caused by tachycardia, a biventricular pacemaker with or without defibrillator capability should be considered. Upgrading to a biventricular device should be considered for patients with chronic HF and a right ventricular pacing system who have undergone atrioventricular node ablation.[73]

NEW DEVELOPMENTS IN NONPHARMACOLOGIC VENTRICULAR RATE CONTROL OF AF IN HF

Diverse alternatives to permanent complete atrioventricular block have been studied to avoid lifelong pacemaker dependency and to allow native electrical conduction. However, these techniques have not yet found their way into daily clinical practice.

Selective atrioventricular node vagal stimulation is one technique under investigation. In animal models, the feasibility of selective vagal stimulation of the epicardial atrioventricular nodal fat pad that is located at the junction of the inferior vena cava and left atrium to achieve acute[74,75] and sustained (up to 6 weeks)[76] and reversible lowering of the ventricular response has been reported. It has been shown to be feasible in humans, using an endocardial neurostimulator.[77,78] Recently, research has been expanded to chronic HF whereby the vagal tone is reduced. Zhang and colleagues[79] demonstrated, in a canine model of pacing-induced HF and AF, that selective atrioventricular node vagal stimulation led to a decrease in ventricular rate and improvement in LVEF and remained present during 6 months of follow-up.

As an extension to selective atrioventricular node vagal stimulation, several other techniques of increasing vagal tone are under investigation, such as right cervical vagal nerve stimulation. Although right cervical vagal nerve stimulation seems to have beneficial effects in HF (eg, improvements in LVEF and left ventricular systolic volume, NYHA functional class, quality of life, and exercise tolerance), these effects were observed without a significant change the ventricular rate. Whether this approach is of use for ventricular rate control in patients with AF and HF is, therefore, uncertain.[80,81]

SUMMARY

Ventricular rate control in patients with AF and chronic HF is recommended as the first-line therapy in the acute phase. The decision for long-term ventricular rate control should be based on patient symptoms and the cause of heart failure. If ventricular rate control is adopted, a target of less than 110 bpm is appropriate for most patients. Stricter rate control may be indicated in patients with persisting AF-related symptoms under lenient rate control or in the setting of HF with ongoing ischemia, severe diastolic dysfunction, hypertrophic cardiomyopathy, hypotension, or signs of pulmonary congestion, although the beneficial effects of stricter rate control have not yet been proven. In general, rate control is easy to achieve with beta-blockers and digoxin alone or in combination. If unsuccessful, amiodarone or atrioventricular node ablation can be considered.

REFERENCES

1. Wang TJ, Larson MG, Levy D, et al. Temporal relations of atrial fibrillation and congestive heart failure and their joint influence on mortality: the Framingham Heart Study. Circulation 2003;107:2920–5.

2. Smit MD, Moes ML, Maass AH, et al. The importance of whether atrial fibrillation or heart failure develops first. Eur J Heart Fail 2012;14:1030–40.

3. Cleland JG, Swedberg K, Follath F, et al. The Euro-Heart Failure survey programme– a survey on the quality of care among patients with heart failure in Europe. Part 1: patient characteristics and diagnosis. Eur Heart J 2003;24:442–63.

4. Neuberger HR, Mewis C, van Veldhuisen DJ, et al. Management of atrial fibrillation in patients with heart failure. Eur Heart J 2007;28:2568–77.

5. Maisel WH, Stevenson LW. Atrial fibrillation in heart failure: epidemiology, pathophysiology, and rationale for therapy. Am J Cardiol 2003;91:2D–8D.

6. McManus DD, Shaikh AY, Abhishek F, et al. Atrial fibrillation and heart failure parallels: lessons for atrial fibrillation prevention. Crit Pathw Cardiol 2011;10:46–51.

7. Dries DL, Exner DV, Gersh BJ, et al. Atrial fibrillation is associated with an increased risk for mortality and heart failure progression in patients with asymptomatic and symptomatic left ventricular systolic dysfunction: a retrospective analysis of the solvd trials. Studies of left ventricular dysfunction. J Am Coll Cardiol 1998;32:695–703.

8. Shinbane JS, Wood MA, Jensen DN, et al. Tachycardia-induced cardiomyopathy: a review of animal models and clinical studies. J Am Coll Cardiol 1997;29:709–15.

9. Clark DM, Plumb VJ, Epstein AE, et al. Hemody-namic effects of an irregular sequence of ventricu-lar cycle lengths during atrial fibrillation. J Am Coll Cardiol 1997;30:1039–45.

10. Van Den Berg MP, Tuinenburg AE, Crijns HJ, et al. Heart failure and atrial fibrillation: current concepts and controversies. Heart 1997;77:309–13.

11. Naito M, David D, Michelson EL, et al. The hemody-namic consequences of cardiac arrhythmias: evaluation of the relative roles of abnormal atrio-ventricular sequencing, irregularity of ventricular rhythm and atrial fibrillation in a canine model. Am Heart J 1983;106:284–91.

12. Daoud EG, Weiss R, Bahu M, et al. Effect of an irregular ventricular rhythm on cardiac output. Am J Cardiol 1996;78:1433–6.

13. Grogan M, Smith HC, Gersh BJ, et al. Left ventric-ular dysfunction due to atrial fibrillation in patients initially believed to have idiopathic dilated cardio-myopathy. Am J Cardiol 1992;69:1570–3.

14. Pozzoli M, Cioffi G, Traversi E, et al. Predictors of primary atrial fibrillation and concomitant clinical and hemodynamic changes in patients with chronic heart failure: a prospective study in 344 pa-tients with baseline sinus rhythm. J Am Coll Cardiol 1998;32:197–204.

15. Li D, Fareh S, Leung TK, et al. Promotion of atrial fibrillation by heart failure in dogs: atrial remodeling of a different sort. Circulation 1999;100:87–95.

16. Li D, Shinagawa K, Pang L, et al. Effects of angiotensin-converting enzyme inhibition on the development of the atrial fibrillation substrate in dogs with ventricular tachypacing-induced congestive heart failure. Circulation 2001;104: 2608–14.

17. Shinagawa K, Shi YF, Tardif JC, et al. Dynamic na-ture of atrial fibrillation substrate during develop-ment and reversal of heart failure in dogs. Circulation 2002;105:2672–8.

18. Van Gelder IC, Groenveld HF, Crijns HJ, et al. Lenient versus strict rate control in patients with atrial fibrillation. N Engl J Med 2010;362:1363–73.

19. Fuster V, Ryden LE, Cannom DS, et al. 2011 ACCF/AHA/HRS focused updates incorporated into the ACC/AHA/ESC 2006 guidelines for the manage-ment of patients with atrial fibrillation: a report of the american college of cardiology foundation/american heart association task force on practice guidelines. Circulation 2011;123:e269–367.

20. Wyse DG, Waldo AL, DiMarco JP, et al. A comparison of rate control and rhythm control in patients with atrial fibrillation. N Engl J Med 2002;347:1825–33.

21. Van Gelder IC, Hagens VE, Bosker HA, et al. A comparison of rate control and rhythm control in patients with recurrent persistent atrial fibrillation. N Engl J Med 2002;347:1834–40.

22. Hohnloser SH, Kuck KH, Lilienthal J. Rhythm or rate control in atrial fibrillation Pharmacological Intervention in Atrial Fibrillation (PIAF): a rando-mised trial. Lancet 2000;356:1789–94.

23. Carlsson J, Miketic S, Windeler J, et al. Random-ized trail of rate-control versus rhythm-control in persistent atrial fibrillation: the Strategies of Treat-ment of Atrial Fibrillation (STAF) study. J Am Coll Cardiol 2003;41:1690–6.

24. Opolski G, Torbicki A, Kosior DA, et al. Rate control vs rhythm control in patients with nonvalvular persistent atrial fibrillation: the results of the Polish How to Treat Chronic Atrial Fibrillation (HOT CAFE) study. Chest 2004;126:476–86.

25. Ogawa S, Yamashita T, Yamazaki T, et al. Optimal treatment strategy for patients with paroxysmal atrial fibrillation: J-RHYTHM study. Circ J 2009;73:242–8.

26. Roy D, Talajic M, Nattel S, et al. Rhythm control versus rate control for atrial fibrillation and heart failure. N Engl J Med 2008;358:2667–77.

27. Suman-Horduna I, Roy D, Frasure-Smith N, et al. Quality of life and functional capacity in patients with atrial fibrillation and congestive heart failure. J Am Coll Cardiol 2013;61:455–60.

28. Henrard V, Ducharme A, Khairy P, et al. Cardiac re-modeling with rhythm versus rate control strategies for atrial fibrillation in patients with heart failure: in-sights from the AF-CHF echocardiographic sub-study. Int J Cardiol 2013;165(3):430–6.

29. Lazzari JO, Gonzalez J. Reversible high rate atrial fibrillation dilated cardiomyopathy. Heart 1997;77: 486.

30. Hagens VE, Crijns HJ, van Veldhuisen DJ, et al. Rate control versus rhythm control for patients with persistent atrial fibrillation with mild to moder-ate heart failure: results from the Rate Control versus Electrical Cardioversion (RACE) study. Am Heart J 2005;149:1106–11.

31. Hagens VE, van Veldhuisen DJ, Kamp O, et al. Ef-fect of rate and rhythm control on left ventricular function and cardiac dimensions in patients with persistent atrial fibrillation: results from the Rate Control versus Electrical Cardioversion for Persis-tent Atrial Fibrillation (RACE) study. Heart Rhythm 2005;2:19–24.

32. Groenveld HF, Crijns HJ, Van den Berg MP, et al. The effect of rate control on quality of life in patients with permanent atrial fibrillation: data from the RACE II (Rate Control Efficacy in Permanent Atrial Fibrillation II) study. J Am Coll Cardiol 2011;58: 1795–803.

33. Smit MD, Crijns HJ, Tijssen JG, et al. Effect of lenient versus strict rate control on cardiac remod-eling in patients with atrial fibrillation data of the RACE II (Rate Control Efficacy in Permanent Atrial Fibrillation II) study. J Am Coll Cardiol 2011;58: 942–9.

34. Mulder B, Tijssen J, Hillege H, et al. Stringency of rate control in patients with atrial fibrillation and heart failure: data of the Rate Control Efficacy in Permanent Atrial Fibrillation: a comparison between lenient versus strict rate control II (RACE II) study. Circulation 2010;122:A16829.

35. Khand AU, Rankin AC, Martin W, et al. Carvedilol alone or in combination with digoxin for the management of atrial fibrillation in patients with heart failure? J Am Coll Cardiol 2003;42:1944–51.

36. Silvet H, Hawkins LA, Jacobson AK. Heart rate control in patients with chronic atrial fibrillation and heart failure. Congest Heart Fail 2013;19:25–8.

37. Rienstra M, van Gelder IC, Van Den Berg MP, et al. A comparison of low versus high heart rate in patients with atrial fibrillation and advanced chronic heart failure: effects on clinical profile, neurohormones and survival. Int J Cardiol 2006;109:95–100.

38. Cooper HA, Bloomfield DA, Bush DE, et al. Relation between achieved heart rate and outcomes in patients with atrial fibrillation (from the Atrial Fibrillation Follow-up Investigation of Rhythm Management [AFFIRM] Study). Am J Cardiol 2004;93:1247–53.

39. Van Gelder IC, Wyse DG, Chandler ML, et al. Does intensity of rate-control influence outcome in atrial fibrillation? An analysis of pooled data from the race and affirm studies. Europace 2006;8:935–42.

40. Groenveld HF, Crijns HJ, Rienstra M, et al. Does intensity of rate control influence outcome in persistent atrial fibrillation? Data of the race study. Am Heart J 2009;158:785–91.

41. Castagno D, Skali H, Takeuchi M, et al. Association of heart rate and outcomes in a broad spectrum of patients with chronic heart failure: results from the CHARM (Candesartan in Heart Failure: Assessment of Reduction in Mortality and morbidity) program. J Am Coll Cardiol 2012;59:1785–95.

42. Connolly SJ, Camm AJ, Halperin JL, et al. Dronedarone in high-risk permanent atrial fibrillation. N Engl J Med 2011;365:2268–76.

43. Camm AJ, Kirchhof P, Lip GY, et al. Guidelines for the management of atrial fibrillation: the Task Force for the Management of Atrial Fibrillation of the European Society of Cardiology (ESC). Eur Heart J 2010;31:2369–429.

44. Hunt SA, Abraham WT, Chin MH, et al. 2009 focused update incorporated into the ACC/AHA 2005 guidelines for the diagnosis and management of heart failure in adults: a report of the American College of Cardiology Foundation/American Heart Association Task Force on Practice Guidelines: developed in collaboration with the International Society for Heart and Lung Transplantation. Circulation 2009;119:e391–479.

45. Olshansky B, Rosenfeld LE, Warner AL, et al. The Atrial Fibrillation Follow-up Investigation of Rhythm Management (AFFIRM) study: approaches to control rate in atrial fibrillation. J Am Coll Cardiol 2004;43:1201–8.

46. Weerasooriya R, Davis M, Powell A, et al. The Australian Intervention Randomized Control of Rate in Atrial Fibrillation Trial (AIRCRAFT). J Am Coll Cardiol 2003;41:1697–702.

47. Rienstra M, Damman K, Mulder B, et al. Beta-blockers and outcome in heart failure and atrial fibrillation: a meta-analysis. J Am Coll Cardiol HF 2013;1:21–8.

48. Segal JB, McNamara RL, Miller MR, et al. The evidence regarding the drugs used for ventricular rate control. J Fam Pract 2000;49:47–59.

49. Tamariz LJ, Bass EB. Pharmacological rate control of atrial fibrillation. Cardiol Clin 2004;22:35–45.

50. Mason DA, Moore JD, Green SA, et al. A gain-of-function polymorphism in a g-protein coupling domain of the human beta1-adrenergic receptor. J Biol Chem 1999;274:12670–4.

51. Joseph SS, Lynham JA, Grace AA, et al. Markedly reduced effects of (-)-isoprenaline but not of (-)-cgp12177 and unchanged affinity of beta-blockers at gly389-beta1-adrenoceptors compared to arg389-beta1-adrenoceptors. Br J Pharmacol 2004;142:51–6.

52. Parvez B, Chopra N, Rowan S, et al. A common beta1-adrenergic receptor polymorphism predicts favorable response to rate-control therapy in atrial fibrillation. J Am Coll Cardiol 2012;59:49–56.

53. Rau T, Dungen HD, Edelmann F, et al. Impact of the beta1-adrenoceptor Arg389Gly polymorphism on heart-rate responses to bisoprolol and carvedilol in heart-failure patients. Clin Pharmacol Ther 2012;92:21–8.

54. Kao DP, Davis G, Aleong R, et al. Effect of bucindolol on heart failure outcomes and heart rate response in patients with reduced ejection fraction heart failure and atrial fibrillation. Eur J Heart Fail 2013;15(3):324–33.

55. Corley SD, Epstein AE, DiMarco JP, et al. Relationships between sinus rhythm, treatment, and survival in the Atrial Fibrillation Follow-up Investigation of Rhythm Management (AFFIRM) study. Circulation 2004;109:1509–13.

56. Friberg L, Hammar N, Rosenqvist M. Digoxin in atrial fibrillation: report from the Stockholm cohort study of atrial fibrillation (SCAF). Heart 2010;96: 275–80.

57. Hou ZY, Chang MS, Chen CY, et al. Acute treatment of recent-onset atrial fibrillation and flutter with a tailored dosing regimen of intravenous amiodarone. A randomized, digoxin-controlled study. Eur Heart J 1995;16:521–8.

58. Brignole M, Gianfranchi L, Menozzi C, et al. Assessment of atrioventricular junction ablation and DDDR mode- switching pacemaker versus pharmacological treatment in patients with

severely symptomatic paroxysmal atrial fibrillation: a randomized controlled study. Circulation 1997; 90.2017–24.

59. Brignole M, Menozzi C, Gianfranchi L, et al. Assessment of atrioventricular junction ablation and VVIR pacemaker versus pharmacological treatment in patients with heart failure and chronic atrial fibrillation: a randomized, controlled study. Circulation 1998;98:953–60.

60. Kay GN, Ellenbogen KA, Giudici M, et al. The Ablate and Pace trial: a prospective study of catheter ablation of the AV conduction system and permanent pacemaker implantation for treatment of atrial fibrillation. APT investigators. J Interv Card Electrophysiol 1998;2:121–35.

61. Wood MA, Brown-Mahoney C, Kay GN, et al. Clinical outcomes after ablation and pacing therapy for atrial fibrillation: a meta-analysis. Circulation 2000; 101:1138–44.

62. Moss AJ, Zareba W, Hall WJ, et al. Prophylactic implantation of a defibrillator in patients with myocardial infarction and reduced ejection fraction. N Engl J Med 2002;346:877–83.

63. Wilkoff BL, Cook JR, Epstein AE, et al. Dual-chamber pacing or ventricular backup pacing in patients with an implantable defibrillator: the Dual Chamber and VVI Implantable Defibrillator (DAVID) trial. JAMA 2002;288:3115–23.

64. Hohnloser SH, Kuck KH, Dorian P, et al. Prophylactic use of an implantable cardioverter-defibrillator after acute myocardial infarction. N Engl J Med 2004;351:2481–8.

65. Smit MD, Van Dessel PF, Nieuwland W, et al. Right ventricular pacing and the risk of heart failure in implantable cardioverter-defibrillator patients. Heart Rhythm 2006;3:1397–403.

66. Vernooy K, Dijkman B, Cheriex EC, et al. Ventricular remodeling during long-term right ventricular pacing following his bundle ablation. Am J Cardiol 2006;97:1223–7.

67. Tops LF, Schalij MJ, Holman ER, et al. Right ventricular pacing can induce ventricular dyssynchrony in patients with atrial fibrillation after atrioventricular node ablation. J Am Coll Cardiol 2006;48:1642–8.

68. Tan ES, Rienstra M, Wiesfeld AC, et al. Long-term outcome of the atrioventricular node ablation and pacemaker implantation for symptomatic refractory atrial fibrillation. Europace 2008;10:412–8.

69. Simantirakis EN, Vardakis KE, Kochiadakis GE, et al. Left ventricular mechanics during right ventricular apical or left ventricular-based pacing in patients with chronic atrial fibrillation after atrioventricular junction ablation. J Am Coll Cardiol 2004; 43:1013–8.

70. Puggioni E, Brignole M, Gammage M, et al. Acute comparative effect of right and left ventricular pacing in patients with permanent atrial fibrillation. J Am Coll Cardiol 2004;43:234–8.

71. Brignole M, Gammage M, Puggioni E, et al. Comparative assessment of right, left, and biventricular pacing in patients with permanent atrial fibrillation. Eur Heart J 2005;26:712–22.

72. Doshi RN, Daoud EG, Fellows C, et al. Left ventricular-based cardiac stimulation post AV nodal ablation evaluation (the PAVE study). J Cardiovasc Electrophysiol 2005;16:1160–5.

73. Leon AR, Greenberg JM, Kanuru N, et al. Cardiac resynchronization in patients with congestive heart failure and chronic atrial fibrillation: effect of upgrading to biventricular pacing after chronic right ventricular pacing. J Am Coll Cardiol 2002;39: 1258–63.

74. Wallick DW, Zhang Y, Tabata T, et al. Selective AV nodal vagal stimulation improves hemodynamics during acute atrial fibrillation in dogs. Am J Physiol Heart Circ Physiol 2001;281:H1490–7.

75. Zhuang S, Zhang Y, Mowrey KA, et al. Ventricular rate control by selective vagal stimulation is superior to rhythm regularization by atrioventricular nodal ablation and pacing during atrial fibrillation. Circulation 2002;106:1853–8.

76. Zhang Y, Yamada H, Bibevski S, et al. Chronic atrioventricular nodal vagal stimulation: first evidence for long-term ventricular rate control in canine atrial fibrillation model. Circulation 2005; 112:2904–11.

77. Mischke K, Zarse M, Schmid M, et al. Chronic augmentation of the parasympathetic tone to the atrioventricular node: a nonthoracotomy neurostimulation technique for ventricular rate control during atrial fibrillation. J Cardiovasc Electrophysiol 2010;21:193–9.

78. Schauerte P, Mischke K, Plisiene J, et al. Catheter stimulation of cardiac parasympathetic nerves in humans: a novel approach to the cardiac autonomic nervous system. Circulation 2001;104:2430–5.

79. Zhang Y, Popovic ZB, Kusunose K, et al. Therapeutic effects of selective atrioventricular node vagal stimulation in atrial fibrillation and heart failure. J Cardiovasc Electrophysiol 2013;24:86–91.

80. Zhang Y, Popovic ZB, Bibevski S, et al. Chronic vagus nerve stimulation improves autonomic control and attenuates systemic inflammation and heart failure progression in a canine high-rate pacing model. Circ Heart Fail 2009;2:692–9.

81. Field ME, Hamdan MH. AV nodal fat pad stimulation for rate control in atrial fibrillation and heart failure: a better solution? J Cardiovasc Electrophysiol 2013;24:92–3.

Rhythm Control of Atrial Fibrillation in Heart Failure

Jordi Heijman, PhD[a], Niels Voigt, MD[a,b],
Issam H. Abu-Taha, PhD[a], Dobromir Dobrev, MD[a,b,c],*

KEYWORDS

- Antiarrhythmic drugs • Atrial fibrillation • Heart failure • Rhythm control

KEY POINTS

- Atrial fibrillation (AF) and heart failure (HF) are common cardiovascular pathologies with severe prognostic implications that show bidirectional interactions.
- Current rhythm-control strategies using antiarrhythmic drugs in patients with HF do not improve outcome, which may at least be partly due to the lack of safe and effective antiarrhythmic drugs for rhythm control of AF in HF.
- Amiodarone and dofetilide are the only antiarrhythmic drugs currently available for patients with HF but their success is limited by extracardiovascular toxicity and drug-induced proarrhythmia, respectively.
- Novel atrial-specific antiarrhythmic drugs or drugs targeting common arrhythmogenic pathways between AF and HF, and improved patient selection based on recent genetic data, may help to improve rhythm control of AF in HF.

INTRODUCTION

Atrial fibrillation (AF) and heart failure (HF) affect at least 2.7 and 5.1 million people in the United States alone,[1] figures which are expected to rise with the aging of the population, posing a significant burden on health care in the developed world. Both conditions are individually associated with increased morbidity and mortality.[1]

AF and HF frequently coexist and show bidirectional interactions. HF is a more powerful risk factor for AF than advanced age, hypertension, valvular heart disease, diabetes, or prior myocardial infarction, increasing the risk for AF by 4.5-fold to 5.9-fold.[2] The reported prevalence of AF in HF ranges from 13% to 27% and correlates with the severity of the left ventricular (LV) dysfunction.[3] Initial studies failed to determine whether AF is an independent risk factor associated with worse outcome in HF or simply reflects increased overall risk. However, more recent studies and studies in larger populations, such

Funding Sources: The authors' work is supported by the European Network for Translational Research in Atrial Fibrillation (EUTRAF, No. 261057), the German Federal Ministry of Education and Research (AF Competence Network [01Gi0204] and DZHK [German Center for Cardiovascular Research]), the Deutsche Forschungsgemeinschaft (Do 769/1-3), and by a grant from Fondation Leducq (European-North American Atrial Fibrillation Research Alliance, ENAFRA, 07CVD03).
Conflicts of Interest: DD is an advisor and lecturer for Sanofi, Merck-Sharp-Dohme, Biotronik, Boehringer Ingelheim, and Boston Scientific. The other authors have no conflicts of interest to disclose.
a Institute of Pharmacology, Faculty of Medicine, University Duisburg-Essen, Hufelandstrasse 55, Essen 45122, Germany; b Division of Experimental Cardiology, Medical Faculty Mannheim, Heidelberg University, Theodor-Kutzer-Ufer 1-3, 68167 Mannheim, Germany; c DZHK (German Centre for Cardiovascular Research) Partner Site Mannheim/Heidelberg, Theodor-Kutzer-Ufer 1-3, 68167 Mannheim, Germany
* Corresponding author. Institute of Pharmacology, Faculty of Medicine, University Duisburg-Essen, Hufelandstrasse 55, Essen 45122, Germany.
E-mail address: dobromir.dobrev@uk-essen.de

Heart Failure Clin 9 (2013) 407–415
http://dx.doi.org/10.1016/j.hfc.2013.06.001
1551-7136/13/$ – see front matter © 2013 Elsevier Inc. All rights reserved.

as the Studies of Left Ventricular Dysfunction (SOLVD)[4] and Valsartan in Acute Myocardial Infarction (VALIANT)[5] trials, have suggested that AF is independently associated with worse outcome in HF.[3] Moreover, even studies where baseline AF was not predictive of increased morbidity and mortality, such as the Carvedilol or Metroprolol European Trial (COMET), found that new-onset AF was associated with a particularly negative impact on HF prognosis.[6] In agreement, Smit and colleagues[7] have recently shown that despite the bidirectional interaction between AF and HF, the order in which both conditions develop matters. In particular, they showed that HF patients developing AF had a worse prognosis than AF patients who developed HF.

The severity and prevalence of both conditions make the treatment of AF in the setting of HF, including the associated risk of stroke, of critical importance. However, current therapeutic options for AF have important limitations including limited safety and efficacy,[8–10] a situation that is exacerbated in the presence of HF. A better understanding of the basic mechanisms underlying both pathologies and their interactions is required to facilitate the development of novel therapeutics.

RATE CONTROL VERSUS RHYTHM CONTROL

Rate control and rhythm control are the 2 predominant treatment strategies for AF. In the former (reviewed elsewhere in this edition), only the ventricular response is controlled, whereas in the latter the goal is to achieve normal sinus rhythm. Most clinical studies have failed to show a clear survival benefit in patients with pharmacologic rhythm control. In particular, the Atrial Fibrillation Follow-up Investigation of Rhythm Management (AFFIRM) and RAte Control versus Electrical cardioversion (RACE) trials found no benefit or even a trend toward harm with rhythm control of AF.[11,12] These findings were confirmed in the setting of HF by the Atrial Fibrillation and Congestive Heart Failure (AF-CHF) trial, where no differences in overall survival, cardiovascular death, worsened HF, or stroke were found between rate and rhythm control at 37 months' follow-up.[13] As such, rhythm control is currently only recommended in patients who remain symptomatic despite adequate rate control.[14,15] However, it is likely that the performance of rhythm control in these studies is negatively affected by the limited success to maintain sinus rhythm in patients, with success rates ranging from 26% to 64%.[16] Moreover, subsequent analysis of the data from the AFFIRM trial has shown that maintenance of sinus rhythm was associated with a survival benefit that was offset by the risk associated with antiarrhythmic drug therapy.[17] On the other hand, it cannot be ruled out that patients able to maintain sinus rhythm are simply healthier.[2] Safer and more effective antiarrhythmic drugs for the maintenance of sinus rhythm may help to determine whether rhythm control is indeed the preferred strategy for patients with AF and HF.

BASIC MECHANISMS UNDERLYING AF

Conceptually, AF is determined by factors controlling abnormal impulse formation and propagation (**Fig. 1**).[9,18] HF and AF share various risk factors, including age, hypertension, diabetes mellitus, valvular heart disease, and genetic factors, which create a vulnerable substrate for the initiation of atrial and ventricular arrhythmias. In the atria, impulse formation outside of the sinoatrial node (ectopic/triggered activity), particularly around the pulmonary veins (PV), can maintain AF when occurring repetitively ("driver") or can trigger reentry in a vulnerable substrate. Substantial experimental research has provided important insights into the molecular factors contributing to these arrhythmia mechanisms in AF and the contributing role of HF.

Ectopic Activity

In the atrial myocyte, the Na^+ current (I_{Na}) rapidly depolarizes the membrane potential, creating the upstroke of the atrial action potential (AP). Subsequent activation of voltage-gated L-type Ca^{2+} current ($I_{Ca,L}$) results in Ca^{2+} entry into the atrial myocyte, promoting a much larger Ca^{2+} release from the sarcoplasmic reticulum (SR) stores through the ryanodine receptor channel (RyR2), giving rise to the systolic Ca^{2+} transient, which controls myocyte contraction. The influx of Ca^{2+} is tightly controlled by inactivation of $I_{Ca,L}$, which, together with the activation of a complement of K^+ currents, is also responsible for the repolarization of the AP, determining AP duration.

Triggered activity is generally mediated by early or delayed afterdepolarizations. Early afterdepolarizations (EADs) are secondary depolarizations of the membrane potential that occur before final repolarization of the AP. They generally occur in the setting of AP prolongation, for example, due to loss-of-function mutations or pharmacologic inhibition of repolarizing K^+ currents. Prolongation of the AP allows $I_{Ca,L}$ to recover from nonconducting inactivated states, thereby depolarizing the membrane potential and causing the EAD upstroke.

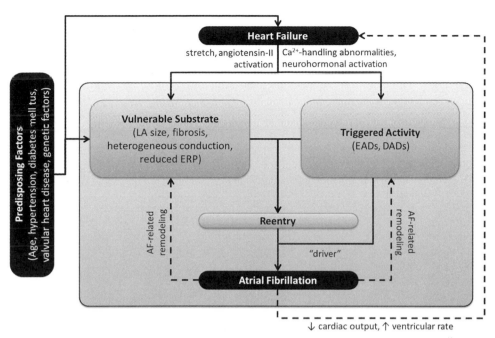

Fig. 1. Conceptual overview of the mechanisms underlying atrial fibrillation and the bidirectional interaction between atrial fibrillation and heart failure. LA, left atrium.

Delayed afterdepolarizations (DADs) occur after full repolarization of the AP and are caused by abnormalities in subcellular Ca^{2+} handling. Recent research has shown that dysfunction of RyR2 plays a critical role in AF, resulting in increased Ca^{2+} leak from the SR and spontaneous SR Ca^{2+}-release events.[19] Phosphorylation of RyR2 by Ca^{2+}/calmodulin-dependent protein kinase II (CaMKII) has been identified as an important contributor to this RyR2 dysfunction.[19] The Ca^{2+} released into the cytosol during spontaneous SR Ca^{2+}-release events is partly extruded via the Na^{+}/Ca^{2+} exchanger (NCX1), which brings in 3 Na^{+} for every Ca^{2+} extruded, thereby causing a depolarizing transient-inward current (I_{NCX}), generating a DAD. The balance between I_{NCX} and the repolarizing inward-rectifier K^{+} currents determines the DAD amplitude. If this amplitude is sufficiently large, Na^{+} channels will be activated, giving rise to a triggered AP.

Reentry

Reentry is a central mechanism for maintaining AF, although the exact presentation remains a subject of debate and may vary from patient to patient.[20] Sustained reentry can occur in the presence or absence ("functional reentry") of fixed anatomic obstacles.[21] The leading circle and spiral wave concepts have been proposed as conceptual models of functional reentry. Although conceptually different, both models share several notions, including the predicted effects of K^{+} channel alterations.[21] The spiral wave concept more accurately predicts the effect of I_{Na} blockade.[21] An advantage of the leading circle model is its definition by simple, clinically relevant electrophysiological concepts.[21] Leading circle reentry establishes itself in the smallest pathway that can support reentry such that all points in the reentrant path regain excitability before the arrival of the next impulse. As such, reentry is promoted by slow conduction velocity (CV) and a short effective refractory period (ERP), the product of which has been termed wavelength (wavelength = CV × ERP).[20,21] CV is largely determined by the availability of I_{Na} to overcome the electrotonic load of the surrounding myocardium, the number of electrical connections (gap junctions) between myocytes, and the composition of the extracellular matrix, notably the amount of fibrosis.[9] ERP is determined by AP duration and the post-repolarization refractoriness, which is predominantly due to the recovery kinetics of I_{Na}.

AF-related Remodeling

When a rapid atrial rate is maintained, AF-related electrical and structural remodeling occur, further stabilizing the arrhythmia, contributing to the progression from paroxysmal to permanent AF, and making AF more difficult to treat.[22] Electrical remodeling is characterized by shortening of atrial ERP and abnormal Ca^{2+} handling, promoting reentry and ectopic activity, respectively.[23,24] Shortening of atrial ERP predominantly results from reduced $I_{Ca,L}$, increased basal inward-rectifier current (I_{K1}), and development of a "constitutively active" acetylcholine-dependent inward-rectifier K^+ current ($I_{K,AChc}$) that is active in the absence of muscarinic receptor agonists. Increased inward-rectifier K^+ currents cause hyperpolarization of the resting membrane potential, which has been shown to stabilize reentrant circuits ("rotors") by promoting recovery of I_{Na} from inactivation.[25] Abnormal Ca^{2+} handling plays a critical role in ectopic activity-promoting DAD formation. Chronic AF is associated with increased CaMKII expression, RyR2 hyperphosphorylation, and more spontaneous SR Ca^{2+}-release events, which lead to DADs and triggered APs.[19]

Structural remodeling of the atria can occur in various pathologic conditions, including HF, or can be a direct result of AF. Increased atrial fibrosis is a hallmark of structural atrial remodeling.[22] It contributes to conduction slowing and heterogeneous conduction, thereby promoting reentry. Proliferation of fibroblasts and differentiation into collagen-secreting myofibroblasts are main profibrotic mechanisms activated by a wide range of stimuli including myocardial injury, oxidative stress, inflammation, and stretch.[22] Angiotensin II and transforming growth factor-β1 are well-established profibrotic signaling molecules, and recent evidence also suggests roles for platelet-derived growth factor and connective tissue growth factor.[22] Interestingly, recent evidence suggests that AF may also promote ventricular remodeling. In particular, Ling and colleagues[26] found that AF was independently associated with increased LV interstitial fibrosis in patients.

The Role of HF in AF

HF and AF share numerous risk factors. In addition, various studies have highlighted pathways through which HF can directly promote AF. Congestive HF and the associated increased hemodynamic load cause abnormal atrial stretch, contributing to atrial dilatation and atrial myocyte hypertrophy.[27] Activation of stretch-sensitive ion channels may affect atrial electrophysiology, and Ca^{2+}-handling. Congestive HF is also associated with a pronounced increase in atrial fibrosis[3] and is accompanied by neurohormonal activation, which can promote atrial ectopic activity through abnormal Ca^{2+} handling and further amplify atrial fibrosis via increased angiotensin-II levels.[3] Together, these processes create a large vulnerable substrate with slow, heterogeneous conduction and spatially heterogeneous electrophysiological

properties, strongly promoting atrial reentry. Congestive HF causes atrial ionic remodeling that is different from atrial tachycardia-related remodeling. Atrial AP duration is not substantially reduced by HF-related remodeling, with some reports of increased AP duration in animal models of congestive HF, although this may depend on the duration of HF.[28,29] Patients with HF-dependent AF will experience both HF- and AF-related remodeling. Due to cross-talk between both processes, the resulting remodeling is more complex and different from the sum of the individual processes.[22]

There are several interesting parallels between the ventricular remodeling observed in HF and chronic AF-related remodeling, notably with regard to abnormal Ca^{2+} handling.[29] The increased CaMKII-dependent RyR2 phosphorylation, increased SR Ca^{2+} leak, and spontaneous SR Ca^{2+}-release events had already been identified in HF before their discovery in AF.[19,29] In addition, both pathologies share an upregulation of NCX1, contributing to larger DAD amplitudes for a given Ca^{2+} release. Both conditions also result in reduced CV and increase conduction heterogeneity, promoting reentry.

ANTIARRHYTHMIC DRUGS FOR RHYTHM CONTROL IN AF IN THE PRESENCE OF HF

The class Ic drugs flecainide and propafenone predominantly inhibit voltage-gated Na^+ channels, thereby reducing atrial excitability, without affecting AP duration. They were shown to delay the first occurrence of AF and reduce the portion of time in AF in the structurally normal heart.[30,31] However, in patients with previous myocardial infarction or structural heart disease, class Ic antiarrhythmics have been associated with increased mortality[32] and are therefore contraindicated in patients with coronary artery disease or HF.[14,15] It is likely that under these conditions, the reentry-promoting effects of ventricular conduction slowing due to Na^+ channel inhibition outweigh antiarrhythmic effects due to reduced excitability.

Class III Drugs

Commonly used pure class III antiarrhythmic drugs include ibutilide, sotalol, and, in the United States, dofetilide.[30,31] These drugs predominantly block the rapidly activating delayed-rectifier K^+ current (I_{Kr}), thereby prolonging ERP and reducing the likelihood of reentry. The Danish Investigators of Arrhythmia and Mortality on Dofetilide trial (DIAMOND-CHF)[33] showed that dofetilide significantly reduced the risk of hospitalization for woroening HF, was more effective than placebo in maintaining sinus rhythm, and was not associated with increased mortality in patients with congestive HF. As such, dofetilide is an option for the maintenance of sinus rhythm in patients with HF in the United States.[15] However, in general all class III drugs can cause QT prolongation, carrying the risk of EADs and drug-induced torsades de pointes arrhythmias. Therefore, dofetilide dosage has to be personalized for each patient based on renal function, weight, and other clinical variables to prevent excessive QT prolongation.[15]

Multichannel Blockers

Although not officially approved for AF in the United States, amiodarone is the most-employed and most-successful antiarrhythmic drug for the maintenance of normal sinus rhythm in AF patients with and without HF.[30,31] Its reported efficacy for the maintenance of sinus rhythm lies between 50% and 78%.[31] Amiodarone is a class III antiarrhythmic drug, potently inhibiting I_{Kr}, but together with its active metabolite N-desethylamiodarone has a wide range of additional targets including I_{Na} and $I_{Ca,L}$ and also acts as a noncompetitive antagonist of α- and β-adrenoceptors, thereby showing actions of all 4 drug classes.[10,30] In addition, amiodarone and N-desethylamiodarone both cause venodilation,[34,35] potentially reducing preload, an effect that might contribute to its efficacy, especially in patients with HF. The Congestive Heart Failure Survival Trial of Antiarrhythmic Therapy (CHF-STAT) has shown that patients with congestive HF and AF treated with amiodarone were more likely to convert to sinus rhythm and had a reduced incidence of new-onset AF. However, the AF-CHF study has shown that this does not translate into improved survival compared with rate control.[13] Although amiodarone can cause QT-interval prolongation, it is not generally associated with development of torsades de pointes arrhythmias. Amiodarone has been associated with hepatotoxicity, photosensitivity, and pulmonary dysfunction (pneumonitis, fibrosis). Due to the iodine moieties, amiodarone frequently causes thyroid dysfunction, ranging from laboratory test abnormalities and thyreoiditis to hypothyreoidism and hyperthyreoidism. Treatment includes discontinuation of amiodarone, although due to its long half-time, thyroid dysfunction may persist for months after discontinuation. Overall, the substantial extracardiac side effects of amiodarone limit its use in a large proportion of patients.

Dronedarone was recently developed by altering the structure of amiodarone in an attempt to reduce its extracardiovascular toxicity. Like amiodarone, it blocks a wide range of ion channels and exhibits actions of all 4 drug classes.[36] Dronedarone was approved for the treatment of AF based on the results of the ATHENA (A Trial With Dronedarone to Prevent Hospitalization or Death in Patients With Atrial Fibrillation) trial, which showed that dronedarone reduced the rate of hospitalizations and cardiovascular death. In contrast, the ANDROMEDA (European Trial of Dronedarone in Moderate to Severe Congestive Heart Failure) trial found that dronedarone was associated with increased mortality in patients with severe HF.[37] Similarly, the Permanent Atrial Fibrillation Outcome Study Using Dronedarone on Top of Standard Therapy (PALLAS) trial, in which more than half of the patients had New York Heart Association class II or III congestive HF, was recently halted because of excess risk of stroke and cardiovascular death.[38] Overall, dronedarone is less effective compared with amiodarone and is not recommended for rhythm control of AF in patients with HF, except perhaps those with stable class I HF. Dronedarone is also not appropriate for patients with persistent/permanent AF.

Multichannel blockers have shown promise for the treatment of AF. Intravenous vernakalant was recently approved for the rapid conversion of recent-onset AF in Europe. Vernakalant targets multiple K^+-currents including the atrial-selective ultrarapid delayed-rectifier K^+ current (I_{Kur}) and $I_{K,ACh}$, which do not contribute to the ventricular AP, and uses differences between atrial and ventricular Na^+-channel properties to achieve an atrial-predominant action, thereby preventing ventricular proarrhythmia.[8] The safety and efficacy of vernakalant was evaluated in the AVRO and ACT trials, showing improved conversion to sinus rhythm compared with placebo and the slow-acting amiodarone, without ventricular arrhythmia.[31,39] However, the efficacy of vernakalant is substantially lower in patients with HF compared with hemodynamically stable patients.[39] Oral vernakalant has been evaluated for the long-term prevention of AF recurrence and has shown potential in several trials.[31] However, further development of oral vernakalant has recently been halted, likely because of low efficacy to maintain normal sinus rhythm.

Ranolazine is a multichannel blocker approved for the treatment of chronic angina. It is a potent inhibitor of I_{Na}, including its persistent (late) component ($I_{Na,late}$) and also inhibits I_{Kr} and RyR2 at clinically relevant concentrations.[10,40] Ranolazine has been shown to have antiarrhythmic properties at both the atrial and the ventricular level, including in dogs with HF, but is not yet approved for the treatment of AF.[40,41]

NONANTIARRHYTHMIC RHYTHM CONTROL OF AF IN HF

Several nonantiarrhythmic ("upstream") pharmacologic interventions including angiotensin-II converting enzyme inhibitors, angiotensin-II receptor blockers, β-adrenoceptor blockers, and statins are routinely used in the treatment of patients with AF (reviewed elsewhere in this edition) and have been suggested to be antiarrhythmic by limiting the deleterious effects of neurohormonal hyperactivity, oxidative stress, and inflammation.[3,42,43]

Catheter and surgical ablation of AF are the main nonpharmacologic approaches for rhythm control. Catheter ablation strategies aim to isolate the PV electrically, which is often sufficient to achieve sinus rhythm in patients with paroxysmal AF, whereas patients with persistent AF require additional lesions.[2,16] Surgical ablation techniques are advancing and might be used alone or in combination with endocardial catheter procedures. Adverse effects are more frequent with antiarrhythmic drugs than ablation. Hunter and colleagues[44] have recently shown that restoration of sinus rhythm by catheter ablation of AF is associated with a reduced incidence of stroke and death compared with predominantly pharmacologically treated patients from the Euro Heart Survey on AF. In patients with HF, Hsu and colleagues[45] have shown that AF ablation resulted in improved LV function, reduced LV dimensions, and increased exercise capacity. However, in a different cohort of patients with advanced HF, ablation restored long-term sinus rhythm in only 50% of patients and did not significantly improve LV ejection fraction assessed by cardiac magnetic resonance imaging.[46] Because of the paucity of available antiarrhythmic drugs for rhythm control of AF in patients with HF, ablation is recommended as a first-line treatment for patients with New York Heart Association class III and class IV HF in the European guidelines.[14] However, more data about the long-term efficacy of ablation from prospective studies are required.[16] Moreover, the complexity of the procedure, the frequent requirement of additional ablations, and the costs involved prohibit the use of ablation for the large number of AF patients. As such, careful patient selection, better antiarrhythmic drugs, and advances in ablation technology remain a requirement for optimal rhythm control.

Antiarrhythmic drugs may be used in conjunction with ablation procedures to prevent AF recurrence (**Fig. 2**). The PABA-CHF (Pulmonary Vein Antrum Isolation vs AV Node Ablation With Biventricular Pacing for Treatment of Atrial Fibrillation in Patients With Congestive Heart Failure) trial reported maintenance of sinus rhythm in 71% of HF patients following PV isolation alone and in 88% of HF patients with PV isolation and antiarrhythmic drug therapy at 6 months' follow-up.[47] Moreover, because catheter ablation and surgical ablation modify the arrhythmogenic substrate, previously ineffective antiarrhythmic drugs may be reevaluated following ablation procedures.[48] Finally, the performance of antiarrhythmic, ablative, and combined rhythm-control strategies

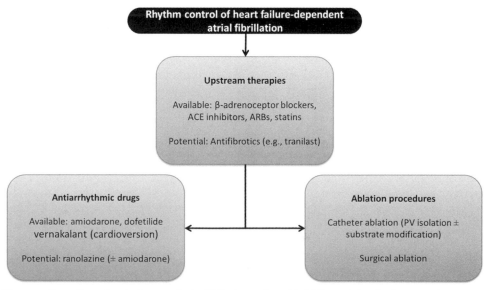

Fig. 2. Therapeutic options for rhythm control of HF -dependent AF. ACE, angiotensin-II converting enzyme; ARB, angiotensin-II type-1 receptor blockers; PV, pulmonary veins.

may be supported by upstream therapy to limit AF-related and HF-related remodeling.

FUTURE PERSPECTIVES
Novel Antiarrhythmic Strategies and Agents

Patients with HF often take multiple medications, making unwanted drug interactions likely and further necessitating the development of safe atrial-specific and pathology-specific antiarrhythmics for rhythm control of AF. Novel atrial-specific antiarrhythmic drugs targeting I_{Kur} and $I_{K,ACh}$ and/or showing atrial-predominant I_{Na} inhibition may facilitate rhythm control of AF without ventricular proarrhythmia.[9,10] A recent study found that bolus injection of the novel I_{Kur} inhibitor MK-0448 could abolish AF in a canine HF model, but had no effect on atrial or ventricular refractoriness in human subjects,[49] suggesting that I_{Kur} inhibition alone may not be sufficient to prevent AF in patients.

An alternative strategy for rhythm control of AF in patients with HF is to target pathologic processes or arrhythmogenic mechanisms common to AF and HF. Recent research strongly suggests that abnormal Ca^{2+} handling is a prime candidate for such dual antiarrhythmic therapy.[9,19] For example, the dual antiarrhythmic actions of ranolazine[40] may at least partly be due to its effects on Ca^{2+} handling, by both direct RyR2 inhibition and lowering intracellular Ca^{2+} through $I_{Na,late}$ inhibition, thereby reducing Na^+ load and promoting Ca^{2+} extrusion via NCX. In addition, several lead compounds that stabilize RyR2 and reduce SR Ca^{2+} leak have been identified and shown to have antiarrhythmic properties in several preclinical models.[9,10] Of particular interest in this group is the β-adrenoceptor blocker carvedilol, which was shown to be more effective than $β_1$-adrenoceptor selective blockers in reducing all-cause mortality in patients with HF in a recent meta-analysis.[50] Carvedilol and its newer analogues also inhibit RyR2 and this may importantly contribute to their antiarrhythmic action.[9]

Recent research has shown that gene transfer of connexin gap-junction proteins responsible for cell-to-cell communication improves atrial conduction and reduces AF occurrence in a large-animal model of rapid atrial pacing.[51] HF-dependent AF is also associated with changes in connexins,[51] suggesting that pharmacologic or gene therapy for connexins may have potential in the treatment of HF-dependent AF.[9] Finally, the transforming growth factor-β1 blocker tranilast prevents pro-fibrotic atrial remodeling and suppresses AF development in a canine model of tachycardiomyopathy, highlighting the clinical potential of antifibrotic drugs for the treatment of AF in the context of HF.[52]

Patient Selection and Personalized Treatment

Genome-wide association studies have identified several genetic polymorphisms that influence the risk of AF in the general population. Interestingly, Smith and colleagues[53] have recently shown that at least one of these polymorphisms in the ZFHX3 gene on chromosome 16q22 also associated with an increased risk for AF in patients with HF. Moreover, Parvez and colleagues[54] recently discovered that successful rhythm control of AF partly depends on a common variant on chromosome 4q25 near the PITX2 gene. In the future, such genetic information may help to identify patients that are likely to benefit from rhythm control and may suggest which approach to use.

SUMMARY

AF and HF are prevalent conditions with serious prognostic implications that frequently coexist. Although it remains unclear whether AF is an independent risk factor for worse outcomes in patients with HF and whether rhythm control is superior to rate control, it is clear that there is a dire need for safer and more effective antiarrhythmic drugs for AF in patients with and without HF. Amiodarone and dofetilide are currently the only antiarrhythmic drugs available for rhythm control in HF patients but their success is limited by extracardiovascular toxicity and substantial risk of proarrhythmia, respectively. Recent antiarrhythmic drugs such as ranolazine show promising results and an improved understanding of AF and HF pathophysiology has facilitated the development of several interesting lead compounds for atrial antiarrhythmic drugs. However, more extensive experimental testing and long-term follow-up in patients with HF of different causes is required to assess their safety and efficacy.

REFERENCES

1. Go AS, Mozaffarian D, Roger VL, et al. Heart disease and stroke statistics–2013 update a report from the American Heart Association. Circulation 2012;127(1):e6–245.
2. Darby AE, Dimarco JP. Management of atrial fibrillation in patients with structural heart disease. Circulation 2012;125(7):945–57.
3. Anter E, Jessup M, Callans DJ. Atrial fibrillation and heart failure: treatment considerations for a dual epidemic. Circulation 2009;119(18):2516–25.
4. Dries DL, Exner DV, Gersh BJ, et al. Atrial fibrillation is associated with an increased risk for mortality and

heart failure progression in patients with asymptom-
atic and symptomatic left ventricular dysfunction: a retrospective analysis of the SOLVD
trials. Studies of Left Ventricular Dysfunction. J Am
Coll Cardiol 1998;32(3):695–703.

5. Køber L, Swedberg K, McMurray JJ, et al. Previously known and newly diagnosed atrial fibrillation:
a major risk indicator after a myocardial infarction
complicated by heart failure or left ventricular
dysfunction. Eur J Heart Fail 2006;8(6):591–8.

6. Swedberg K, Olsson LG, Charlesworth A, et al.
Prognostic relevance of atrial fibrillation in patients
with chronic heart failure on long-term treatment
with beta-blockers: results from COMET. Eur Heart
J 2005;26(13):1303–8.

7. Smit MD, Moes ML, Maass AH, et al. The importance of whether atrial fibrillation or heart failure
develops first. Eur J Heart Fail 2012;14(9):1030–40.

8. Dobrev D, Nattel S. New antiarrhythmic drugs
for treatment of atrial fibrillation. Lancet 2010;
375(9721):1212–23.

9. Dobrev D, Carlsson L, Nattel S. Novel molecular
targets for atrial fibrillation therapy. Nat Rev Drug
Discov 2012;11(4):275–91.

10. Heijman J, Voigt N, Dobrev D. New directions in
antiarrhythmic drug therapy for atrial fibrillation.
Future Cardiol 2013;9(1):71–88.

11. Van Gelder IC, Hagens VE, Bosker HA, et al.
A comparison of rate control and rhythm control
in patients with recurrent persistent atrial fibrillation.
N Engl J Med 2002;347(23):1834–40.

12. Wyse DG, Waldo AL, DiMarco JP, et al.
A comparison of rate control and rhythm control
in patients with atrial fibrillation. N Engl J Med
2002;347(23):1825–33.

13. Roy D, Talajic M, Nattel S, et al. Rhythm control
versus rate control for atrial fibrillation and heart
failure. N Engl J Med 2008;358(25):2667–77.

14. Camm AJ, Kirchhof P, Lip GY, et al. Guidelines for
the management of atrial fibrillation: the Task Force
for the Management of Atrial Fibrillation of the
European Society of Cardiology (ESC). Europace
2010;12(10):1360–420.

15. Fuster V, Ryden LE, Cannom DS, et al. ACC/AHA/
ESC 2006 guidelines for the management of patients
with atrial fibrillation: a report of the American College
of Cardiology/American Heart Association Task
Force on Practice Guidelines and the European Society of Cardiology Committee for Practice Guidelines
(Writing Committee to Revise the 2001 Guidelines for
the Management of Patients With Atrial Fibrillation):
developed in collaboration with the European Heart
Rhythm Association and the Heart Rhythm Society.
Circulation 2006;114(7):e257–354.

16. Chinitz JS, Halperin JL, Reddy VY, et al. Rate or
rhythm control for atrial fibrillation: update and
controversies. Am J Med 2012;125(11):1049–56.

17. Corley SD, Epstein AE, DiMarco JP, et al. Relationships between sinus rhythm, treatment, and
survival in the Atrial Fibrillation Follow-Up Investigation of Rhythm Management (AFFIRM) Study.
Circulation 2004;109(12):1509–13.

18. Wakili R, Voigt N, Kaab S, et al. Recent advances in
the molecular pathophysiology of atrial fibrillation.
J Clin Invest 2011;121(8):2955–68.

19. Voigt N, Li N, Wang Q, et al. Enhanced sarcoplasmic
reticulum Ca^{2+} leak and increased Na^+-Ca^{2+}
exchanger function underlie delayed afterdepolarizations in patients with chronic atrial fibrillation.
Circulation 2012;125(17):2059–70.

20. Atienza F, Martins RP, Jalife J. Translational
research in atrial fibrillation: a quest for mechanis-
tically based diagnosis and therapy. Circ Arrhythm
Electrophysiol 2012;5(6):1207–15.

21. Comtois P, Kneller J, Nattel S. Of circles and
spirals: bridging the gap between the leading
circle and spiral wave concepts of cardiac reentry.
Europace 2005;7(Suppl 2):10–20.

22. Nattel S, Burstein B, Dobrev D. Atrial remodeling
and atrial fibrillation: mechanisms and implications.
Circ Arrhythm Electrophysiol 2008;1(1):62–73.

23. Dobrev D. Electrical remodeling in atrial fibrillation.
Herz 2006;31(2):108–12 [quiz: 142–143].

24. Nattel S, Dobrev D. The multidimensional role of
calcium in atrial fibrillation pathophysiology: mechanistic insights and therapeutic opportunities. Eur
Heart J 2012;33(15):1870–7.

25. Pandit SV, Berenfeld O, Anumonwo JM, et al. Ionic
determinants of functional reentry in a 2-D model of
human atrial cells during simulated chronic atrial
fibrillation. Biophys J 2005;88(6):3806–21.

26. Ling LH, Kistler PM, Ellims AH, et al. Diffuse ventricular fibrosis in atrial fibrillation: noninvasive
evaluation and relationships with aging and systolic dysfunction. J Am Coll Cardiol 2012;60(23):
2402–8.

27. De Jong AM, Maass AH, Oberdorf-Maass SU,
et al. Mechanisms of atrial structural changes
caused by stretch occurring before and during
early atrial fibrillation. Cardiovasc Res 2011;89(4):
754–65.

28. Rankin AC, Workman AJ. Duration of heart failure
and the risk of atrial fibrillation: different mechanisms at different times? Cardiovasc Res 2009;
84(2):180–1.

29. Nattel S, Maguy A, Le Bouter S, et al. Arrhythmogenic ion-channel remodeling in the heart: heart
failure, myocardial infarction, and atrial fibrillation.
Physiol Rev 2007;87(2):425–56.

30. Zimetbaum P. Antiarrhythmic drug therapy for atrial
fibrillation. Circulation 2012;125(2):381–9.

31. Camm J. Antiarrhythmic drugs for the maintenance
of sinus rhythm: risks and benefits. Int J Cardiol
2012;155(3):362–71.

32. Akiyama T, Pawitan Y, Greenborg H, et al. Increased risk of death and cardiac arrest from encainide and flecainide in patients after non-Q-wave acute myocardial infarction in the Cardiac Arrhythmia Suppression Trial. CAST Investigators. Am J Cardiol 1991;68(17):1551–5.

33. Torp-Pederson C, Moller M, Bloch-Thomsen PE, et al. Dofetilide in patients with congestive heart failure and left ventricular dysfunction. Danish Investigations of Arrhythmia and Mortality on Dofetilide Study Group. N Engl J Med 1999;341(12): 857–65.

34. Grossmann M, Dobrev D, Kirch W. Amiodarone causes endothelium-dependent vasodilation in human hand veins in vivo. Clin Pharmacol Ther 1998;64:302–11.

35. Grossmann M, Dobrev D, Himmel HM, et al. Local venous response to N-desethylamiodarone in humans. Clin Pharmacol Ther 2000;67(1):22–31.

36. Patel C, Yan GX, Kowey PR. Dronedarone. Circulation 2009;120(7):636–44.

37. Køber L, Torp-Pedersen C, McMurray JJ, et al. Increased mortality after dronedarone therapy for severe heart failure. N Engl J Med 2008;358(25): 2678–87.

38. Connolly SJ, Camm AJ, Halperin JL, et al. Dronedarone in high-risk permanent atrial fibrillation. N Engl J Med 2011;365(24):2268–76.

39. Dobrev D, Hamad B, Kirkpatrick P. Vernakalant. Nat Rev Drug Discov 2010;9(12):915–6.

40. Verrier RL, Kumar K, Nieminen T, et al. Mechanisms of ranolazine's dual protection against atrial and ventricular fibrillation. Europace 2013;15(3):317–24. http://dx.doi.org/10.1093/europace/eus380.

41. Frommeyer G, Schmidt M, Clauss C, et al. Further insights into the underlying electrophysiological mechanisms for reduction of atrial fibrillation by ranolazine in an experimental model of chronic heart failure. Eur J Heart Fail 2012; 14(12):1322–31.

42. Savelieva I, Kakouros N, Kourliouros A, et al. Upstream therapies for management of atrial fibrillation: review of clinical evidence and implications for European Society of Cardiology guidelines. Part I: primary prevention. Europace 2011;13(3): 308–28.

43. Goette A, Bukowska A, Dobrev D, et al. Acute atrial tachyarrhythmia induces angiotensin II type 1 receptor-mediated oxidative stress and microvascular flow abnormalities in the ventricles. Eur Heart J 2009;30(11):1411–20.

44. Hunter RJ, McCready J, Diab I, et al. Maintenance of sinus rhythm with an ablation strategy in patients with atrial fibrillation is associated with a lower risk of stroke and death. Heart 2012;98(1):48–53.

45. Hsu LF, Jais P, Sanders P, et al. Catheter ablation for atrial fibrillation in congestive heart failure. N Engl J Med 2004;351(23):2373–83.

46. MacDonald MR, Connelly DT, Hawkins NM, et al. Radiofrequency ablation for persistent atrial fibrillation in patients with advanced heart failure and severe left ventricular systolic dysfunction: a randomised controlled trial. Heart 2011;97(9):740–7.

47. Khan MN, Jais P, Cummings J, et al. Pulmonary-vein isolation for atrial fibrillation in patients with heart failure. N Engl J Med 2008;359(17):1778–85.

48. Naccarelli GV, Gonzalez MD. Atrial fibrillation and the expanding role of catheter ablation: do antiarrhythmic drugs have a future? J Cardiovasc Pharmacol 2008;52(3):203–9.

49. Pavri BB, Greenberg HE, Kraft WK, et al. MK-0448, a specific Kv1.5 inhibitor: safety, pharmacokinetics, and pharmacodynamic electrophysiology in experimental animal models and humans. Circ Arrhythm Electrophysiol 2012;5(6):1193–201.

50. Dinicolantonio JJ, Lavie CJ, Fares H, et al. Meta-analysis of carvedilol versus beta 1 selective beta-blockers (atenolol, bisoprolol, metoprolol, and nebivolol). Am J Cardiol 2013;111(5):765–9.

51. Kato T, Iwasaki YK, Nattel S. Connexins and atrial fibrillation: filling in the gaps. Circulation 2012; 125(2):203–6.

52. Nakatani Y, Nishida K, Sakabe M, et al. Tranilast prevents atrial remodeling and development of atrial fibrillation in a canine model of atrial tachycardia and left ventricular dysfunction. J Am Coll Cardiol 2013;61(5):582–8.

53. Smith JG, Melander O, Sjogren M, et al. Genetic polymorphisms confer risk of atrial fibrillation in patients with heart failure: a population-based study. Eur J Heart Fail 2012;15(3):250–7.

54. Parvez B, Vaglio J, Rowan S, et al. Symptomatic response to antiarrhythmic drug therapy is modulated by a common single nucleotide polymorphism in atrial fibrillation. J Am Coll Cardiol 2012; 60(6):539–45.

Upstream Therapy for Atrial Fibrillation in Heart Failure

Andreas Goette, MD

KEYWORDS

- Atrial fibrillation • Heart failure • Upstream therapy • Statins • Prevention

KEY POINTS

- Heart failure is a major factor that increases the likelihood for atrial fibrillation (AF).
- Several aspects of the morphologic and electrophysiologic alterations promoting AF in heart failure (congestive heart failure [CHF]) have been studied in animal models and in patients with CHF; under these conditions, ectopic activity originating from the pulmonary veins or other sites is more likely to occur and to trigger longer episodes of AF.
- Angiotensin-converting enzyme inhibitors, angiotensin receptor blockers, and spironolactone may help to reduce the occurrence of AF.
- Statins are indicated if patients have an indication for their use, such as increased low-density lipoprotein levels or established coronary artery disease.
- Results for secondary prevention are very heterogeneous, and the effect of upstream therapy is less well established in this clinical setting.

PATHOPHYSIOLOGY OF ATRIAL FIBRILLATION IN HEART FAILURE

Atrial fibrillation (AF) is the most common sustained arrhythmia in humans, causing an increasing number of complications and deaths.[1–3] Reports suggest that approximately 1% of the total population is affected.[4] The number of patients with AF is likely to double or triple within the next 2 to 3 decades.[5] The prevalence of AF is clearly age dependent. Patients with AF usually seek medical attention because of AF-related symptoms, and the treatment of these symptoms has been the main motivation for AF therapy in the past. However, even the presence of asymptomatic AF markedly decreases quality of life.[2,6] AF also doubles mortality independently of other known disease-causing factors and is one of the most common causes for stroke. Left ventricular function, the best-validated clinical parameter for cardiac prognosis, can be markedly impaired in patients with AF and improves when sinus rhythm is maintained for a longer period of time.[2,7] Heart failure with dyspnea on exertion (New York Heart Association [NYHA] classes II–IV) is found in 30% of patients with AF,[8] and AF is found in 30% to 40% of patients with heart failure.[2,9] Heart failure and AF seem to promote each other, with AF compromising left ventricular function and left ventricular dysfunction causing atrial dilation and pressure overload. Treatment of heart failure is able to prevent AF,[2,10] adding to the evidence that AF is promoted by these conditions.

In order to investigate how congestive heart failure (CHF) promotes AF, experimental models of CHF have been described.[11] When CHF was induced by pacing with a ventricular pacemaker at a high rate (>200 beats per minute) for 5 weeks, atrial fibrosis was dramatically increased in dogs with CHF,[11] with large areas of connective tissue. These structural abnormalities were accompanied

Disclosures: The author has nothing to disclose.
Department of Cardiology and Intensive Care Medicine, St. Vincenz Hospital Paderborn GmbH, EUTRAF Working Group, University Hospital Magdeburg, Am Busdorf 2, Paderborn 33098, Germany
E-mail address: andreas.goette@med.ovgu.de

Heart Failure Clin 9 (2013) 417–425
http://dx.doi.org/10.1016/j.hfc.2013.07.010
1551-7136/13/$ – see front matter © 2013 Elsevier Inc. All rights reserved.

by regional conduction heterogeneity. Studies have supported the role of atrial fibrosis in the promotion of AF in CHF.[2,12,13] Atrial damage in the CHF model occurs rapidly, with a peak in inflammation, apoptosis, and necrosis within 24 hours after activation of the ventricular pacemaker.[2,14] The renin-angiotensin system is an important mediator in the development of an AF substrate in CHF. Inhibition of angiotensin II (AT II) production by the angiotensin-converting enzyme (ACE) blocker enalapril not only attenuated CHF-induced atrial fibrosis but also reduced conduction heterogeneity and AF stability.[2,15,16] Atrial fibrosis and increased AF stability in the canine CHF model can also be inhibited by simvastatin,[17] pirfenidone,[18] polyunsaturated ω-3 fatty acids,[19] and sprionolactone.[20] The peroxisome proliferator-activated receptor α (PPARα) activator fenofibrate was not effective in this model[17]; but in rabbits with tachycardiomyopathy-induced CHF, the PPARγ activator pioglitazone did reduce atrial structural remodeling and AF stability.[2,21]

MOLECULAR DRUG TARGETS FOR UPSTREAM THERAPY

Chronic atrial stretch seems to be one of the most prominent trigger mechanisms for signaling changes involved in the pathogenesis of AF. Atria seem to react much faster and more strongly to increased wall stress caused by atrial dilatation than ventricular myocardium.[14] The induction of heart failure by rapid ventricular pacing induces the development of apoptosis and increased collagen synthesis in the atria within a couple of days, whereas the degree of such changes is substantially smaller and the time course much slower in the ventricles.[2,11] At the molecular level, the development of atrial fibrosis caused by pressure and/or volume overload is mediated by both angiotensin II-dependent and independent mechanisms.[2,15,17] Left ventricular failure increases atrial synthesis of angiotensin II, and thereby atrial fibrosis is induced via activation of mitogen-activated protein (MAP) kinases.[2,22] Signaling pathways mediated by angiotensin II type 1 receptors (AT-1 receptors) are linked to G proteins. Studies have shown a linear correlation between angiotensin II, MAP kinase activation, and the degree of atrial fibrosis.[15] Another tyrosine kinase that is activated by angiotensin II is Janus kinase 2 (JAK2).[22] JAK2 initiates the activation of transcription factors signal transducer and activator of transcription (STAT)-1 and STAT-3. A recent study demonstrated that the angiotensin II/Rac1/STAT3 pathway is an important signaling pathway involved in atrial structural remodeling.[23]

In addition to angiotensin II, pacing-induced ventricular failure also increases atrial transforming growth factor (TGF)-β and platelet-derived growth factor (PDGF) levels. TGF-β operates predominantly by autocrine and paracrine mechanisms. Binding of a TGF-β homodimer to 2 TGF-β type II receptors causes phosphorylation of signaling molecules belonging to the family known as SMADs. When phosphorylated, SMADs aggregate and enter the nucleus to induce myocardial fibrosis.[24] In addition, TGF-β1 can redirect protein synthesis to favor expression of fetal genes as described in fibrillating atria.[25] Atrial fibroblasts are activated significantly faster than ventricular fibroblasts in the CHF models, explaining the rapid and more severe degree of interstitial fibrosis in the atria.[26]

Another important contributor to atrial remodeling in CHF is oxidative stress.[27] The PPARγ activator pioglitazone antagonizes angiotensin II actions and possesses antiinflammatory and antioxidant properties. Pioglitazone attenuated CHF-induced atrial structural remodeling and AF vulnerability.[2] In the same study, both pioglitazone and candesartan reduced TGF-β, tumor necrosis factor α, and MAP kinase, but neither affected p38 kinase or c-Jun N-terminal kinase activation. In contrast, ω-3 polyunsaturated fatty acids attenuate CHF-related phosphorylation of the MAP kinases ERK and p38.[2,19] In failing human myocardium, NADPH oxidase-related reactive oxygen species (ROS) production increases, with enhanced expression and activity of Rac1. The application of 3-hydroxy-3-methylglutaryl coenzyme A reductase inhibitors (statins) like simvastatin inhibits myocardial Rac1-GTPase activity.[17] The small GTPase Rac1 regulates NADPH oxidase activity. Statins downregulate Rac1-GTPase activity by reducing isoprenylation and translocation of Rac1 to the cell membrane.[28] The inhibition of Rac1 by statins decreases NADPH oxidase-related reactive oxygen species production in cardiac myocytes and reduces myocardial hypertrophy. Furthermore, simvastatin reduces human atrial myofibroblast proliferation via a RhoA pathway.[29] In addition, simvastatin, but not fenofibrate (PPARα agonist), inhibits canine atrial fibroblast proliferation, which paralleled collagen-synthetic fibroblast function.[2] Thus, statins and PPARα agonists have very different efficacy in preventing CHF-related atrial structural remodeling.

In addition to cellular effects, atrial stretch is also associated with an altered expression of matrix metalloproteinases (MMP). In patients with AF with congestive heart failure, an increased collagen I fraction seems to be associated with upregulation of MMP-2 and downregulation of tissue inhibitor of metalloprotease-1.[2,30,31] In addition to MMPs,

ADAMs (a disintegrin and metalloprotelnase) also influence interstitial matrix composition and cell-cell and cell-matrix interactions. ADAMs form a large family of membrane-bound glycoproteins that function in proteolysis, signaling, cell adhesion, and cleavage-secretion of membrane-bound proteins.[2] Arndt and colleagues[32] described the effect of AF in patients with concomitant heart diseases on the regulation of ADAMs. Atrial tissue of patients with permanent AF shows increased levels of ADAM10 and ADAM15. Membrane expression of ADAM15 is significantly upregulated during AF, whereas most ADAM15 is retarded in the cytoplasm during sinus rhythm. The ADAM15/integrin $\beta 1$ ratio is significantly increased in fibrillating tissue and correlates with the left atrial diameter and the duration of fibrillation. Thus, the regulation of MMPs and ADAMs influences the composition of interstitial matrix and contributes to geometric changes and dilatation of the atria and ventricles.[2,33]

Although atrial fibrosis is proarrhythmic in some animal models,[2,34,35] the quantitative association between atrial fibrosis and AF is not very strong. Some but not all human studies have found that atrial fibrosis is more pronounced in patients with chronic AF than in patients in sinus rhythm.[2,36] The degree of atrial fibrosis and fibrogenic activity correlates with the persistence of AF.[2,37] However, from these studies, it is unclear whether increased fibrosis is caused by underlying structural disease or by AF itself.[2]

UPSTREAM THERAPY FOR AF

As described, the treatment of CHF has been shown to reduce the incidence of AF in experimental models and clinical studies. Animal studies showed that the antiarrhythmic effects of ACE inhibitors and angiotensin receptor blockers (ARB) are related to their effect on atrial morphology.[38,39] The results are supported by analyses of several clinical trials: Valsartan Heart Failure Trial (Val-HeFT), Studies of Left Ventricular Dysfunction (SOLVD), and Candesartan in Heart Failure: Assessment of Reduction in Mortality and Morbidity (CHARM).[40] Furthermore, the Randomized Aldactone Evaluation Study (RALES) trial showed that spironolactone (an aldosterone antagonist) reduces circulating procollagen I and III levels in patients with CHF, which was associated with an improved survival.[11] Other targets and drugs for upstream therapy like statins, polyunsaturated fatty acids are less well studied in clinical trials so far. Of note, the results for primary prevention are significantly better than data for secondary prevention of AF in patients with CHF.

RENIN-ANGIOTENSIN-ALDOSTERONE SYSTEM INHIBITION IN CHF

In patients, several post hoc analyses of clinical trials suggest that therapy with ACE inhibitors, AT-1-receptor blocker, statins, and polyunsaturated fatty acids (PUFAs) are useful to prevent AF (Table 1). CHF is one of the most important risk factors for AF and, as evidenced by multivariate analysis from the Framingham Study, increases the risk of AF by 4.5-fold in men and 5.9-fold in women.[42,43] Diastolic left ventricular dysfunction is associated with a 5.26-fold increased risk of AF.[43,44] The occurrence of CHF in middle age confers an 8% risk of developing AF over a 10-year period if the patient's age at the time of CHF diagnosis was 55 to 64 years, which increases to 30% if CHF was diagnosed at 45 to 54 years of age.[43,45] Furthermore, the presence of CHF not only increases the likelihood of developing AF but is also the leading independent predictor of progression to permanent AF, with an odds ratio of 2.2.[46] New-onset AF in CHF is associated with clinical deterioration and poor prognosis.[43,47] There are reports that the absence of AF is associated with fewer symptoms and better functional status and left ventricular function in patients with CHF.[43,48,49] The true benefit of preserving sinus rhythm in patients with CHF in the AF-CHF and other secondary prevention studies might have been offset by the relatively low efficacy and adverse effects of antiarrhythmic drugs. Thus, upstream therapies (eg, renin-angiotensin-aldosterone system [RAAS] inhibitors) that target both the underlying condition and the substrate formation for AF may offer a greater benefit than specific antiarrhythmic drugs.[43,50]

The first large study to report the beneficial effect of RAAS inhibition on the occurrence of new-onset AF was the Trandolapril Cardiac Evaluation (TRACE) study in patients with recent myocardial infarction and an ejection fraction of 35% or less.[10] Patients who received trandolapril were less likely to develop new-onset AF during 2 to 4 years of follow-up compared with the placebo group (2.8% vs 5.3%). The report from the TRACE study was followed by similar retrospective analysis of the single-center results from the SOLVD trial, which also demonstrated less AF occurrence in patients with CHF and an ejection fraction of 35% or less with enalapril as opposed to placebo after 2.9 years of follow-up (5.4% vs 24.0%).[43] Later studies with ARBs yielded similar results.

In the Val-HeFT study, in 4395 patients with symptomatic CHF, therapy with valsartan was associated with a 37% reduction in relative risk of newly detected AF compared with placebo

Table 1
Clinical trials of renin-angiotensin systems inhibition to prevent new-onset AF in patients with CHF or AMI (primary prevention)

References	Study Design	Patients	Intervention	Primary Outcome
Pedersen et al,[10] 1999	TRACE study (post hoc analysis)	1577 with AMI and reduced LVEF	Trandolapril vs placebo Follow-up: 2–4 y	Reduced incidence of new-onset AF
Pizetti et al	GISSI-3 study (post hoc analysis)	17,749 with AMI	Lisinopril vs no lisinopril Follow-up: 4 y	No difference in new-onset AF
Vermes et al	SOLVD study (post hoc analysis)	347 with LV dysfunction	Enalapril vs placebo Follow-up: 2.9 y	Reduced incidence of new-onset AF
Alsheikh-Ali et al	SOLVD study (post hoc analysis)	6797 with LV dysfunction	Enalapril vs placebo Follow-up: 34 mo	Reduced incidence of hospitalization with AF
Maggioni et al	Val-HeFT study (post hoc analysis)	4395 with chronic symptomatic HF	Valsartan vs placebo Follow-up: 23 mo	Reduced incidence of new-onset AF
Ducharme et al,[52] 2006	CHARM study (prespecified secondary end point)	6379 with symptomatic CHF	Candesartan vs placebo Follow-up: 37.7 mo	Reduced incidence of new-onset AF
Hansson et al	CAPPP study (randomized, open label [analysis on adverse event reports])	10,985 with hypertension	Captopril vs diuretics ± beta-blocker Follow-up: 6.1 y	No difference in new-onset AF
Hansson et al	STOP-2 study (randomized, open label)	6628 with hypertension	Enalapril/lisinopril vs CCB vs diuretics ± beta-blocker Study duration: 4 y	No difference in new-onset AF
Lh'Allier et al	Retrospective longitudinal cohort study	10,926 with hypertension	ACEI vs CCB Average follow-up: 4.5 y	Reduced incidence of new-onset AF
Wachtell et al,[64] 2005	LIFE study (randomized, double blind)	8851 with hypertension + ECG LVH	Losartan vs atenolol Follow-up: 4.8 y	Reduced incidence of new-onset AF

Abbreviations: ACEI, ACE inhibitor; AMI, acute myocardial infarction; CCB, calcium channel blockers; ECG, electrocardiogram; GISSI, Gruppo Italiano per lo Studio della Sopravvivenza nell'Insufficienza cardiaca; HF, heart failure; LIFE, Losartan Intervention For End Point Reduction in Hypertension; LV, left ventricular; LVEF, left ventricular ejection fraction; LVH, left ventricular hypertrophy.

Adapted from Savelieva I, Kakouros N, Kourliouros A, et al. Upstream therapies for management of atrial fibrillation. Part I: primary prevention. Europace 2011;13:308–28; with permission.

(5.12% vs 7.95%) during 1.9 years.[43,51] This benefit from an ARB was present despite a high (93%) rate of concomitant use of ACE inhibitors (ACEIs). This study has also demonstrated that the occurrence of AF was independently associated with adverse major outcomes, such as all-cause death and combined mortality and morbidity, which increased by 40% and 38%, respectively, in the presence of AF. However, whether valsartan therapy improved the outcome within the new-onset AF group compared with placebo has not been reported.[43]

One of the limitations of these retrospective analyses was that AF was not a prespecified end point, and a significant proportion of asymptomatic or mildly symptomatic episodes might not have been reported. The CHARM program designated AF as one of the secondary end points.[43] The AF substudy from the CHARM trials has shown that adding candesartan to conventional CHF therapy in 6379 patients with symptomatic CHF and without a history of AF at enrollment led to a lower incidence of new-onset AF compared with placebo, albeit this reduction was not as significant as in the previous reports (5.55% vs 6.74%).[43,52] Of note, the magnitude of the preventative effect of RAAS inhibition varies in patients according to the degree of impairment of left ventricular function. Thus, although statistically there was no heterogeneity of the effect of candesartan on AF between the 3 component trials in the CHARM program, the greatest benefit was seen in patients with impaired systolic function and without the concurrent use of ACEIs enrolled in the CHARM-alternative study and the least in patients with CHF and preserved systolic function.[51]

Similarly, irbesartan did not influence the incidence of AF reported as an adverse event in the Irbesartan in Patients with Heart Failure and Preserved Ejection Fraction trial.[53] Four meta-analyses have shown that the risk of new-onset AF in patients with CHF was reduced by 30% to 48%, suggesting that ACEIs and ARBs may be effective in the primary prevention of AF in this clinical setting.[38,54–56] This finding is consistent with experimental evidence of atrial fibrosis as the leading mechanism of AF in CHF models and evidence of antifibrotic effects of RAAS inhibition. It is unclear whether therapy with ACEIs and ARBs can prevent or delay the occurrence of AF in patients with CHF and preserved systolic function. There is no direct evidence that upstream therapies with RAAS inhibitors can reduce morbidity and mortality in patients with CHF by deterring AF.[43]

STATINS IN CHF

Retrospective analyses from randomized controlled trials (RCTs) and registries in patients with CHF have suggested a modest reduction in the incidence of AF, mainly newly detected AF, although the differentiation between truly new-onset AF and recurrent AF has not always been possible.[43,57–59] In the AdvancentSM registry of 25,268 patients with an ejection fraction of 40% or less and left ventricular dysfunction of an ischemic cause in 72%, lipid-lowering therapy (mostly statins or combination therapy) was associated with a 31% reduction in relative risk of developing AF compared with no therapy.[57] This effect was greater than that of beta-blockers and RAAS inhibitors. The Sudden Cardiac Death in Heart Failure Trial investigators reported a similar 28% reduction in relative risk of AF, which was comparable with that of amiodarone.[43,58]

The GISSI-HF (Gruppo Italiano per lo Studio della Sopravvivenza nell'Insufficienza cardiaca Heart Failure) study enrolled 3690 patients with sinus rhythm. Therapy with rosuvastatin reduced the risk of any AF during the study by only 13%. The difference with the placebo arm became statistically significant only after adjustment for clinical variables, laboratory findings, and concomitant therapy.[59] In the prespecified subgroup of patients with no history of paroxysmal AF, the incidence of new-onset AF was 9.8% in the rosuvastatin arm and 11.6% in the placebo arm. Patients in whom AF was present on the baseline electrocardiogram (19.3%) were excluded, but it could not be ascertained whether all patients who developed AF in the course of the study had new-onset AF.[43] There was a nonsignificant difference between the rosuvastatin and placebo arms in the proportion of patients with AF at study entry who were excluded from analysis (18.8% vs 19.8%). During the study, AF occurred in 15% patients: 13.9% in the rosuvastatin group and 16.0% in the placebo group (absolute difference 2.1%). It is possible that more patients in the rosuvastatin arm may have had unrecognized AF at baseline and, hence, a greater likelihood of recurrent AF.[43] Because of the retrospective nature of these reports, much important information is not available. One brief report from a large cohort of patients with CHF who were prescribed statins has suggested that the intensity of treatment might play a role; thus, in this study, AF was less common in those who received high doses (atorvastatin 80 mg, simvastatin 80 mg, and lovastatin 40 mg) as opposed to lower doses of the same agent.[43,60]

Table 2
Clinical trials of statins to prevent new-onset and progression of AF (primary and secondary prevention)

References	Study Design	Patients	Intervention	Primary Outcome
Hanna et al	Retrospective	25,268 with CHF	Lipid-lowering drug use vs no use	Reduced incidence of new onset AF
Adabag et al	Retrospective	13,783 with CHD	Statins vs no statins Average follow-up: 4.8 y	No difference in new-onset AF

Abbreviation: CHD, coronary heart diseases.
Adapted from Savelieva I, Kakouros N, Kourliouros A, et al. Upstream therapies for management of atrial fibrillation. Part I: primary prevention. Europace 2011;13:308–28; with permission.

Table 3
Clinical trials of ω-3 (omega-3) polyunsaturated fatty acids to prevent AF in patients without CHF

References	Study Design	Patients	Intervention	Primary Outcome
Mozaffarian et al	Cardiovascular Health Study (population-based, prospective cohort)	4815	Dietary intake assessment Follow-up: 12 y	Reduced incidence of AF
Frost et al	Danish Diet, Cancer and Health study (population-based, prospective cohort)	47,949	Dietary intake assessment Mean follow-up: 5.4 y	No difference in incidence of AF
Brouwer et al	Rotterdam study: (population-based, prospective cohort)	5184	Dietary intake assessment Follow-up: 6.4 y	No difference in incidence of AF

Adapted from Savelieva I, Kakouros N, Kourliouros A, et al. Upstream therapies for management of atrial fibrillation. Part I: primary prevention. Europace 2011;13:308–28; with permission.

META-ANALYSES OF STATIN TRIALS

Other meta-analyses of the efficacy of statins for primary prevention of AF in different clinical settings have yielded controversial results (**Table 2**).[43,60,61] The first meta-analysis by Fauchier and colleagues,[60] which included 3 RCTs of primary prevention (one in ACS and 2 in postoperative AF) in 3101 patients, has shown a nonsignificant trend toward fewer AF events. In a meta-analysis by Liu and colleagues,[61] statin treatment was associated with a reduction in new-onset AF both after cardiac surgery and in the nonsurgical setting but only in the observational studies. No effect on AF was seen when the results of RCTs were analyzed. The most recent meta-analysis, which has not yet been published in full, has confirmed the previous findings by showing a 30% reduction in relative risk of new-onset or recurrent AF with statins compared with control in 7 hypothesis-generating relatively small and short-term studies in mixed populations, including patients with acute coronary syndrome (ACS), cardiac surgery, and after electrical cardioversion (411 events in 3609 patients).[62] However, in 15 (1514 events in 68,504 patients) hypothesis-testing long-term prospective RCTs in large patient populations with and without cardiovascular pathologic conditions, the use of statins had no effect on the occurrence of (mainly) new-onset AF compared with control or placebo.[43] Further analysis revealed no difference in the effects of statins in patients with coronary artery disease (CAD) versus other underlying cardiovascular pathology. Thus, the value of statins for the primary prevention of AF has not been sufficiently demonstrated, except perhaps for patients undergoing cardiac surgery. Nevertheless, several positive reports suggest some benefit of statins in patients with underlying heart disease, particularly CHF.[43,63]

SUMMARY

CHF induces substantial molecular alteration in atrial tissue. These changes are proarrhythmic and increase the likelihood for AF. Thus, aggressive therapy for CHF has been shown to be useful for the primary prevention of AF in these patients; in particular, ACE inhibitors, ARBs, and spironolactone may help to reduce the occurrence of AF. Statins are indicated if patients have an indication for their use, such as increased low-density lipoprotein levels or established CAD. Results for secondary prevention are very heterogeneous, and the effect of upstream therapy is less well established in this clinical setting. This point may be explained by the fact that an established proarrhythmic atrial fibrosis is not reversible; therefore, the burden of AF cannot be decreased by such therapies. The impact of PUFA therapy is not established in patients with CHF (**Table 3**). Although there are experimental data showing antiarrhythmic effects, the true clinical benefit of long-term PUFA application is very vague in patients with CHF.[2,43,47,64–70]

There is a good deal of supporting evidence for the use of upstream therapies, mostly in favor of modification of the RAAS axis. It is, therefore, entirely appropriate that drugs acting beneficially on the RAAS are prescribed in the heart failure population using the additional benefit on the predisposition to AF to provide supporting arguments.

REFERENCES

1. Fuster V, Ryden LE, Cannom DS, et al. ACC/AHA/ESC 2006 guidelines for the management of patients with atrial fibrillation-executive summary: A report of the American College of Cardiology/American Heart Association Task Force on practice

guidelines and the European Society of Cardiology Committee for Practice Guidelines (Writing Committee to Revise the 2001 Guidelines for the Management of Patients with Atrial Fibrillation) developed in collaboration with the European Heart Rhythm Association and the Heart Rhythm Society. Eur Heart J 2006;27:1979–2030.

2. Schotten U, Verheule S, Kirchhof P, et al. Pathophysiological mechanisms of atrial fibrillation: a translational appraisal. Physiol Rev 2011;91(1): 265–325.

3. Kirchhof P, Auricchio A, Bax J, et al. Outcome parameters for trials in atrial fibrillation: executive summary: recommendations from a consensus conference organized by the German Atrial Fibrillation Competence NETwork (AFNET) and the European Heart Rhythm Association (EHRA). Eur Heart J 2007;28:2803–17.

4. Kannel WB, Wolf PA, Benjamin EJ, et al. Prevalence, incidence, prognosis, and predisposing conditions for atrial fibrillation: population-based estimates. Am J Cardiol 1998;82:2N–9N.

5. Hobbs FD, Fitzmaurice DA, Mant J, et al. A randomised controlled trial and cost-effectiveness study of systematic screening (targeted and total population screening) versus routine practice for the detection of atrial fibrillation in people aged 65 and over. The SAFE study. Health Technol Assess 2005;9:1–74, iii–iv, ix–x.

6. Wilhelmsen L, Rosengren A, Lappas G. Hospitalizations for atrial fibrillation in the general male population: morbidity and risk factors. J Intern Med 2001;250:382–9.

7. Khan MN, Jaïs P, Cummings J, et al. Pulmonary-vein isolation for atrial fibrillation in patients with heart failure. N Engl J Med 2008;359:1778–85.

8. Nieuwlaat R, Capucci A, Camm AJ, et al. Atrial fibrillation management: a prospective survey in ESC member countries: the Euro Heart Survey on Atrial Fibrillation. Eur Heart J 2005;26:2422–34.

9. Cleland JG, Swedberg K, Follath F, et al. The Euro-Heart Failure survey programme: a survey on the quality of care among patients with heart failure in Europe. Part 1: patient characteristics and diagnosis. Eur Heart J 2003;24:442–63.

10. Pedersen OD, Bagger H, Kober L, et al. Trandolapril reduces the incidence of atrial fibrillation after acute myocardial infarction in patients with left ventricular dysfunction. Circulation 1999;100:376–80.

11. Li D, Fareh S, Leung TK, et al. Promotion of atrial fibrillation by heart failure in dogs: atrial remodeling of a different sort. Circulation 1999;100:87–95.

12. Cha TJ, Ehrlich JR, Zhang L, et al. Dissociation between ionic remodeling and ability to sustain atrial fibrillation during recovery from experimental congestive heart failure. Circulation 2004;109: 412–8.

13. Shinagawa K, Shi Y, Tardif JC, et al. Dynamic nature of atrial fibrillation substrate during development and reversal of heart failure in dogs. Circulation 2002;105:2672–8.

14. Hanna N, Cardin S, Leung TK, et al. Differences in atrial versus ventricular remodeling in dogs with ventricular tachypacing-induced congestive heart failure. Cardiovasc Res 2004;63(2):236 44.

15. Li D, Shinagawa K, Pang L, et al. Effects of angiotensin-converting enzyme inhibition on the development of the atrial fibrillation substrate in dogs with ventricular tachypacing-induced congestive heart failure. Circulation 2001;104:2608–14.

16. Shi Y, Li D, Tardif JC, et al. Enalapril effects on atrial remodeling and atrial fibrillation in experimental congestive heart failure. Cardiovasc Res 2002;54: 456–61.

17. Shiroshita-Takeshita A, Brundel BJ, Burstein B, et al. Effects of simvastatin on the development of the atrial fibrillation substrate in dogs with congestive heart failure. Cardiovasc Res 2007; 74:75–84.

18. Lee KW, Everett TH, Rahmutula D, et al. Pirfenidone prevents the development of a vulnerable substrate for atrial fibrillation in a canine model of heart failure. Circulation 2006;114:1703–12.

19. Sakabe M, Shiroshita-Takeshita A, Maguy A, et al. Omega-3 polyunsaturated fatty acids prevent atrial fibrillation associated with heart failure but not atrial tachycardia remodeling. Circulation 2007;116: 2101–9.

20. Yang SS, Han W, Zhou HY, et al. Effects of spironolactone on electrical and structural remodeling of atrium in congestive heart failure dogs. Chin Med J 2008;121:38–42.

21. Shimano M, Tsuji Y, Inden Y, et al. Pioglitazone, a peroxisome proliferator-activated receptor-gamma activator, attenuates atrial fibrosis and atrial fibrillation promotion in rabbits with congestive heart failure. Heart Rhythm 2008;5(3):451–9.

22. Goette A, Staack T, Röcken C, et al. Increased expression of extracellular-signal regulated kinase and angiotensin-converting enzyme in human atria during atrial fibrillation. J Am Coll Cardiol 2000;35: 1669–77.

23. Tsai CT, Lai LP, Kuo KT, et al. Angiotensin II activates signal transducer and activators of transcription 3 via Rac1 in atrial myocytes and fibroblasts: implication for the therapeutic effect of statin in atrial structural remodeling. Circulation 2008; 117(3):344–55.

24. Brand T, Schneider MD. Transforming growth factor-β signal transduction. Circ Res 1996;78:173–9.

25. Parker TG, Packer SE, Schneider MD. Peptide growth factors can provoke fetal contractile proteins gene expression in rat cardiac myocytes. J Clin Invest 1990;85:507–14.

26. Burstein B, Libby E, Calderone A, et al. Differential behaviors of atrial versus ventricular fibroblasts: a potential role for platelet-derived growth factor in atrial-ventricular remodeling differences. Circulation 2008;117(13):1630–41.

27. Cha YM, Shen WK, Jahangir A, et al. Failing atrial myocardium: energetic deficits accompany structural remodeling and electrical instability. Am J Physiol Heart Circ Physiol 2003;284(4):H1313–20.

28. Adam O, Neuberger HR, Böhm M, et al. Prevention of atrial fibrillation with 3-hydroxy-3-methylglutaryl coenzyme A reductase inhibitors. Circulation 2008;118:1285–93.

29. Porter KE, O'Regan DJ, Balmforth AJ, et al. Simvastatin reduces human atrial myofibroblast proliferation independently of cholesterol lowering via inhibition of RhoA. Cardiovasc Res 2004;61:745–55.

30. Cooradi D, Callegari S, Benussi S, et al. Regional left atrial interstitial remodeling in patients with chronic atrial fibrillation undergoing mitral-valve surgery. Virchows Arch 2004;445(5):498–505.

31. Xu J, Cui G, Esmailian F, et al. Atrial extracellular matrix remodeling and the maintenance of atrial fibrillation. Circulation 2004;109:363–8.

32. Arndt M, Röcken C, Nepple K, et al. Altered expression of ADAMs (a disintegrin and metalloproteinase) in fibrillating human atria. Circulation 2002;105:720–5.

33. Hunt MJ, Aru GM, Hayden MR, et al. Induction of oxidative stress and disintegrin metalloproteinase in human heart end-stage failure. Am J Physiol Lung Cell Mol Physiol 2002;283:L239–45.

34. Burstein B, Nattel S. Atrial fibrosis: mechanisms and clinical relevance in atrial fibrillation. J Am Coll Cardiol 2008;51:802–9.

35. Everett TH, Olgin JE. Atrial fibrosis and the mechanisms of atrial fibrillation. Heart Rhythm 2007;4: S24–7.

36. Boldt A, Wetzel U, Lauschke J, et al. Fibrosis in left atrial tissue of patients with atrial fibrillation with and without underlying mitral valve disease. Heart 2004;90:400–5.

37. Gramley F, Lorenzen J, Plisiene J, et al. Decreased plasminogen activator inhibitor and tissue metalloproteinase inhibitor expression may promote increased metalloproteinase activity with increasing duration of human atrial fibrillation. J Cardiovasc Electrophysiol 2007;18:1076–82.

38. Healey JS, Baranchuk A, Crystal E, et al. Prevention of atrial fibrillation with angiotensin-converting enzyme inhibitors and angiotensin receptor blockers: a meta-analysis. J Am Coll Cardiol 2005;45(11):1832–9.

39. Hammwöhner M, D'Alessandro A, Dobrev D, et al. New antiarrhythmic drugs for therapy of atrial fibrillation: II. Non-ion channel blockers. Herzschrittmacherther Elektrophysiol 2006;17(2):73–80.

40. Ehrlich JR, Hohnloser SH, Nattel S. Role of angiotensin system and effects of its inhibition in atrial fibrillation: clinical and experimental evidence. Eur Heart J 2006;27(5):512–8.

41. Zannad F, Alla F, Dousset B, et al. Limitation of excessive extracellular matrix turnover may contribute to survival benefit of spironolactone therapy in patients with congestive heart failure: insights from the randomized Aldactone evaluation study (RALES). Rales Investigators. Circulation 2000;102(22):2700–6.

42. Benjamin EJ, Levy D, Vaziri SM, et al. Independent risk factors for atrial fibrillation in a population-based cohort: the Framingham Heart Study. JAMA 1994;271:840–4.

43. Savelieva I, Kakouros N, Kourliouros A, et al. Upstream therapies for management of atrial fibrillation. Part I: primary prevention. Europace 2011; 13:308–28.

44. Tsang TS, Gersh BJ, Appleton CP, et al. Left ventricular diastolic dysfunction as a predictor of the first diagnosed nonvalvular atrial fibrillation in 840 elderly men and women. J Am Coll Cardiol 2002; 40:1636–44.

45. Schnabel RB, Sullivan LM, Levy D, et al. Development of a risk score for atrial fibrillation (Framingham Heart Study): a community-based cohort study. Lancet 2009;373:739–45.

46. De Vos CB, Pisters R, Nieuwlaat R, et al. Progression from paroxysmal to persistent atrial fibrillation clinical correlates and prognosis. J Am Coll Cardiol 2010;55:725–31.

47. Wang TJ, Larson MG, Levy D, et al. Temporal relations of atrial fibrillation and congestive heart failure and their joint influence on mortality: the Framingham Heart Study. Circulation 2003;107(23):2920–5.

48. Shelton RJ, Clark AL, Goode K, et al. A randomised, controlled study of rate versus rhythm control in patients with chronic atrial fibrillation and heart failure: (CAFE-II Study). Heart 2009; 95:924–30.

49. Guglin M, Chen R, Curtis AB. Sinus rhythm is associated with fewer heart failure symptoms: insights from the AFFIRM trial. Heart Rhythm 2010; 7:596–601.

50. Savelieva I, Camm AJ. Atrial fibrillation and heart failure: natural history and pharmacological treatment. Europace 2004;5:S5–19.

51. Maggioni AP, Latini R, Carson PE, et al. Valsartan reduces the incidence of atrial fibrillation in patients with heart failure: results from the Valsartan Heart Failure Trial (Val-HeFT). Am Heart J 2005;149: 548–57.

52. Ducharme A, Swedberg K, Pfeffer MA, et al. Prevention of atrial fibrillation in patients with symptomatic chronic heart failure by candesartan in the Candesartan in Heart failure: Assessment of

Reduction in Mortality and Morbidity (CHARM) program. Am Heart J 2006;152:86–92.

53. Massie BM, Carson PE, McMurray JJ, et al. Irbesartan in patients with heart failure and preserved ejection fraction. N Engl J Med 2008;359:2456–67.

54. Anand K, Mooss AN, Hee TT, et al. Meta-analysis: inhibition of renin–angiotensin system prevents new-onset atrial fibrillation. Am Heart J 2006;152:217–22.

55. Jibrini MB, Molnar J, Arora RR. Prevention of atrial fibrillation by way of abrogation of the renin–angiotensin system: a systematic review and meta-analysis. Am J Ther 2008;15:36–43.

56. Schneider MP, Hua TA, Boehm M, et al. Prevention of atrial fibrillation by renin–angiotensin system inhibition a meta-analysis. J Am Coll Cardiol 2010; 55:2299–307.

57. Hanna IR, Heeke B, Bush H, et al. Lipid-lowering drug use is associated with reduced prevalence of atrial fibrillation in patients with left ventricular systolic dysfunction. Heart Rhythm 2006;3:881–6.

58. Dickinson MG, Hellkamp AS, Ip JH, et al. Statin therapy was associated with reduced atrial fibrillation and flutter in heart failure patients in SCD-HEFT [abstract]. Heart Rhythm 2006;3:S49.

59. Maggioni AP, Fabbri G, Lucci D, et al. Effects of rosuvastatin on atrial fibrillation occurrence: ancillary results of the GISSI-HF trial. Eur Heart J 2009;19: 2327–36.

60. Fauchier L, Pierre B, de Labriolle A, et al. Antiarrhythmic effect of statin therapy and atrial fibrillation a meta-analysis of randomized controlled trials. J Am Coll Cardiol 2008;51:828–35.

61. Liu T, Li G, Korantzopoulos P, et al. Statin use and development of atrial fibrillation: a systematic review and meta-analysis of randomized clinical trials and observational studies. Int J Cardiol 2008;126: 160–70.

62. Rahimi K, Emberson J, Mcgale P, et al. Effect of statins on atrial fibrillation: a collaborative meta-analysis of randomised controlled trials. Eur Heart J 2009 [abstract 2782].

63. Savelieva I, Camm J. Statins and polyunsaturated fatty acids for treatment of atrial fibrillation. Nat Clin Pract Cardiovasc Med 2008;5:30–41.

64. Wachtell K, Lehto M, Gerdts E, et al. Angiotensin II receptor blockade reduces new-onset atrial fibrillation and subsequent stroke compared to atenolol: the Losartan Intervention For End Point Reduction in Hypertension (LIFE) study. J Am Coll Cardiol 2005;45(5):712–9.

65. Ueng KC, Tsai TP, Yu WC, et al. Use of enalapril to facilitate sinus rhythm maintenance after external cardioversion of long-standing persistent atrial fibrillation. Results of a prospective and controlled study. Eur Heart J 2003;24(23):2090–8.

66. Heckbert SR, Wiggins KL, Glazer NL, et al. Antihypertensive treatment with ACE inhibitors or beta-blockers and risk of incident atrial fibrillation in a general hypertensive population. Am J Hypertens 2009;22(5):538–44.

67. Dagres N, Karatasakis G, Panou F, et al. Pre-treatment with Irbesartan attenuates left atrial stunning after electrical cardioversion of atrial fibrillation. Eur Heart J 2006;27(17):2062–8.

68. Verdecchia P, Reboldi G, Gattobigio R, et al. Atrial fibrillation in hypertension: predictors and outcome. Hypertension 2003;41(2):218–23.

69. Hammwöhner M, Smid J, Lendeckel U, et al. New drugs for atrial fibrillation. J Interv Card Electrophysiol 2008;35:55–62.

70. Goette A, Schön N, Kirchhof P, et al. Angiotensin II-antagonist in paroxysmal atrial fibrillation (ANTI-PAF) trial. Circ Arrhythm Electrophysiol 2012;5(1): 43–51.

Stroke Prevention in Atrial Fibrillation in Heart Failure

Eduard Shantsila, PhD, Gregory Y.H. Lip, MD*

KEYWORDS

- Heart failure • Atrial fibrillation • Anticoagulation • Stroke • Prevention

KEY POINTS

- Patients with atrial fibrillation associated with heart failure have a high risk of stroke.
- Oral anticoagulation with vitamin K antagonists or novel licensed medicines should be considered in all such patients unless contraindicated.
- A risk of anticoagulation-related bleeding should be assessed and regularly reviewed.
- Possible benefits of sinus rhythm maintenance for stroke prevention in heart failure are not entirely clear and may need to be explored further as new treatment options emerge.
- Relatively scarce data are available on stroke prevention in atrial fibrillation in heart failure with preserved ejection fraction, which requires further research.

INTRODUCTION

Heart failure (HF) and atrial fibrillation (AF) represent two major problems of modern cardiology with important clinical, prognostic, and socioeconomic implications. Each of these clinical entities poses high morbidity, impaired quality of life, and poor outcome, including increased risk of stroke. Of importance, these two conditions share several common pathophysiological mechanisms and risk factors (ie, hypertension, cardiac ischemia), which potentiate the associated health risks.

AF and HF often coexist. The prevalence of AF in patients with HF ranges from 13% to 40%, showing comparable rates in systolic HF and HF with preserved ejection fraction (HFpEF).[1–3] The recent EuroHeart Failure Survey II (EHFS II) confirmed the role of AF as one of the most common underlying conditions among patients admitted with acute HF.[4] Among patients with HF, those with AF have worse functional class, quality of life, and lower exercise tolerance.[5]

These conditions contribute to the pathogenesis of each other. AF promotes HF development and progression, primarily via triggering tachycardia-induced cardiomyopathy, loss of effective atrial systole, irregularity of ventricular contractions, and impairment of cardiac filling. In a large population of 360,000 subjects, AF was independently associated with a doubled risk of HF development.[6] Atrial systole can contribute up to 25% of the cardiac output, and as much as 50% in patients with preexisting valvular disease or ventricular dysfunction.[7,8]

In addition, a drastic shift in cardiac hemodynamics in HF provides a background for AF development. HF can increase the risk for the development of AF in several ways, including elevation of cardiac filling pressures with mechanical stretching of the atria, dysregulation of intracellular calcium, and neurohormonal changes, linked to atrial remodeling and fibrosis.[9,10] In the Framingham Study, HF was the strongest predictor for AF onset, with an increased risk of almost

Disclosures: The authors have nothing to disclose.
University of Birmingham Centre for Cardiovascular Sciences, City Hospital, Birmingham B18 7QH, UK
* Corresponding author.
E-mail address: g.y.h.lip@bham.ac.uk

Heart Failure Clin 9 (2013) 427–435
http://dx.doi.org/10.1016/j.hfc.2013.07.008
1551-7136/13/$ – see front matter © 2013 Elsevier Inc. All rights reserved.

fivefold in men and sixfold in women.[11] A third of HF patients free of AF developed the arrhythmia within the following 4 years.[12] Of note, the prevalence of AF in patients with HF increased in parallel with the severity of the disease, ranging from 4% in patients with mild HF to 50% in the most severe forms of HF.[13] In those with AF, the presence of HF predicts progression to more persistent patterns of AF.[14]

In the Candesartan in Heart Failure-Assessment of Reduction in Mortality and morbidity (CHARM) program, which covered 7599 patients with symptomatic HF with a 3-year follow-up, AF predicted a high risk of cardiovascular morbidity and mortality and all-cause mortality regardless of baseline cardiac contractility.[2] In an even larger population of almost 100,000 patients admitted with HF and enrolled in Get With The Guidelines-Heart Failure program, AF was independently associated with adverse outcomes.[15] Indeed, a meta-analysis of clinical trials of patients with AF confirmed a significantly higher risk of death with AF compared with subjects in sinus rhythm.[16]

Importantly, HF is a major risk factor of stroke in patients with AF. Its presence almost doubles the risk of ischemic stroke and systemic embolism.[17] Independent risk factors for stroke in AF include recent cardiac failure or moderately-to-severely impaired left ventricular ejection fraction (LVEF).[17] As an example, Pozzoli and colleagues[18] prospectively followed patients with mild HF in sinus rhythm and confirmed that the onset of AF was linked with a significant predisposition to systemic thromboembolism, as well as an increased incidence of clinical and hemodynamic complications and a poorer outlook. Of note, accumulating data point toward prognostic relevance of both systolic HF and HFpEF as risk factors for future strokes. In a recent, relatively small study, rates of ischemic stroke over 3-year follow-up were about threefold higher in patients with AF with HFpEF than in those with AF without HF (hazard ratio 3.29; 95% CI 1.58–6.86; $P = .001$).[19]

THE PROTHROMBOTIC STATE IN AF AND HF

Both AF and HF predispose to thrombogenesis. The association between AF and the risk of stroke has been recognized for decades and recently similar links have been established for HF. Both conditions present components of Virchow's triad for thrombus formation (ie, abnormal blood stasis, endothelial or endocardial damage, or dysfunction), and abnormal hemostasis.

The left atrial appendage is a small but long sack located on the lateral aspect of the left atrium. Having a relatively narrow inlet, this structure clearly predisposes to blood stasis and represents the usual site of intra atrial thrombus generation, particularly in patients with AF.[20,21] Additionally, AF is often associated with an increased left atrial size, further predisposing to stasis and cardiac thrombus formation.[22] The implication of left atrial enlargement in thrombogenesis is supported by evidence of a significant and independent association between the left atrial size, adjusted for body surface area and risk of stroke.[23,24]

It is important to emphasize that the pathogenesis of thrombogenesis in AF is multifactorial and is not solely related to blood stasis in a poorly contractile left atrium and left atrial appendage.[25] Endothelial and endocardial damage and/or dysfunction are also well documented in both AF and HF.[26,27] Small areas of endothelial denudation and thrombotic aggregation have been noted in patients with AF and cerebral embolism. The diverse and complex pattern of endothelial dysfunction in HF has been extensively documented and discussed in detail elsewhere.[28] Also, AF and HF can be considered as conditions characterized by systemic and local cardiac inflammation.[25,29] The final component of Virchow's triad in AF and HF is the presence of abnormal hemostasis and coagulation (eg, elevated levels of fibrin turnover products).[25,27,30,31]

ANTICOAGULATION IN AF WITH HF

Given the high prevalence of AF in patients with HF and its implications for the management of HF, patients' peripheral pulses should be checked during each visit. If AF is suspected, the diagnosis of AF needs to be documented by an ECG. Pharmacologic thromboembolism prophylaxis is of paramount importance for stroke prevention in AF with HF.

According to current guidelines, risk assessment for stroke in such patients should be based on the CHA$_2$DS$_2$-VASc score (**Table 1**).[32,33] It is crucial to appreciate that chronic oral anticoagulation is preferable in most AF patients with systolic HF (score $\geq$1) because most have a firm indication for the treatment (ie, score $\geq$2). In parallel to HF as an important risk factor of stroke in AF, such patients often have other comorbidities, such as coronary artery disease, hypertension, valvular heart disease, renal dysfunction, and diabetes, which further increase the risk of AF-related stroke.[34,35] In fact, both European and American guidelines on the management of HF advocate routine use of oral anticoagulation in all patients with HF and a history of AF.[32,36]

In addition to universal contraindications to oral anticoagulants, such therapy in subjects with HF

Table 1
The CHA₂DS₂-VASc stroke risk score

Letter	Risk Factor	Points
C	Congestive HF or left ventricular dysfunction	1
H	Hypertension	1
A	Age >75 y	2
D	Diabetes mellitus	1
S	Stroke, transient ischemic attack, or thromboembolism	2
V	Vascular disease	1
A	Age 65–74 y	1
S	Sex category (ie, female sex)	1

Maximum 9 points.

Adapted from Lip GY, Frison L, Halperin JL, et al. Identifying patients at high risk for stroke despite anticoagulation: a comparison of contemporary stroke risk stratification schemes in an anticoagulated atrial fibrillation cohort. Stroke 2010;41:2731–8; with permission.

may be restricted by a high bleeding risk. Consequently, every patient with AF and HF considered for anticoagulation should have a formal bleeding risk estimation based on the validated HAS-BLED score (**Table 2**).[32,37,38] Careful considerations of the initiation and regular review of anticoagulant therapy should be ensured in patients with HF with a HAS-BLED score greater than or equal to 3 and modifiable risk factors of bleeding have to be addressed.

All patients receiving oral anticoagulation with vitamin K antagonists (VKAs) should have regular monitoring of the degree of anticoagulation based on international normalized ratio (INR), which is the ratio of the actual prothrombin time and of a standardized control serum. The suggested optimal range of INR in nonvalvular AF is 2.0 to 3.0 to allow optimal balance of effective stroke prevention and small risk of bleeding.[39,40]

The early period following initiation of anticoagulation with VKA bears considerable risk for both over- and under-coagulation despite following established protocols of initiation of VKA.[41] Given the complicated pharmacologic features of warfarin and other VKAs, all patients should be given advice on the importance of INR monitoring due to high interindividual and intraindividual variations in response to medications. The patients must also be advised on lifestyle, food, alcohol consumption, and relevant drug interactions. The need to seek immediate medical help in cases of bleeding should be emphasized.

Of note, at present there is little role for aspirin in stroke prevention in patients with AF and HF. In the minority of patients not suitable for oral

Table 2
The HAS-BLED bleeding risk score

Letter	Clinical Characteristic	Points	Definition
H	Hypertension	1	Systolic blood pressure >160 mm Hg
A	Abnormal renal	1	Presence of chronic dialysis or renal transplantation or serum creatinine ≥200 mmol/L
	Abnormal liver function	1	Chronic hepatic disease (eg, cirrhosis) or biochemical evidence of significant hepatic derangement (eg, bilirubin .2 × upper limit of normal, in association with aspartate aminotransferase-alanine aminotransferase-alkaline phosphatase .3 × upper limit normal)
S	Stroke	1	History of stroke
B	Bleeding	1	Previous bleeding history and/or predisposition to bleeding (eg, bleeding diathesis, anemia)
L	Labile INRs	1	Unstable or high INRs or poor time in therapeutic range (eg, 60%).
E	Elderly	1	Age >65 y, frail condition
D	Drugs or alcohol (1 point each)	1 or 2	Concomitant use of drugs (eg, antiplatelet agents, nonsteroidal antiinflammatory drugs, or alcohol abuse)

Maximum 9 points.

Abbreviation: INRs, international normalized ratios.

Adapted from Pisters R, Lane DA, Nieuwlaat R, et al. A novel user-friendly score (HAS-BLED) to assess 1-year risk of major bleeding in patients with atrial fibrillation: the euro heart survey. Chest 2010;138:1093–1100; with permission.

anticoagulation due to contraindications or high risk of bleeding. Aspirin is unlikely to provide adequate stroke prevention and bears a risk of bleeding comparable to warfarin. The efficacy and clinical place of interventional percutaneous left atrial appendage closure is insufficiently established in AF patients with HF.

Of note, although discontinuation of oral anticoagulation may be required in patients undergoing surgery it can usually be continued at modified doses in most patients undergoing cardiac catheterization, especially if the radial approach is used. Catheter ablation for AF and the implantation of cardiac electronic devices are now widely performed on uninterrupted warfarin with an INR within the therapeutic range.

ORAL ANTICOAGULANTS FOR USE IN AF WITH HF

Oral anticoagulation is effective through inhibition of different coagulation factors. VKAs such as warfarin have been used for more than 50 years, providing effective stroke prevention in AF. The pharmacologic effects of VKAs are based on their ability to downregulate the levels of factors II (prothrombin), VII, IX, and X by interrupting carboxylation of these vitamin K-dependent factors.[42] Vitamin K availability depends on normal activity of the enzyme vitamin K epoxide reductase. Its inhibition by warfarin results in vitamin K depletion and production of functionally inactive factors, thus disrupting coagulation cascades mediated by these factors. However, the usefulness of VKAs is complicated by the need for cumbersome monitoring and numerous food and drug interactions leading to substantial variability in their oral absorption and bioavailability. Warfarin is mainly bound to albumin in the plasma and is metabolized by the liver. It has a relatively long half-life of around 40 hours, which means it often takes several days to reach the therapeutic level. Foods that contain a high level of vitamin K, such as broccoli, reduce the effect of warfarin. Excessive use of alcohol interferes with function of liver enzymes and affects the metabolism of VKAs.[43]

Novel oral anticoagulants have recently focused on selective inhibitors of coagulation factor. Inhibition of the two key factors of the coagulation cascade, factor Xa and factor IIa (thrombin), blocks both extrinsic and intrinsic coagulation cascades (**Table 3**). These two factors are considered the most promising targets for novel anticoagulants.

To ensure effective anticoagulation, it is desirable to block activity of both free and fibrin-bound thrombin. This can be achieved using direct thrombin inhibitors that provide potent inhibition of both forms of thrombin and prevent generation of fibrin from fibrinogen. Dabigatran etexilate, a second-generation, reversible, direct thrombin inhibitor, has been recently licensed for thromboembolism prevention in AF.[44] Dabigatran etexilate possesses the desirable qualities of effective anticoagulant with predictable pharmacokinetics and pharmacodynamics. The drug is rapidly absorbed with therapeutic concentrations achieved within 2 hours, with estimated half-lives of 14 to 17 hours when administered regularly. The drug shows an average bioavailability of 6.5%, thus it requires high doses to maintain therapeutic plasma levels. Simultaneous administration of proton pump inhibitors reduced the absorption of the drug by 20% to 25%.[44] About 80% of dabigatran etexilate is eliminated by the kidneys without biotransformation; therefore, its use is restricted in patients with severe renal dysfunction. These novel oral anticoagulants are usually well tolerated by patients AF with bleeding complications being the most serious reported side-effect.

Direct factor Xa inhibitors, rivaroxaban, and apixaban reversibly inhibit free plasma factor Xa and block factor Xa bound to platelets as part of

Table 3			
Mode of action and characteristics of new oral anticoagulants			
	Dabigatran	**Rivaroxaban**	**Apixaban**
Mode of action	Direct thrombin inhibitor	Direct factor Xa inhibitor	Direct factor Xa inhibitor
Prodrug	Yes	No	No
Dosing	Twice daily	Once daily	Twice daily
Time to peak drug level	2 h	3 h	3 h
Bioavailability	6.5%	60%–80%	>50%
Half-life	14–17 h	9 h	9–14 h
Elimination	80% renal	65% renal, 35% liver	25% renal, 75% fecal
Interaction	Proton pump inhibitors	Potent CYP3A4 inhibitors	Potent CYP3A4 inhibitors

the prothrombinase complex.[45] Both rivaroxaban and apixaban are selective oral direct factor Xa inhibitors with favorable pharmacokinetic profile. Rivaroxaban has a bioavailability of 60% to 80% and its peak plasma levels are reached within 3 hours after administration. The medication has a half-life of 9 hours in young subjects, but it can be longer (about 12 hours) in the older age typical of patients with AF and HF; therefore, it has a potential for one-daily administration. Rivaroxaban is metabolized by the liver via CYP3A4 with about 65% of the metabolite cleared out by the kidneys and the rest eliminated by the liver.[46] Apixaban is a potent and highly selective inhibitor of factor Xa with bioavailability of more than 50% and a half-life of 9 to 14 hours. The drug is metabolized in the liver via CYP3A4 and predominantly excreted by the intestines with about 25% eliminated by the kidneys.[45]

All three novel anticoagulants do not need monitoring of parameters of coagulation but require monitoring of renal function, especially given that there are no established protocols to reverse their anticoagulant action.

The use of dabigatran, rivaroxban, or apixaban for thromboembolism prevention in AF has been tested in large, multicenter, randomized clinical trials. Three key clinical trials, RE-LY (the Randomized Evaluation of Long-Term Anticoagulation Therapy), ROCKET-AF (the Rivaroxaban Once Daily Oral Direct Factor Xa Inhibition Compared with Vitamin K Antagonism for Prevention of Stroke and Embolism Trial in Atrial Fibrillation), and

ARISTOTLE (Apixaban for reduction in stroke and other ThromboemboLic events in atrial fibrillation), confirmed the efficacy and good safety profiles of the new drugs, which were at least noninferior to VKAs in thromboprophylaxis and had lower risk of intracranial hemorrhage than warfarin (**Table 4**).[47–49] Moreover, compared with VKAs, twice-daily apixaban and dabigatran 150 mg significantly reduced risk of stroke.[47,49] In addition, treatment with apixaban was associated with lower mortality compared with warfarin.[49] Finally, lower rates of major bleedings were seen in patients receiving dabigatran 110 mg twice daily or apixaban.[47,49] Although these trial were not specifically devoted to patients with HF, such subjects represented a sizable proportion of the participants and subgroup analyses of these three trials have not found any significant detrimental effect of coexisting HF on the treatment effects.[47–49]

The 2012 focused update of the European Society of Cardiology guidelines on the management of AF highlights dabigatran, apixaban, and rivaroxaban as first-line choices of oral anticoagulation.[38] However, their cost is high and this needs to be weighed against the benefits, such as clinical safety, efficacy, and convenience of use. One special consideration relates to patients with renal dysfunction, which is common in HF. The currently approved new oral anticoagulant drugs are contraindicated in severe renal impairment (ie, creatinine clearance <30 mL/min) and lowering of the dose was required in RE-LY, ROCKET-AF, and ARISTOTLE trials in subjects

Table 4
Major clinical trial on new oral anticoagulants in AF

	RE-LY	ROCKET-AF	ARISTOTLE
Active medication	Dabigatran	Rivaroxaban	Apixaban
Participant number	18,113	14,264	18,201
Age	72 ± 9 y	73 (65–78) y	70 (63–76) y
Follow-up duration	2.1 y	3.5 y	2.1 y
Mean CHADS$_2$ score	2.1 ± 1.1	3.5 ± 0.9	2.1 ± 1.1
Paroxysmal AF	32.8%	17.6%	15.3%
Subjects with HF	5793 (32%)	8908 (63%)	6451 (35%)
HF criteria	LVEF <40%, NYHA class ≥II HF symptoms within 6 mo before screening	Symptomatic HF or LVEF ≤35%	Symptomatic HF within the previous 3 mo or LVEF ≤40%
Stroke or systemic thromboembolism	1.5% for 110 mg dose 1.1% for 150 mg dose	2.1%	1.3%
Major bleeding	2.7% for 110 mg dose 3.1% for 150 mg dose	3.6%	1.8%
Interaction with HF	No ($P = .42$ or $P = .33$)	No	No ($P = .50$)

Data from Refs.[47–49]

with moderate kidney dysfunction (creatinine clearance 30–50 mL/min).[17,19]

RATE CONTROL VERSUS RHYTHM CONTROL: DOES IT MATTER FOR STROKE PREVENTION IN HF?

The main clinical trials, which directly compared rate control versus rhythm control strategy for stroke prevention in AF generally failed to prove superiority of one strategy over another. However, these trials provide limited specific evidence in relation to patients with HF. In the Atrial Fibrillation Follow-up Investigation of Rhythm Management (AFFIRM) study,[50,51] only 26% of subjects had evidence of reduced LVEF, and 23% of participants had a history of congestive HF, but only 9% of the subjects had symptoms compatible with New York Heart Association (NYHA) functional class of II or greater. Overall LVEF in the AFFIRM study was relatively good (ie, 55 ± 14%). Of interest, the rhythm control approach was associated with a higher risk of death than the rate control approach only in subjects without congestive HF, with no difference seen in those having HF.

Subjects with HF were better represented in the RAte Control versus Electrical cardioversion for Persistent Atrial Fibrillation (RACE)[52,53] trial with about half of the 512 participants having a history of symptomatic HF and with average left ventricular fractional shortening of 30%. After a mean 2.3-year follow-up, the composite primary end point of death from cardiovascular causes, HF, thromboembolic complications, bleeding, implantation of a pacemaker, and severe adverse effects of drugs developed in 17.2% of those randomized for the rate control strategy and 22.6% of those aiming to maintain sinus rhythm. Although there was a numerical trend toward lower HF rates in the rate control group (3.5% vs 4.5% in the rhythm control group), the difference was not statistically significant, perhaps due to the relatively small study population. Unfortunately, the published data do not provide specific information on how the observed trends could affect risk of stroke in subjects with HF.

According to the results of the How to Treat Chronic Atrial Fibrillation (HOT CAFE) trial,[54] all participants had a certain degree of congestive HF at baseline, although almost half of the subjects had only mild HF symptoms equivalent to NYHA class I. NYHA class 2 to 3 was present in 53% of those randomized to the rate control approach versus 71% of those subjected to the rhythm control strategy, with overall average left ventricular fractional shortening of 31%. In the rhythm control arm only, a significant improvement in exercise tolerance was noticed with a rise in maximal workload (P<.001). In addition, rhythm control was linked favorably with left and right atrial remodeling and improvement in left ventricular contractility. However, this did not translate into any significant benefits for stroke or death prevention.

A comparison of the two strategies of AF management in HF was performed in the randomized Atrial Fibrillation and Congestive Heart Failure (AF-CHF) trial[55] of 1376 patients with LVEF <35% (mean LVEF 27 ± 6%) followed for an average for 3 years. Amiodarone was the predominant pharmacologic agent used to achieve rhythm control. There was no difference in mortality or HF-related hospitalizations between the groups. In addition, there was no difference in stroke rates (P = .68), but the number of such events was low: 9 (1%) in rhythm control group and 11 (2%) in the rate control group.

It is important to acknowledge that all of these studies have certain limitations requiring cautious interpretation of their results. For example, potential benefits of maintenance of sinus rhythm could have been masked by side effects of currently available treatments. In addition, a sizable proportion of subjects assigned for rhythm control failed to preserve sinus rhythm during the study period.[56] Finally, conditions of strict rate control under the clinical trial environment may not be entirely applicable in real-life settings. Indeed, according to a large population-based observational study of over 40,000 subjects with AF (30% of whom had HF, stroke, or TIA), incidence rate was lower in patients treated with rhythm control than in those on rate control therapy.[57] This was particularly true in patients with moderate-to-high-risk of stroke and the association remained significant in multivariate analysis. In addition, in a substudy from the Danish Investigations of Arrhythmia and Mortality on Dofetilide (DIAMOND) trials, in subjects with AF or atrial flutter and severe systolic left ventricular dysfunction, restoration of sinus rhythm was associated with a significant reduction in mortality.[58] Accordingly, available data on clinical potential of sinus rhythm preservation in patients with AF and HF for stroke prevention are inconclusive and merit further investigation.

SUMMARY

Patients with AF associated with HF have a high risk of stroke. Oral anticoagulation with VKAs or novel licensed medicines should be considered in all such patients unless contraindicated. A risk of anticoagulation-related bleeding should be assessed and regularly reviewed. Possible benefits of sinus rhythm maintenance for stroke prevention in HF are not entirely clear and may need to be explored further as new treatment options emerge. Relatively scarce data are available in relation to HFpEF with further research needed on this clinically and socially important problem.

REFERENCES

1. Linssen GC, Rienstra M, Jaarsma T, et al. Clinical and prognostic effects of atrial fibrillation in heart failure patients with reduced and preserved left ventricular ejection fraction. Eur J Heart Fail 2011; 13:1111–20.

2. Olsson LG, Swedberg K, Ducharme A, et al. Atrial fibrillation and risk of clinical events in chronic heart failure with and without left ventricular systolic dysfunction: results from the Candesartan in Heart Failure-Assessment of Reduction in Mortality and morbidity (CHARM) program. J Am Coll Cardiol 2006;47:1997–2004.

3. Carson PE, Johnson GR, Dunkman WB, et al. The influence of atrial fibrillation on prognosis in mild to moderate heart failure. The V-HeFT Studies. The V-HeFT VA Cooperative Studies Group. Circulation 1993;87:VI102–10.

4. Nieminen MS, Brutsaert D, Dickstein K, et al. Euro-Heart Failure Survey II (EHFS II): a survey on hospitalized acute heart failure patients: description of population. Eur Heart J 2006;27:2725–36.

5. Fung JW, Sanderson JE, Yip GW, et al. Impact of atrial fibrillation in heart failure with normal ejection fraction: a clinical and echocardiographic study. J Card Fail 2007;13:649–55.

6. Goyal A, Norton CR, Thomas TN, et al. Predictors of incident heart failure in a large insured population: a one million person-year follow-up study. Circ Heart Fail 2010;3:698–705.

7. Leonard JJ, Shaver J, Thompson M. Left atrial transport function. Trans Am Clin Climatol Assoc 1981;92:133–41.

8. Rahimtoola SH, Ehsani A, Sinno MZ, et al. Left atrial transport function in myocardial infarction. Importance of its booster pump function. Am J Med 1975;59:686–94.

9. Cha YM, Dzeja PP, Shen WK, et al. Failing atrial myocardium: energetic deficits accompany structural remodeling and electrical instability. Am J Physiol Heart Circ Physiol 2003;284:H1313–20.

10. Li D, Shinagawa K, Pang L, et al. Effects of angiotensin-converting enzyme inhibition on the development of the atrial fibrillation substrate in dogs with ventricular tachypacing-induced congestive heart failure. Circulation 2001;104:2608–14.

11. Benjamin EJ, Levy D, Vaziri SM, et al. Independent risk factors for atrial fibrillation in a population-based cohort. The Framingham Heart Study. JAMA 1994;271:840–4.

12. Chamberlain AM, Redfield MM, Alonso A, et al. Atrial fibrillation and mortality in heart failure: a community study. Circ Heart Fail 2011;4:740–6.

13. Maisel WH, Stevenson LW. Atrial fibrillation in heart failure: epidemiology, pathophysiology, and rationale for therapy. Am J Cardiol 2003;91:2D–8D.

14. Camm AJ, Breithardt G, Crijns H, et al. Real-life observations of clinical outcomes with rhythm- and rate-control therapies for atrial fibrillation RECORDAF (Registry on Cardiac Rhythm Disorders Assessing the Control of Atrial Fibrillation). J Am Coll Cardiol 2011;58:493–501.

15. Mountantonakis SE, Grau-Sepulveda MV, Bhatt DL, et al. Presence of atrial fibrillation is independently associated with adverse outcomes in patients hospitalized with heart failure: an analysis of get with the guidelines-heart failure. Circ Heart Fail 2012; 5:191–201.

16. Wasywich CA, Pope AJ, Somaratne J, et al. Atrial fibrillation and the risk of death in patients with heart failure: a literature-based meta-analysis. Intern Med J 2010;40:347–56.

17. Risk factors for stroke and efficacy of antithrombotic therapy in atrial fibrillation. Analysis of pooled data from five randomized controlled trials. Arch Intern Med 1994;154:1449–57.

18. Pozzoli M, Cioffi G, Traversi E, et al. Predictors of primary atrial fibrillation and concomitant clinical and hemodynamic changes in patients with chronic heart failure: a prospective study in 344 patients with baseline sinus rhythm. J Am Coll Cardiol 1998;32:197–204.

19. Jang SJ, Kim MS, Park HJ, et al. Impact of heart failure with normal ejection fraction on the occurrence of ischaemic stroke in patients with atrial fibrillation. Heart 2013;99(1):17–21.

20. Blackshear JL, Odell JA. Appendage obliteration to reduce stroke in cardiac surgical patients with atrial fibrillation. Ann Thorac Surg 1996;61:755–9.

21. Pollick C, Taylor D. Assessment of left atrial appendage function by transesophageal echocardiography. Implications for the development of thrombus. Circulation 1991;84:223–31.

22. Sanfilippo AJ, Abascal VM, Sheehan M, et al. Atrial enlargement as a consequence of atrial fibrillation. A prospective echocardiographic study. Circulation 1990;82:792–7.

23. Predictors of thromboembolism in atrial fibrillation: II. Echocardiographic features of patients at risk. The Stroke Prevention in Atrial Fibrillation Investigators. Ann Intern Med 1992;116:6–12.

24. Di Tullio MR, Sacco RL, Sciacca RR, et al. Left atrial size and the risk of ischemic stroke in an ethnically mixed population. Stroke 1999;30:2019–24.

25. Watson T, Shantsila E, Lip GY. Mechanisms of thrombogenesis in atrial fibrillation: Virchow's triad revisited. Lancet 2009;373:155–66.

26. Masawa N, Yoshida Y, Yamada T, et al. Diagnosis of cardiac thrombosis in patients with atrial fibrillation in the absence of macroscopically visible thrombi. Virchows Arch A Pathol Anat Histopathol 1993;422:67–71.

27. Marin F, Roldan V, Climent VE, et al. Plasma von Willebrand factor, soluble thrombomodulin, and fibrin D-dimer concentrations in acute onset non-rheumatic atrial fibrillation. Heart 2004;90:1162–6.

28. Shantsila E, Wrigley BJ, Blann AD, et al. A contemporary view on endothelial function in heart failure. Eur J Heart Fail 2012;14:873–81.

29. Vaduganathan M, Greene SJ, Butler J, et al. The immunological axis in heart failure: importance of the leukocyte differential. Heart Fail Rev 2013; 99(1):17–21.

30. Watson T, Shantsila E, Lip GY. Fibrin d-dimer levels and thromboembolic events in patients with atrial fibrillation. Int J Cardiol 2007;120:123–4 [author reply 125–6].

31. Lip GY, Lowe GD, Rumley A, et al. Increased markers of thrombogenesis in chronic atrial fibrillation: effects of warfarin treatment. Br Heart J 1995; 73:527–33.

32. McMurray JJ, Adamopoulos S, Anker SD, et al. ESC guidelines for the diagnosis and treatment of acute and chronic heart failure 2012: the Task Force for the Diagnosis and Treatment of Acute and Chronic Heart Failure 2012 of the European Society of Cardiology. Developed in collaboration with the Heart Failure Association (HFA) of the ESC. Eur Heart J 2012;33:1787–847.

33. Lip GY, Nieuwlaat R, Pisters R, et al. Refining clinical risk stratification for predicting stroke and thromboembolism in atrial fibrillation using a novel risk factor-based approach: the euro heart survey on atrial fibrillation. Chest 2010;137:263–72.

34. Gheorghiade M, Pang PS. Acute heart failure syndromes. J Am Coll Cardiol 2009;53:557–73.

35. Gheorghiade M, Abraham WT, Albert NM, et al. Systolic blood pressure at admission, clinical characteristics, and outcomes in patients hospitalized with acute heart failure. JAMA 2006;296:2217–26.

36. Jessup M, Abraham WT, Casey DE, et al. 2009 focused update: ACCF/AHA Guidelines for the Diagnosis and Management of Heart Failure in Adults: a report of the American College of Cardiology Foundation/American Heart Association Task Force on Practice Guidelines: developed in collaboration with the International Society for Heart and Lung Transplantation. Circulation 2009;119: 1977–2016.

37. Pisters R, Lane DA, Nieuwlaat R, et al. A novel user-friendly score (HAS-BLED) to assess 1-year risk of major bleeding in patients with atrial fibrillation: the Euro Heart survey. Chest 2010;138:1093–100.

38. Camm AJ, Lip GY, De Caterina R, et al. 2012 focused update of the ESC Guidelines for the management of atrial fibrillation: an update of the 2010 ESC Guidelines for the management of atrial fibrillation. Developed with the special contribution of the European Heart Rhythm Association. Eur Heart J 2012;33:2719–47.

39. Camm AJ, Kirchhof P, Lip GY, et al. Guidelines for the management of atrial fibrillation: the Task Force for the Management of Atrial Fibrillation of the European Society of Cardiology (ESC). Eur Heart J 2010;31:2369–429.

40. You JJ, Singer DE, Howard PA, et al. Antithrombotic therapy for atrial fibrillation: antithrombotic therapy and prevention of thrombosis, 9th ed: American college of chest physicians evidence-based clinical practice guidelines. Chest 2012; 141:e531S–75S.

41. Roberts GW, Helboe T, Nielsen CB, et al. Assessment of an age-adjusted warfarin initiation protocol. Ann Pharmacother 2003;37:799–803.

42. Ansell J, Hirsh J, Poller L, et al. The pharmacology and management of the vitamin k antagonists: the Seventh ACCP Conference on Antithrombotic and Thrombolytic Therapy. Chest 2004;126:204S–33S.

43. Holbrook AM, Pereira JA, Labiris R, et al. Systematic overview of warfarin and its drug and food interactions. Arch Intern Med 2005;165: 1095–106.

44. Stangier J, Rathgen K, Stahle H, et al. The pharmacokinetics, pharmacodynamics and tolerability of dabigatran etexilate, a new oral direct thrombin inhibitor, in healthy male subjects. Br J Clin Pharmacol 2007;64:292–303.

45. Khoo CW, Tay KH, Shantsila E, et al. Novel oral anticoagulants. Int J Clin Pract 2009;63:630–41.

46. Kubitza D, Becka M, Voith B, et al. Safety, pharmacodynamics, and pharmacokinetics of single doses of bay 59-7939, an oral, direct factor xa inhibitor. Clin Pharmacol Ther 2005;78:412–21.

47. Connolly SJ, Ezekowitz MD, Yusuf S, et al. Dabigatran versus warfarin in patients with atrial fibrillation. N Engl J Med 2009;361:1139–51.

48. Granger CB, Alexander JH, McMurray JJ, et al. Apixaban versus warfarin in patients with atrial fibrillation. N Engl J Med 2011;365:981–92.

49. Patel MR, Mahaffey KW, Garg J, et al. Rivaroxaban versus warfarin in nonvalvular atrial fibrillation. N Engl J Med 2011;365:883–91.

50. Wyse DG, Waldo AL, DiMarco JP, et al. A comparison of rate control and rhythm control in patients with atrial fibrillation. N Engl J Med 2002;347:1825–33.

51. Corley SD, Epstein AE, DiMarco JP, et al. Relationships between sinus rhythm, treatment, and survival in the Atrial Fibrillation Follow-Up Investigation of

Rhythm Management (AFFIRM) Study. Circulation 2004;109:1509–13.

52. Van Gelder IC, Hagens VE, Bosker HA, et al. A comparison of rate control and rhythm control in patients with recurrent persistent atrial fibrillation. N Engl J Med 2002;347:1834–40.

53. Hagens VE, Crijns HJ, Van Veldhuisen DJ, et al. Rate control versus rhythm control for patients with persistent atrial fibrillation with mild to moderate heart failure: results from the RAte Control versus Electrical cardioversion (RACE) study. Am Heart J 2005;149:1106–11.

54. Opolski G, Torbicki A, Kosior DA, et al. Rate control vs rhythm control in patients with nonvalvular persistent atrial fibrillation: the results of the Polish How to Treat Chronic Atrial Fibrillation (HOT CAFE) Study. Chest 2004;126:476–86.

55. Roy D, Talajic M, Nattel S, et al. Rhythm control versus rate control for atrial fibrillation and heart failure. N Engl J Med 2008;358:2667–77.

56. Humphries KH, Kerr CR, Steinbuch M, et al. Limitations to antiarrhythmic drug use in patients with atrial fibrillation. CMAJ 2004;171:741–5.

57. Isadok MA, Jackevicius CA, Essebag V, et al. Rhythm versus rate control therapy and subsequent stroke or transient ischemic attack in patients with atrial fibrillation. Circulation 2012;126:2680–7.

58. Pedersen OD, Bagger H, Keller N, et al. Efficacy of dofetilide in the treatment of atrial fibrillation-flutter in patients with reduced left ventricular function: a Danish investigations of arrhythmia and mortality on dofetilide (diamond) substudy. Circulation 2001;104:292–6.

Impact of Atrial Fibrillation on Outcomes in Heart Failure

Eugene C. DePasquale, MD, Gregg C. Fonarow, MD*

KEYWORDS

- Atrial fibrillation • Heart failure treatment • Prognosis • Antiarrhythmic therapy
- Antithrombotic therapy • Catheter ablation

KEY POINTS

- The presence of atrial fibrillation (AF) is a marker of worse prognosis in patients with heart failure (HF), associated with increased morbidity and mortality.
- Management strategies are aimed at limiting symptoms through rate or rhythm control as well as anticoagulation to prevent systemic embolization and stroke, avoiding therapies that increase mortality in the population with HF.
- Current data suggest that pharmacologic rhythm control has no advantage over rate control.
- It remains unknown whether prompt restoration of sinus rhythm or aggressive rate control in patients hospitalized with new-onset AF is beneficial; further study is required.
- Improvements in invasive strategies to restore sinus rhythm have resulted in increased efficacy and safety; however, further data are warranted to determine their role in the treatment of AF in HF.
- New anticoagulants have emerged and present their unique advantages and challenges.
- Advances in pharmacotherapy, nonpharmacologic therapies, and treatment strategies have benefited patients with AF and heart failure.

Atrial fibrillation (AF) affects many patients with heart failure (HF). The prevalence of both AF and HF increases with advancing age, and the 2 conditions can precipitate one another. It is estimated that the annual incidence of AF in the general HF population is approximately 5%, whereas as many as 40% of patients with advanced HF have AF. Like the general population of patients with AF, the main goals of therapy in patients with HF and AF are symptom control and prevention of arterial thromboembolism. The adverse hemodynamic events of AF may quickly lead to symptom deterioration and reduced exercise capacity, providing significant management challenges.[1–3] This review addresses the impact of AF on HF outcomes as they pertain to prognosis and management.

EPIDEMIOLOGY

AF and HF are both major causes of cardiovascular morbidity and mortality. Decompensated HF may be precipitated by loss of atrial contraction and rapid irregular heart rates, whereas HF progression may lead to AF through increased left atrial stretch. The incidence of AF was examined in a Framingham Heart Study (n = 1470) in which 22% of 708 patients who developed HF without previous AF subsequently developed AF (incidence rate 5.4% per year).[4,5] A subsequent study

Disclosures: None (E.C. DePasquale). NHLBI, research, significant; AHRQ, research, significant; Novartis, consultant, significant; Medtronic, consultant, modest (G.C. Fonarow).
Ahmanson-UCLA Cardiomyopathy Center, Division of Cardiology, David Geffen School of Medicine, 100 UCLA Medical Plaza, Suite 630 East, Los Angeles, CA 90095, USA
* Corresponding author. Ahmanson-UCLA Cardiomyopathy Center, Ronald Reagan UCLA Medical Center, 10833 LeConte Avenue, Room 47-123 CHS, Los Angeles, CA 90095-1679.
E-mail address: gfonarow@mednet.ucla.edu

Heart Failure Clin 9 (2013) 437–449
http://dx.doi.org/10.1016/j.hfc.2013.07.009

from Framingham reported that the odds ratio (OR) for developing AF among patients with HF was 4.5 for men and 4.9 for women over a 2-year period[6,7] compared with patients without HF.

The prevalence of AF in the HF population increases with advancing age and has been reported from less than 10% up to 50%, with variations depending on New York Heart Association (NYHA) class and severity of HF.[8–13] A direct relationship between NYHA class and the occurrence of AF has been shown, with prevalence increasing from 4% to 40% with progression from NYHA I to NYHA IV.[14–22]

DOES AF INDEPENDENTLY PREDICT MORTALITY?

Data conflict as to whether AF is an independent predictor of mortality in patients with HF. Three-year follow-up of the SOLVD (Studies of Left Ventricular Dysfunction) trial (n = 6517), which consisted of patients with asymptomatic left ventricular dysfunction or NYHA class II to III HF, showed that AF (present in 6.4%) was a significant predictor of all-cause mortality (34 vs 23%) and was maintained after multivariate analysis.[14,23] In CHARM (Candesartan in Heart Failure Assessment of Reduction in Mortality and Morbidity), 7599 patients with symptomatic HF with either reduced or preserved ejection fraction were enrolled, of which baseline AF was present in approximately 18%. AF was shown to be an independent predictor of all-cause mortality in this population in both HF with reduced ejection

fraction (37 vs 28% in patients without AF) or preserved ejection fraction (34 vs 14%).[24,25]

However, the V-HeFT (Vasodilator Heart Failure Trial) trials of 1427 patients with NYHA class II to III, of whom 14% had AF, did not show a significant difference in 2-year mortality or hospitalization for HF.[9,26] Similarly, a study examining the prognostic effect of AF on HF in both a national population in New Zealand (n = 55,106) and a cohort of 197 patients recruited after HF admission into the Auckland Heart Failure Management Study reported that the presence of AF in these 2 populations was not associated with an adverse prognosis.[27,28]

However, more recent data from the Get With The Guidelines Heart Failure Registry suggest otherwise. In 99,810 patients with HF enrolled in the registry between 2005 and 2010, patients with AF on admission (31.4%) were compared with those in sinus rhythm. In this cohort, AF was found to be independently associated with adverse hospital outcomes (hospital mortality 4.0% vs 2.6%, $P<.001$) and increased length of stay (>4 days: 48.8% vs 41.5%, $P<.001$). Analysis also showed that hospital outcomes were worse in those with newly diagnosed AF (adjusted OR for mortality [95% confidence internal (CI)] 1.29 [1.10–1.52] vs 1.17 [1.05–1.29]) (**Fig. 1**).[26,29] It remains unknown whether the association between new-onset AF and mortality is causative or whether the development of AF is a marker of more advanced disease. Despite conflicting reports in the literature, more recent data show that AF is at minimum a marker of adverse

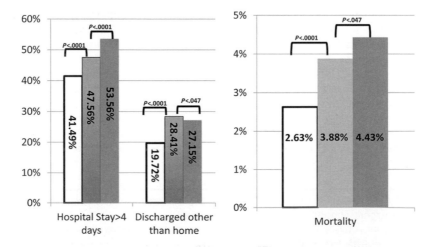

☐ Sinus Rhythm   ▨ Pre-Existing Atrial Fibrillation   ▪ New Onset Atrial Fibrillation

Fig. 1. Hospital outcomes stratified by AF groups. (*From* Mountantonakis SE, Grau-Sepulveda MV, Bhatt DL, et al. Presence of atrial fibrillation is independently associated with adverse outcomes in patients hospitalized with heart failure. Circ Heart Fail 2012;5(2):198; with permission.)

outcomes in this population, if not a mediator of adverse outcomes.

AF MANAGEMENT IN THE SETTING OF HF

AF can lead to worsening symptoms in patients with HF, and uncontrolled HF may precipitate or accelerate the ventricular response of AF or result in AF in those in sinus rhythm. It is critical that all reversible causes of both AF and HF be identified and corrected. Symptomatic patients with AF with rapid ventricular rates may require therapy to slow the ventricular response before any considerations of rate versus rhythm control strategies.

Rhythm Versus Rate Control

Rate and rhythm control strategies have been tested in various studies with the hypothesis that restoration and maintenance of sinus rhythm allow HF symptoms to be more easily controlled. The AF and Congestive Heart Failure (AF-CHF) trial was designed to determine whether long-term rhythm control is superior to rate control in patients with HF with reduced ejection fraction and AF. In this trial, 1376 patients with left ventricular dysfunction were randomized to a strategy of rhythm control (amiodarone, sotalol, or dofetilide) or rate control. No significant difference was observed between groups in the primary outcome of cardiovascular death or outcome of event-free survival (mean follow-up 37 months) (**Fig. 2**).[30-32] There was also no difference in quality of life with similar

6-minute walk distance assessments and NYHA class.[33-36] However, evidence from subsets of patients with HF in the AFFIRM (Atrial Fibrillation Follow-Up Investigation of Rhythm Management), RACE (Rate Control vs Electrical Cardioversion for Persistent Atrial Fibrillation Study) and DIAMOND (Danish Investigations of Arrhythmia and Mortality ON Dofetilide) trials have presented conflicting data on mortality, thromboembolic complications, and hospitalization in patients receiving rhythm control therapy.[24,25,36-41]

Rate Control

Rate control to prevent AF with rapid ventricular response may lead to improvement in symptoms in those with HF. Post hoc analysis of the US Carvedilol Heart Failure Trials (n = 1094) showed the potential benefit of rate control in 136 patients with HF with reduced left ventricular ejection fraction and AF, with resulting improved ejection fraction and a trend toward reduction in the combined end point of death and HF hospitalization.[11,42] It remains unknown if the improved outcomes observed are caused by rate control or the beneficial effect of the β-blocker in HF.

Initiation or increase of β-blockers in patients with decompensated HF is contraindicated.[33,43] In this setting, the use of digoxin for rate control may be beneficial. However, digoxin may be ineffective when used alone, particularly in patients with increased sympathetic tone.[44-46] Nondihydropyridine calcium channel blockers (ie, diltiazem, verapamil) should be used sparingly and

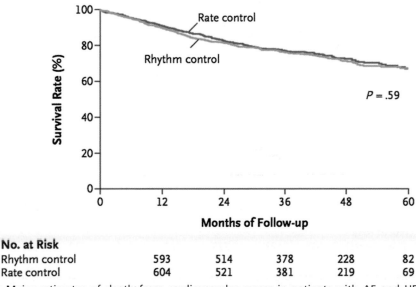

No. at Risk					
	0	12	24	36	48	60
Rhythm control		593	514	378	228	82
Rate control		604	521	381	219	69

Fig. 2. Kaplan-Meier estimates of death from cardiovascular causes in patients with AF and HF treated with rhythm or rate control strategies in the AF-CHF trial. (*From* Roy D, Talajic M, Nattel S, et al. Rhythm control versus rate control for atrial fibrillation and heart failure. N Engl J Med 2008;358(25):2667–77; with permission.)

with caution, because there is significant risk of worsening HF in those with reduced ejection fraction. However, nondihydropyridine calcium channel blockers may be a reasonable choice for rate control of AF in HF with preserved ejection fraction.[4,33,47] Amiodarone may be useful as an adjunct when the use of β-blocker or combination therapy with digoxin does not achieve rate control. Amiodarone is not recommended as a chronic rate control therapy, and therapeutic anticoagulation should be maintained, because there is a possibility of pharmacologically restoring sinus rhythm.[8,33]

The strictness of rate control was examined in RACE II (The Rate Control Efficacy in Permanent Atrial Fibrillation: a Comparison Between Lenient vs Strict Rate Control II trial). In this trial, 614 patients with permanent AF (of whom approximately 10% had history of hospitalization because of HF) were randomized to either a strict (resting heart rate <80 beats per minute [bpm] and heart rate during moderate exercise <110 bpm) or lenient (resting heart rate <110 bpm) rate control strategy. There was no difference in the composite primary outcome of death from cardiovascular causes, hospitalization for HF, and stroke, systemic embolism, bleeding, and life-threatening arrhythmic events (**Fig. 3**).[10,48–50] It is unclear how well this trial applies to the HF population, because there were few patients with HF or reduced ejection fraction in the study. Nevertheless, it may be reasonable to start with a lenient approach and convert to a strict approach in patients who remain symptomatic.

Other strategies for rate control may include a more invasive approach in those in whom pharmacologic rate control has been ineffective or contraindicated. Rate control may be accomplished with radiofrequency ablation of the atrioventricular node and permanent pacemaker placement.[4,51,52] In patients with HF with reduced ejection fraction in whom ventricular pacing may occur greater than 40% of the time, cardiac resynchronization therapy should be strongly considered, because isolated right ventricular pacing may worsen HF and increase frequency of AF, as shown in the DAVID (Dual Chamber and VVI Implantable Defibrillator) and MOST (Mode Selection Trial) trials.[51–54]

The SHIFT trial (Systolic Heart Failure Treatment with the I_f Inhibitor Ivabradine Trial) was a randomized double-blind placebo-controlled parallel group study for patients who were symptomatic with HF with reduced ejection fraction who were in sinus rhythm with heart rate 70 bpm or higher admitted within the previous year for HF on baseline β-blockade in which patients were randomized to ivabradine (n = 3241) or placebo (n = 3264). Although AF was an exclusion criterion for this trial, approximately 8% of patients in each group had history of AF or atrial flutter. The primary end point (composite of cardiovascular death or admission

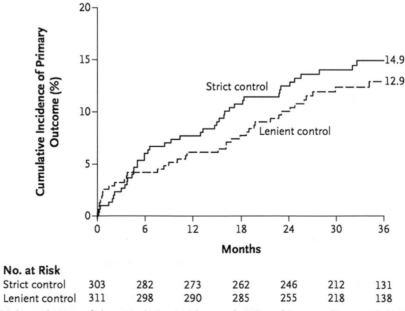

Fig. 3. Kaplan-Meier estimates of the cumulative incidence of major adverse cardiac events in patients with AF treated with either strict or lenient rate control strategies in the RACE II trial. (*From* Van Gelder IC, Groenveld HF, Crijns HJ, et al. Lenient versus strict rate control in patients with atrial fibrillation. N Engl J Med 2010;362(15):1371; with permission.)

for worsening HF) was lower in the ivabradine group (24% compared with 29% in the placebo group). This finding was driven by reduction in HF admissions (16% vs 21%, hazard ratio 0.74, 95% CI 0.66–0.83, P<.001) and deaths caused by HF (3% vs 5%, hazard ratio 0.74, 95% CI 0.58–0.94, P = .014).[55–57] This trial showed that heart rate reduction led to improvement in HF outcomes. These findings are interesting and raise new questions in light of studies showing no significant difference between strict and lenient rate control in RACE II.

Rhythm Control

Rhythm control may be reasonable in patients with HF with AF who are hemodynamically unstable or symptomatic despite rate control.[45] Rhythm control typically commences with direct current cardioversion, particularly in those with sudden-onset HF. Attempts at stabilization and rate control should be pursued before anticipated acute cardioversion. Some practitioners advocate cardioversion without adjunctive antiarrhythmic therapies for an initial episode of AF, and antiarrhythmic therapy in those with recurrent AF episodes. However, in patients with HF, antiarrhythmic agents are typically required to maintain sinus rhythm after cardioversion, especially if there is significant left atrial dilatation.

Rhythm control is usually undertaken with the premise that maintenance of sinus rhythm leads to improved outcomes (eg, reduced symptoms or HF admissions). However, as previously discussed, current evidence suggests no significant difference in mortality or event-free survival between rate or rhythm control approaches. Antiarrhythmic therapies to maintain sinus rhythm are not without risk or side effects and in some cases have raised concerns about increased mortality.[33,58] Current guidelines from the American College of Cardiology (ACC)/American Heart Association (AHA)/Heart Rhythm Society recommend amiodarone and dofetilide as first-line therapy to maintain sinus rhythm in patients with HF and AF.[33,59] However, the European Society of Cardiology (ESC) does not recommend dofetilide (which has limited availability in Europe, anyway) in AF.[60] In addition, dronedarone is not recommended for patients with NYHA class II HF with recent exacerbation and is contraindicated in patients with NYHA class III or IV HF.[60]

Pharmacotherapy

β-blockers
Most patients with HF and AF require a β-blocker to reduce the ventricular rate as well as part of guideline-directed medical therapy for HF with reduced ejection fraction. A meta-analysis of 8680 patients, representing 4 randomized trials, of β-blockade therapy in patients with HF evaluated outcomes in those with AF (n = 1677) and those without AF. No mortality benefit of β-blockers was observed in patients with HF and AF (OR 0.86, 95% CI 0.66–1.13), which may reflect the low event rate in the meta-analysis.[1] However, in general, β-blockade is recommended as guideline-directed medical therapy in HF with reduced ejection fraction.[4]

Amiodarone
Amiodarone at lower doses does not have a negative inotropic effect. In addition, there is a low incidence of QT prolongation and little proarrhythmia, as shown in a meta-analysis (n = 1465) in which 738 patients received low doses of amiodarone. Amiodarone also tends to slow ventricular rates in AF because of its β-blocking and calcium channel–blocking activity.[6] CHF-STAT (Congestive Heart Failure Trial of Antiarrhythmic Therapy) randomized 667 patients with HF with reduced ejection fraction, of whom 15% had AF at baseline, to amiodarone or placebo. This trial reported that amiodarone was able to prevent the development of new-onset AF (4.1% vs 8.3%) and significantly reduce ventricular rate in patients with persistent AF. In addition, amiodarone showed the ability to spontaneously convert AF to sinus rhythm (31% vs 8% in control individuals).[8] However, there are potential adverse events that may occur during the loading phase. In a series of 37 consecutive patients with HF with reduced ejection fraction initiated on amiodarone therapy for AF or atrial flutter,[14] 32% developed bradycardia and 19% required a permanent pacemaker. Amiodarone has many well-documented side effects, including but not limited to pulmonary toxicity, thyroid abnormalities (hypothyroidism and hyperthyroidism), dermatologic manifestations, and gastrointestinal side effects. Amiodarone may be initiated as an outpatient and has low risk of torsades de pointe.[14]

Dofetilide
Dofetilide is a class III antiarrhythmic drug that has been shown to be effective in preventing recurrent AF in patients with HF. In the DIAMOND studies, 506 patients with HF with reduced ejection fraction and baseline AF or atrial flutter were randomized to placebo or dofetilide (n = 234). During the study, those treated with dofetilide were more likely to convert to sinus rhythm (59 vs 34%), with 79% (vs 42%) maintaining sinus rhythm at 1 year.[24] In the larger DIAMOND-CHF trial, in which 1518

patients with HF with reduced ejection fraction (391 with baseline AF) were enrolled and randomized to either dofetilide or placebo, dofetilide showed a significant association with conversion to sinus rhythm at 1 year with no mortality difference at a mean follow-up of 18 months (41 vs 42%). In those with restoration and maintenance of sinus rhythm, mortality was lower independent of therapy. The risk of HF hospitalization was also significantly reduced in the dofetilide treatment group (risk ratio 0.75, 95% CI 0.63–0.89).[26] In addition, a mortality difference was observed when analyzed by baseline corrected QT (QTc) interval. In those with a normal QTc, dofetilide was associated with mortality reduction (risk ratio 0.4, 95% CI 0.3–0.8). However, mortality increased when the QTc was greater than 479 milliseconds (risk ratio 1.3, 95% CI 0.8–1.9). The most clinically important side effect observed was torsades de pointes occurring in 3.3% (n = 25).[27] Patients must be hospitalized to initiate dofetilide to allow for assessment of creatinine clearance and cardiac monitoring, because most episodes of torsades occurred during the initial 3-day period of initiation of therapy.[26]

Dronedarone

Dronedarone has been shown to be effective in maintaining sinus rhythm, reducing ventricular rate during arrhythmia recurrence, and reducing hospitalization caused by cardiovascular events or death in a broad population.[30,32] However, current guidelines do not support the use of dronedarone in patients with NYHA class III to IV HF or HF with reduced ejection fraction.[33,35,36] The US Food and Drug Administration and European Medicines Agency offered similar recommendations in 2011. In ANDROMEDA (Antiarrhythmic Trial with Dronedarone in Moderate to Severe CHF Evaluating Morbidity Decrease),[36] the safety and efficacy of dronedarone (n = 310) was compared with placebo (n = 317) in symptomatic patients with HF with reduced ejection fraction. This trial was discontinued early because of a significant increase in mortality in those assigned to the dronedarone group (8.1% vs 3.8%) at 2 months follow-up related to HF worsening. The safety and efficacy of dronedarone in NYHA class I/II patients with HF are unclear. In addition, there are concerns regarding use of dronedarone in permanent AF. In the PALLAS trial (n = 3236), of which the majority were NYHA class I/II, patients were randomized to dronedarone or placebo. The study was terminated early because of increased rates of HF, stroke, and death from cardiovascular causes.[42]

Sotalol

Sotalol should be used with great caution if at all in patients with HF. Sotalol may increase the risk of torsades de pointes, which is enhanced in the setting of electrolyte abnormalities, reduced ejection fraction, acute-onset or decompensated HF, or renal dysfunction. In 1 large study (n = 3135),[43] 5.0% of patients with HF history experienced torsades with sotalol (compared with 1.7% with no previous history). A meta-analysis examining the safety of sotalol showed that proarrhythmia was associated with HF history, sustained ventricular tachycardia, and myocardial infarction.[44] The SWORD (Survival With Oral D-sotalol) trial reported that sotalol was associated with higher relative risk of mortality than placebo in those with an ejection fraction of 40% or less.[47] ACC/AHA guidelines do not support the use of sotalol in this population.[33]

Class IC antiarrhythmic drugs

Class IC drugs such as flecainide and propafenone are associated with increased risk for proarrhythmias and sudden cardiac death. These medications are not recommended for use in patients with HF. A meta-analysis reported that with increasing HF severity, there was increased risk of spontaneous complex ventricular arrhythmias.[10,48,50]

Angiotensin-converting enzyme inhibitors and angiotensin receptor blockers

Initial studies have suggested that angiotensin-converting enzyme inhibitors (ACEIs) and angiotensin receptor blockers (ARBs) may reduce major adverse cardiovascular events in AF and prevent new-onset and recurrent AF. However, although there are no data to suggest these therapies for this primary purpose, ACEIs and ARBs have been shown to be efficacious in HF, particularly HF with reduced ejection fraction.[4] In the TRACE (Trandolapril Cardiac Evaluation) study of patients with left ventricular dysfunction and sinus rhythm after an acute myocardial infarction,[53] trandolapril was associated with a significant reduction in subsequent development of AF in follow-up at 2 to 4 years compared with placebo. Similar findings were noted in the SOLVD and Val-HeFT (Valsartan Heart Failure Trial) trials.[55,57] However, the ACTIVE I (Atrial Fibrillation Clopidogrel Trial with Irbesartan for Prevention of Vascular Events) trial presented contrary data in 9016 patients with AF history, stroke risk factors, and systolic blood pressure of at least 110 mm Hg randomized to either irbesartan or placebo. Those receiving irbesartan were not more likely to remain in sinus rhythm at baseline, regardless of baseline rhythm (risk ratio

0.97, $P = .61$).[61] Given limited evidence, the guidelines do not support ACEI or ARB therapy for prevention of new-onset AF or secondary prevention of AF, although these agents are recommended for HF and reduced ejection fraction.

Nonpharmacologic Approaches

AF is often triggered by ectopic atrial beats originating from the pulmonary vein ostia. Ablation of these foci or the complete electrical isolation of the pulmonary veins may be accomplished by radiofrequency catheter ablation or surgically.[62,63] This strategy may be beneficial when rate and rhythm control strategies have been unsuccessful. In a matched study of 58 consecutive patients (NYHA class II-IV) with ejection fraction less than 45% who underwent pulmonary vein isolation,[62] successful ablation was achieved without antiarrhythmic therapy in 69% of those with HF (vs 71% without HF) noted at 1 year after the last procedure. NYHA class, quality of life, exercise capacity, and exercise time had significant improvements in both groups. Long-term efficacy in this population remains uncertain.

The Pulmonary Vein Antrum Isolation versus AV Node Ablation with Bi-Ventricular Pacing for Treatment of Atrial Fibrillation in Patients with Congestive Heart Failure Trial (PABA-CHF)[64] examined the efficacy of pulmonary vein isolation ablation compared with atrioventricular node ablation with biventricular pacing for rate control in a randomized trial of 81 patients with NYHA class II/III HF with symptomatic AF refractory to medical therapy. At 6 months, pulmonary vein isolation was associated with significant improvements in quality of life, left ventricular ejection fraction, and 6-minute walk distance. However, longer follow-up periods and larger studies are warranted to confirm these findings.

ANTICOAGULATION

Most patients with AF with HF meet criteria for long-term anticoagulation because of increased risk of embolization, whether or not a rate control or rhythm control strategy is used. There are various risk models that can guide choice of therapy for anticoagulation. A detailed discussion of these models is beyond the scope of this review. However, one of the best validated models is the CHADS2 risk score, which incorporates the presence of HF, hypertension, age greater than 75 years, diabetes, and previous transient ischemic attack or stroke as variables in the model, all of which are weighted with 1 point, except for stroke or transient ischemic attack, which is weighted as 2 points. The more sensitive CHA2DS2-VASc score adds weight to those older than 74 years and incorporates female sex and vascular disease as additional risk factors.[65]

The risks and benefits of anticoagulation must be evaluated before selecting an agent. The HF population have CHADS2 or CHA2DS2-VASc scores of at least 1 by definition. Aspirin therapy (81-325 mg daily) or warfarin (international normalized ratio [INR] 2.0–3.0) is recommended for patients with a CHADS2 score of 1 alone, although this choice may be mitigated by other clinical characteristics (ie, prosthetic valve) as well as physician and patient preference. Patients with CHADS2/CHA2DS2-VASc scores of 2 or greater are at relatively high risk of stroke (annual risk of at least 4%), and anticoagulant therapy is strongly recommended.[33] Warfarin and newer anticoagulants are available to reduce stroke risk in these patients. Warfarin significantly lowers risk of embolism and stroke compared with placebo. Multiple studies have concluded that newer agents (dabigatran, apixaban, rivaroxaban) have similar or lower rates of both ischemic stroke and bleeding, which may support the use of these therapies as alternatives to warfarin.

Warfarin

Several trials with more than 4000 patients randomizing those with nonvalvular/nonrheumatic AF to aspirin, warfarin, or placebo have shown significantly reduced stroke risk with warfarin compared with aspirin or placebo. Mortality was also significantly reduced compared with no antithrombotic therapy with warfarin.[66–69] More recent studies continue to support warfarin efficacy; however, lower absolute levels of stroke risk have been recently observed, which result in a smaller absolute benefit of therapy.[70] In the RE-LY (Randomized Evaluation of Long-Term Anticoagulation Therapy), ROCKET AF (Rivaroxaban Once Daily Oral Direct Factor Xa Inhibition Compared with Vitamin K Antagonism for Prevention of Stroke and Embolism Trial in Atrial Fibrillation), and ARISTOTLE (Apixaban for Reduction in Stroke and Other Thromboembolic Events in Atrial Fibrillation) trials, the risk of stroke or systemic embolism in more than 20,000 patients was 1.7%, 2.2%, and 1.6% per year, respectively. A meta-analysis of 8 randomized trials with more than 55,000 patients treated with warfarin found an annual incidence of stroke or embolism of 1.66%.[71] A major safety concern of warfarin and all anticoagulants is bleeding risk. The absolute rate of major bleeding (bleeding requiring hospitalization, transfusion, surgery, or certain anatomic locations) with warfarin was significantly higher compared with aspirin in a meta-analysis of 6 randomized controlled trials (2.2 vs 1.0 events per 100 patient-years).[70] There is also underutilization of anticoagulation.[65,73] In the ORBIT-AF (Outcomes Registry for Better Informed Treatment of AF) registry of 10,098 patients, more than 70% had CHADS2 scores greater than or equal to 2; however, more than 25% were not treated with systemic anticoagulation (warfarin or dabigatran), despite relative or absolute contraindications in only 14%.[65]

Direct Thrombin and Factor Xa Inhibitors

Dabigatran (direct thrombin inhibitor), apixaban, and rivaroxaban (factor Xa inhibitors) have been compared with warfarin in large randomized trials of intermediate-risk to high-risk patients. These therapies have shown similar or better efficacy and safety compared with warfarin, but do not have the advantage of long-term data. These newer agents do not require INR monitoring. These agents are less affected by dietary and drug interactions. However, these therapies may require twice-daily dosing and may be higher in cost. These agents lack a reversal agent and may require dose adjustment in chronic kidney disease.[74] The ACC/AHA guidelines recommend dabigatran as an alternative to warfarin; however, although approved by the Food and Drug Administration, there are currently no ACC/AHA recommendations regarding the use of apixaban and rivaroxaban.[59] However, the ESC does recommend these 3 agents as alternatives to warfarin in nonvalvular AF.[75] These agents are not recommended in patients with prosthetic valves.

The RE-LY noninferiority trial assessed the safety and efficacy of dabigatran compared with warfarin in 18,113 patients with nonvalvular AF and intermediate risk (mean CHADS2 score of 2.1). The rate of the primary outcome of stroke or systemic embolization was 1.52%, 1.11%, and 1.69% per year in the dabigatran 110 mg, dabigatran 150 mg and warfarin groups, respectively.[76] The risk of major bleeding was significantly lower in the dabigatran 110 mg group compared with warfarin, whereas the dabigatran 150 mg group was equivalent in safety to warfarin.[77–79] Post hoc evaluation of the RE-LY trial reported a nonsignificantly increased rate of myocardial infarction for both doses of dabigatran compared with warfarin.[80] These findings were confirmed in a meta-analysis of 7 trials comparing dabigatran with warfarin, enoxaparin or placebo for either stroke prophylaxis in AF, treatment of deep venous thrombosis, short-term prophylaxis of deep venous thrombosis, or treatment of acute coronary syndrome. Dabigatran was associated with a significantly increased risk of myocardial infarction, cardiac death, or unstable angina compared with the control group (OR 1.27, 95% CI 1.00–1.61).[81] These findings warrant further investigation.

Rivaroxaban was studied in the ROCKET AF trial, in which 14,264 patients with AF at intermediate to high risk of stroke (mean CHADS2 score of 3.5) were randomized to rivaroxaban or warfarin. Similar proportions of patients with HF were in both groups (approximately 62%). Rivaroxaban was shown to be noninferior to warfarin (1.7 vs 2.2% per year, hazard ratio 0.79, 95% CI 0.66–0.96). There was no significant difference in bleeding (major or nonmajor) as well.[82]

Apixaban was studied in the ARISTOTLE trial of 18,201 patients with intermediate risk (mean CHADS2 score 2.1) who were randomized to apixaban or warfarin. There were similar proportions of patients with HF in each group (approximately 36%). Apixaban was shown to be noninferior, because the composite primary end point of stroke and systemic embolism was significantly reduced in the apixaban group (1.3 vs 1.6% per year, hazard ratio 0.79, 95% CI 0.66–0.95). In addition, the rate of major bleeding was significantly lower in the apixaban group, with a significant reduction in the hemorrhagic stroke rate. This trial also showed a significant reduction in the secondary efficacy outcome of all-cause mortality compared with warfarin (3.52 vs 3.94% per year, P = .047).[83]

HF WITH PRESERVED EJECTION FRACTION

AF can impair left ventricular filling in late diastole in HF with preserved ejection fraction, because HF with preserved ejection fraction (HFpEF) may be more dependent on atrial contraction. Rapid ventricular response caused by AF may also impair filling by shortening diastole. Restoration and maintenance of sinus rhythm may be beneficial in this population; however, observational data (n = 382) suggest that there was no survival advantage with this approach.[84] Further study is warranted to assess morbidity and mortality with rate versus rhythm control approaches in a larger randomized cohort. β-blockers and calcium channel blockers are first-line therapies. Digoxin may be beneficial as well.[33] HF with preserved ejection fraction has also been reported to have a higher risk of death, hospitalization from HF, and hospitalization from any cause, although similar to that of patients with reduced ejection fraction in a study of 23,644 patients with HF (HFpEF n = 14,295).[85] However, these findings have not been consistent across all studies.[86–88]

FUTURE DIRECTIONS

Although there is evidence that rate and rhythm control approaches to AF may produce similar outcomes in patients with HF, there are conflicting data with respect to degree of rate control. Lenient and strict rate control were shown to be similar; however, the SHIFT study, although representing differing populations, seemingly indicates that rate control of patients with HF without AF is efficacious. A subset of patients in SHIFT had a history of AF (approximately 8%), and it is unknown if a difference was seen in this population. Data from the Get With The Guidelines Heart Failure Registry have shown that higher admission heart rates are independently associated with worse outcomes in those admitted for HF, irrespective of rhythm. It may be beneficial to further study rate reduction in HF and AF.[89] Long-term follow-up and refinement of patient selection for AF ablation as well as improved algorithms for anticoagulant therapies are needed.[90,91] Cost-effectiveness studies to assess these strategies are also crucial. In addition, further study is warranted in the population with HFpEF, because current therapies may not apply to this cohort of patients, particularly because most standard therapies for HF with reduced ejection fraction have not been efficacious in HFpEF.

SUMMARY

AF affects many patients with HF, and both disorders impose a significant burden on the health care system. The presence of AF is a marker of worse prognosis in this population, associated with increased morbidity and mortality. Management strategies are aimed at limiting symptoms through rate or rhythm control as well as anticoagulation to prevent systemic embolization and stroke, avoiding therapies that increase mortality in the HF population. Current data suggest that pharmacologic rhythm control has no advantage over rate control. It remains unknown whether prompt restoration of sinus rhythm or aggressive rate control in patients hospitalized with new-onset AF is beneficial, and this aspect requires further study. Improvements in invasive strategies to restore sinus rhythm have resulted in increased efficacy and safety; however, further data are warranted to determine their role in the treatment of AF in HF. New anticoagulants have emerged and present their unique advantages and challenges. Advances in pharmacotherapy, nonpharmacologic therapies, and treatment strategies have benefited patients with AF and HF.

REFERENCES

1. Rienstra M, Damman K, Mulder BA, et al. Beta-blockers and outcome in heart failure and atrial fibrillation. JACC Heart Fail 2013;1(1):21–8. http://dx.doi.org/10.1016/j.jchf.2012.09.002.

2. Parthenakis FI, Patrianakos AP, Skalidis EI, et al. Atrial fibrillation is associated with increased neurohumoral activation and reduced exercise tolerance in patients with non-ischemic dilated cardiomyopathy. Int J Cardiol 2007;118(2):206–14. http://dx.doi.org/10.1016/j.ijcard.2006.03.090.

3. Pardaens K, Van Cleemput J, Vanhaecke J, et al. Atrial fibrillation is associated with a lower exercise capacity in male chronic heart failure patients. Heart 1997;78(6):564–8.

4. Yancy CW, Jessup M, Bozkurt B, et al. 2013 ACCF/AHA guideline for the management of heart failure. J Am Coll Cardiol 2013. http://dx.doi.org/10.1016/j.jacc.2013.05.019.

5. Wang TJ, Larson MG, Levy D, et al. Temporal relations of atrial fibrillation and congestive heart failure and their joint influence on mortality. Circulation 2003;107:2920–5.

6. Vorperian VR, Havighurst TC, Miller S, et al. Adverse effects of low dose amiodarone: a meta-analysis. J Am Coll Cardiol 1997;30(3):791–8. http://dx.doi.org/10.1016/S0735-1097(97)00220-9.

7. Benjamin EJ, Levy D, Vaziri SM, et al. Independent risk factors for atrial fibrillation in a population-based cohort. The Framingham Heart Study. JAMA 1994;271(11):840–4. http://dx.doi.org/10.1001/jama.1994.03510350050036.

8. Deedwania PC, Singh BN, Ellenbogen K, et al. Spontaneous conversion and maintenance of sinus rhythm by amiodarone in patients with heart failure and atrial fibrillation: observations from the veterans affairs congestive heart failure survival trial of antiarrhythmic therapy (CHF-STAT). The Department of Veterans Affairs CHF-STAT Investigators. Circulation 1998;98(23):2574–9.

9. Carson PE, Johnson GR, Dunkman WB, et al. The influence of atrial fibrillation on prognosis in mild to moderate heart failure. The V-HeFT Studies. The V-HeFT VA Cooperative Studies Group. Circulation 1993;87(Suppl 6):VI102–10.

10. Stevenson WG, Stevenson LW, Middlekauff HR, et al. Improving survival for patients with atrial fibrillation and advanced heart failure. J Am Coll Cardiol 1996;28(6):1458–63. http://dx.doi.org/10.1016/S0735-1097(96)00358-0.

11. Joglar JA, Acosta AP, Shusterman NH, et al. Effect of carvedilol on survival and hemodynamics in patients with atrial fibrillation and left ventricular dysfunction: retrospective analysis of the US Carvedilol Heart Failure Trials Program. Am Heart J 2001;142(3):498–501. http://dx.doi.org/10.1067/mhj.2001.117318.

12. Mahoney P, Kimmel S, DeNofrio D, et al. Prognostic significance of atrial fibrillation in patients ut a tertiary medical center referred for heart transplantation because of severe heart failure. Am J Cardiol 1999;83(11):1544–7. http://dx.doi.org/10.1016/S0002-9149(99)00144-7.

13. Maisel WH, Stevenson LW. Atrial fibrillation in heart failure: epidemiology, pathophysiology, and rationale for therapy. Am J Cardiol 2003;91(Suppl): 2D–8D. http://dx.doi.org/10.1016/S0002-9149(02)03373-8.

14. Weinfeld MS, Drazner MH, Stevenson WG, et al. Early outcome of initiating amiodarone for atrial fibrillation in advanced heart failure. J Heart Lung Transplant 2000;19(7):638–43.

15. Cohn JN, Johnson G, Ziesche S, et al. A comparison of enalapril with hydralazine-isosorbide dinitrate in the treatment of chronic congestive heart failure. N Engl J Med 1991;325(5):303–10. http://dx.doi.org/10.1056/NEJM199108013250502.

16. Cohn JN, Archibald DG, Ziesche S, et al. Effect of vasodilator therapy on mortality in chronic congestive heart failure. Results of a Veterans Administration Cooperative Study. N Engl J Med 1986;314(24):1547–52. http://dx.doi.org/10.1056/NEJM198606123142404.

17. Doval HC, Nul DR, Grancelli HO, et al. Randomised trial of low-dose amiodarone in severe congestive heart failure. Lancet 1994;344(8921): 493–8. http://dx.doi.org/10.1016/S0140-6736(94)91895-3.

18. Packer M, Poole-Wilson PA, Armstrong PW, et al. Comparative effects of low and high doses of the angiotensin-converting enzyme inhibitor, lisinopril, on morbidity and mortality in chronic heart failure. ATLAS Study Group. Circulation 1999;100(23): 2312–8.

19. Johnstone D, Limacher M, Rousseau M, et al. Clinical characteristics of patients in studies of left ventricular dysfunction (SOLVD). Am J Cardiol 1992; 70(9):894–900. http://dx.doi.org/10.1016/0002-9149(92)90734-G.

20. Singh SN, Fletcher RD, Fisher SG, et al. Amiodarone in patients with congestive heart failure and asymptomatic ventricular arrhythmia. N Engl J Med 1995;333(2):77–82. http://dx.doi.org/10.1056/NEJM199507133330201.

21. Group TCTS. Effects of enalapril on mortality in severe congestive heart failure. Results of the Cooperative North Scandinavian Enalapril Survival Study (CONSENSUS). N Engl J Med 1987; 316(23):1429–35. http://dx.doi.org/10.1056/NEJM198706043162301.

22. Yusuf S, Pepine CJ, Garces C, et al. Effect of enalapril on myocardial infarction and unstable angina in patients with low ejection fractions. Lancet 1992; 340(8829):1173–8.

23. Dries DL, Exner DV, Gersh BJ, et al. Atrial fibrillation is associated with an increased risk for mortality and heart failure progression in patients with asymptomatic and symptomatic left ventricular systolic dysfunction: a retrospective analysis of the SOLVD trials. Studies of Left Ventricular Dysfunction. J Am Coll Cardiol 1998;32(3):695–703.

24. Pedersen OD, Bagger H, Keller N, et al. Efficacy of dofetilide in the treatment of atrial fibrillation-flutter in patients with reduced left ventricular function: a Danish investigations of arrhythmia and mortality on dofetilide (DIAMOND) substudy. Circulation 2001;104(3):292–6.

25. Olsson LG, Swedberg KK, Ducharme AA, et al. Atrial fibrillation and risk of clinical events in chronic heart failure with and without left ventricular systolic dysfunction. J Am Coll Cardiol 2006; 47(10):1997–2004. http://dx.doi.org/10.1016/j.jacc.2006.01.060.

26. Torp-Pedersen C, Møller M, Bloch-Thomsen PE, et al. Dofetilide in patients with congestive heart failure and left ventricular dysfunction. N Engl J Med 1999;341(12):857–65. http://dx.doi.org/10.1056/NEJM199909163411201.

27. Brendorp B, Elming H, Jun L, et al. Qtc interval as a guide to select those patients with congestive heart failure and reduced left ventricular systolic function who will benefit from antiarrhythmic treatment with dofetilide. Circulation 2001;103(10):1422–7.

28. Wasywich CA, Whalley GA, Gamble GD, et al. Does rhythm matter? The prognostic importance of atrial fibrillation in heart failure. Heart Lung Circ 2006;15(6):353–7. http://dx.doi.org/10.1016/j.hlc.2006.07.011.

29. Mountantonakis SE, Grau-Sepulveda MV, Bhatt DL, et al. Presence of atrial fibrillation is independently associated with adverse outcomes in patients hospitalized with heart failure. Circ Heart Fail 2012;5(2):191–201. http://dx.doi.org/10.1161/CIRCHEARTFAILURE.111.965681.

30. Singh BN, Connolly SJ, Crijns HJ, et al. Dronedarone for maintenance of sinus rhythm in atrial fibrillation or flutter. N Engl J Med 2007;357(10):987–99. http://dx.doi.org/10.1056/NEJMoa054686.

31. Roy D, Talajic M, Nattel S, et al. Rhythm control versus rate control for atrial fibrillation and heart failure. N Engl J Med 2008;358(25):2667–77. http://dx.doi.org/10.1056/NEJMoa0708789.

32. Hohnloser SH, Crijns HJ, van Eickels M, et al. Effect of dronedarone on cardiovascular events in atrial fibrillation. N Engl J Med 2009;360(7):668–78. http://dx.doi.org/10.1056/NEJMoa0803778.

33. Fuster V, Ryden LE, Cannom DS, et al. ACC/AHA/ESC 2006 guidelines for the management of patients with atrial fibrillation–executive summary. Circulation 2006;114(7):700–52. http://dx.doi.org/10.1161/CIRCULATIONAHA.106.177031.

34. Suman-Horduna I, Roy D, Frasure Smith N, et al. Quality of life and functional capacity in patients with atrial fibrillation and congestive heart failure. J Am Coll Cardiol 2013;61:455–60. http://dx.doi.org/10.1016/j.jacc.2012.10.031.

35. Hohnloser SH, Crijns HJ, van Eickels M, et al. Dronedarone in patients with congestive heart failure. insights from ATHENA. Eur Heart J 2010;31(14): 1717–21. http://dx.doi.org/10.1093/eurheartj/ehq113.

36. Kober L, Torp-Pedersen C, McMurray JJ, et al. Increased mortality after dronedarone therapy for severe heart failure. N Engl J Med 2008;358(25): 2678–87. http://dx.doi.org/10.1056/NEJMoa0800456.

37. Pozzoli M, Cioffi G, Traversi E, et al. Predictors of primary atrial fibrillation and concomitant clinical and hemodynamic changes in patients with chronic heart failure: a prospective study in 344 patients with baseline sinus rhythm. J Am Coll Cardiol 1998;32(1):197–204. http://dx.doi.org/10.1016/S0735-1097(98)00221-6.

38. Crijns HJ, Tjeerdsma G, de Kam PJ, et al. Prognostic value of the presence and development of atrial fibrillation in patients with advanced chronic heart failure. Eur Heart J 2000;21(15):1238–45. http://dx.doi.org/10.1053/euhj.1999.2107.

39. Khand AU, Rankin AC, Kaye GC, et al. Systematic review of the management of atrial fibrillation in patients with heart failure. Eur Heart J 2000;21(8): 614–32. http://dx.doi.org/10.1053/euhj.1999.1767.

40. Wyse DG, Waldo AL, DiMarco JP, et al. A comparison of rate control and rhythm control in patients with atrial fibrillation. N Engl J Med 2002;347(23):1825–33. http://dx.doi.org/10.1056/NEJMoa021328.

41. Van Gelder IC, Hagens VE, Bosker HA, et al. A comparison of rate control and rhythm control in patients with recurrent persistent atrial fibrillation. N Engl J Med 2002;347(23):1834–40. http://dx.doi.org/10.1056/NEJMoa021375.

42. Connolly SJ, Camm AJ, Halperin JL, et al. Dronedarone in high-risk permanent atrial fibrillation. N Engl J Med 2011;365(24):2268–76. http://dx.doi.org/10.1056/NEJMoa1109867.

43. Lehmann MH, Hardy S, Archibald D, et al. Sex difference in risk of torsade de pointes with d, l-sotalol. Circulation 1996;94(10):2535–41.

44. Soyka LF, Wirtz C, Spangenberg RB. Clinical safety profile of sotalol in patients with arrhythmias. Am J Cardiol 1990;65(2):74A–83A.

45. Cha YM, Redfield MM, Shen WK, et al. Atrial fibrillation and ventricular dysfunction: a vicious electromechanical cycle. Circulation 2004; 109(23):2839–43. http://dx.doi.org/10.1161/01.CIR.0000132470.78896.A8.

46. Gheorghiade M, Fonarow GC, van Veldhuisen DJ, et al. Lack of evidence of increased mortality among patients with atrial fibrillation taking digoxin: findings from post hoc propensity-matched analysis of the AFFIRM trial. Eur Heart J 2013;34(20):1489–97. http://dx.doi.org/10.1093/eurheartj/eht120.

47. Waldo AL, Camm AJ, deRuyter H, et al. Effect of d-sotalol on mortality in patients with left ventricular dysfunction after recent and remote myocardial infarction. The SWORD Investigators. Survival With Oral d-Sotalol. Lancet 1996;348(9019):7–12.

48. Kjekshus J. Arrhythmias and mortality in congestive heart failure. Am J Cardiol 1990;65(19):42I–8I.

49. Van Gelder IC, Groenveld HF, Crijns HJ, et al. Lenient versus strict rate control in patients with atrial fibrillation. N Engl J Med 2010;362(15):1363–73. http://dx.doi.org/10.1056/NEJMoa1001337.

50. Amabile CM, Spencer AP. Keeping your patient with heart failure safe–a review of potentially dangerous medications. Arch Intern Med 2004; 164(7):709–20. http://dx.doi.org/10.1001/archinte.164.7.709.

51. Wilkoff BL, Cook JR, Epstein AE, et al. Dual-chamber pacing or ventricular backup pacing in patients with an implantable defibrillator: the Dual Chamber and VVI Implantable Defibrillator (DAVID) Trial. JAMA 2002;288(24):3115–23. http://dx.doi.org/10.1001/jama.288.24.3115.

52. Sweeney MO, Hellkamp AS, Ellenbogen KA, et al. Adverse effect of ventricular pacing on heart failure and atrial fibrillation among patients with normal baseline QRS duration in a clinical trial of pacemaker therapy for sinus node dysfunction. Circulation 2003;107(23):2932–7. http://dx.doi.org/10.1161/01.CIR.0000072769.17295.B1.

53. Pedersen OD, Bagger H, Kober L, et al. Trandolapril reduces the incidence of atrial fibrillation after acute myocardial infarction in patients with left ventricular dysfunction. Circulation 1999;100(4):376–80.

54. Gasparini M, Regoli F, Galimberti P, et al. Cardiac resynchronization therapy in heart failure patients with atrial fibrillation. Europace 2009;11(Suppl 5):v82–6. http://dx.doi.org/10.1093/europace/eup273.

55. Vermes E, Tardif JC, Bourassa MG, et al. Enalapril decreases the incidence of atrial fibrillation in patients with left ventricular dysfunction: insight from the Studies Of Left Ventricular Dysfunction (SOLVD) trials. Circulation 2003;107(23):2926–31. http://dx.doi.org/10.1161/01.CIR.0000072793.81076.D4.

56. Swedberg K, Komajda M, Böhm M, et al. Ivabradine and outcomes in chronic heart failure (SHIFT): a randomised placebo-controlled study. Lancet 2010;376(9744):875–85. http://dx.doi.org/10.1016/S0140-6736(10)61198-1.

57. Maggioni AP, Latini R, Carson PE, et al. Valsartan reduces the incidence of atrial fibrillation in patients with heart failure: results from the Valsartan Heart Failure Trial (Val-HeFT). Am Heart J 2005;149(3): 548–57. http://dx.doi.org/10.1016/j.ahj.2004.09.033.

58. Flaker GC, Blackshear JL, McBride R, et al. Antiarrhythmic drug therapy and cardiac mortality in atrial fibrillation. The Stroke Prevention in Atrial Fibrillation Investigators. J Am Coll Cardiol 1992;20(3):527–32. http://dx.doi.org/10.1016/0735-1097(92)90003-6.

59. Fuster V, Ryden LE, Cannom DS, et al. 2011 ACCF/AHA/HRS focused updates incorporated into the ACC/AHA/ESC 2006 Guidelines for the management of patients with atrial fibrillation. J Am Coll Cardiol 2011;57(11):e101–98. http://dx.doi.org/10.1016/j.jacc.2010.09.013.

60. European Heart Rhythm Association, European Association for Cardio-Thoracic Surgery, Camm AJ, et al. Guidelines for the management of atrial fibrillation: the Task Force for the Management of Atrial Fibrillation of the European Society of Cardiology (ESC). Eur Heart J 2010;31(19):2369–429. http://dx.doi.org/10.1093/eurheartj/ehq278.

61. Investigators TAI. Irbesartan in patients with atrial fibrillation. N Engl J Med 2011;364(10):928–38. http://dx.doi.org/10.1056/NEJMoa1008816.

62. Hsu LF, Jaïs P, Sanders P, et al. Catheter ablation for atrial fibrillation in congestive heart failure. N Engl J Med 2004;351(23):2373–83. http://dx.doi.org/10.1056/NEJMoa041018.

63. Chen MS, Marrouche NF, Khaykin Y, et al. Pulmonary vein isolation for the treatment of atrial fibrillation in patients with impaired systolic function. J Am Coll Cardiol 2004;43(6):1004–9. http://dx.doi.org/10.1016/j.jacc.2003.09.056.

64. Khan MN, Jaïs P, Cummings J, et al. Pulmonary-vein isolation for atrial fibrillation in patients with heart failure. N Engl J Med 2008;359(17):1778–85. http://dx.doi.org/10.1056/NEJMoa0708234.

65. Cullen MW, Kim S, Piccini JP, et al. Risks and benefits of anticoagulation in atrial fibrillation: insights from the outcomes registry for better informed treatment of atrial fibrillation (ORBIT-AF) registry. Circ Cardiovasc Qual Outcomes 2013;6(4):461–9. http://dx.doi.org/10.1161/CIRCOUTCOMES.113.000127.

66. The Effect of Low-Dose Warfarin on the Risk of Stroke in Patients with Nonrheumatic Atrial Fibrillation. N Engl J Med 1990;323(22):1505–11. http://dx.doi.org/10.1056/NEJM199011293232201.

67. Warfarin versus aspirin for prevention of thromboembolism in atrial fibrillation: stroke prevention in atrial fibrillation II study. Lancet 1994;343:687–91.

68. Petersen P, Boysen G, Godtfredsen J. Placebo-controlled, randomised trial of warfarin and aspirin for prevention of thromboembolic complications in chronic atrial fibrillation. The Copenhagen AFASAK study. Lancet 1989;1:175–9. Available at: http://www.uptodate.com/contents/antithrombotic-therapy-to-prevent-embolization-in-atrial-fibrillation/abstract-text/2563096/pubmed. Accessed July 4, 2013.

69. Ezekowitz MD, Bridgers SL, James KE, et al. Warfarin in the prevention of stroke associated with nonrheumatic atrial fibrillation. N Engl J Med 1992;327:1406–12. http://dx.doi.org/10.1056/NEJM199301143280227.

70. Singer DE, Chang Y, Fang MC, et al. The net clinical benefit of warfarin anticoagulation in atrial fibrillation. Ann Intern Med 2009;151(5):297–305. http://dx.doi.org/10.7326/0003-4819-151-5-200909010-00003.

71. Agarwal S, Hachamovitch R, Menon V. Current trial-associated outcomes with warfarin in prevention of stroke in patients with nonvalvular atrial fibrillation–a meta-analysis. Arch Intern Med 2012;172(8):623–31. http://dx.doi.org/10.1001/archinternmed.2012.121.

72. van Walraven C, Hart RG, Singer DE, et al. Oral anticoagulants vs aspirin in nonvalvular atrial fibrillation–an individual patient meta-analysis. JAMA 2002;288(19):2441–8. http://dx.doi.org/10.1001/jama.288.19.2441.

73. Piccini JP, Hernandez AF, Zhao X, et al. Quality of care for atrial fibrillation among patients hospitalized for heart failure. J Am Coll Cardiol 2009;54(14):1280–9. http://dx.doi.org/10.1016/j.jacc.2009.04.091.

74. Gong IY, Kim RB. Importance of pharmacokinetic profile and variability as determinants of dose and response to dabigatran, rivaroxaban, and apixaban. Can J Cardiol 2013;29(7):S24–33. http://dx.doi.org/10.1016/j.cjca.2013.04.002.

75. Camm AJ, Lip GY, De Caterina R, et al. 2012 focused update of the ESC guidelines for the management of atrial fibrillation: an update of the 2010 ESC guidelines for the management of atrial fibrillation. Developed with the special contribution of the European Heart Rhythm Association. Eur Heart J 2012;33(21):2719–47. http://dx.doi.org/10.1093/eurheartj/ehs253.

76. Connolly SJ, Ezekowitz MD, Yusuf S, et al. Dabigatran versus warfarin in patients with atrial fibrillation. N Engl J Med 2009;361(12):1139–51. http://dx.doi.org/10.1056/NEJMoa0905561.

77. Connolly SJ, Ezekowitz MD, Yusuf S, et al. Newly identified events in the RE-LY trial. N Engl J Med 2010;363(19):1875–6. http://dx.doi.org/10.1056/NEJMc1007378.

78. Ezekowitz MD, Wallentin L, Connolly SJ, et al. Dabigatran and warfarin in vitamin K antagonist-naive and -experienced cohorts with atrial fibrillation. Circulation 2010;122(22):2246–53. http://dx.doi.org/10.1161/CIRCULATIONAHA.110.973735.

79. Eikelboom JW, Wallentin L, Connolly SJ, et al. Risk of bleeding with 2 doses of dabigatran compared with warfarin in older and younger patients with atrial fibrillation: an analysis of the randomized evaluation of long-term anticoagulant therapy (RE-LY) trial. Circulation 2011;123(21):2363–72. http://dx.doi.org/10.1161/CIRCULATIONAHA.110.004747.

80. Hohnloser SH, Oldgren JJ, Yang SS, et al. Myocardial ischemic events in patients with atrial

fibrillation treated with dabigatran or warfarin in the RE-LY (Randomized Evaluation of Long-Term Anticoagulation Therapy) trial. Circulation 2012; 125(5):669–76. http://dx.doi.org/10.1161/CIRCULATIONAHA.111.055970.

81. Uchino K, Hernandez AV. Dabigatran association with higher risk of acute coronary events–meta-analysis of noninferiority randomized controlled trials. Arch Intern Med 2012;172(5):397–402. http://dx.doi.org/10.1001/archinternmed.2011.1666.

82. Patel MR, Mahaffey KW, Garg J, et al. Rivaroxaban versus warfarin in nonvalvular atrial fibrillation. N Engl J Med 2011;365(10):883–91. http://dx.doi.org/10.1056/NEJMoa1009638.

83. Granger CB, Alexander JH, McMurray JJ, et al. Apixaban versus warfarin in patients with atrial fibrillation. N Engl J Med 2011;365(11):981–92. http://dx.doi.org/10.1056/NEJMoa1107039.

84. Kong MH, Shaw LK, O'Connor C, et al. Is rhythm-control superior to rate-control in patients with atrial fibrillation and diastolic heart failure? Ann Noninvasive Electrocardiol 2010;15(3):209–17. http://dx.doi.org/10.1111/j.1542-474X.2010.00365.x.

85. McManus DD, Hsu G, Sung SH, et al. Atrial fibrillation and outcomes in heart failure with preserved versus reduced left ventricular ejection fraction. J Am Heart Assoc 2012;2(1):e005694. http://dx.doi.org/10.1161/JAHA.112.005694.

86. Badheka AO, Rathod A, Kizilbash MA, et al. Comparison of mortality and morbidity in patients with atrial fibrillation and heart failure with preserved versus decreased left ventricular ejection fraction. Am J Cardiol 2011;108(9):1283–8. http://dx.doi.org/10.1016/j.amjcard.2011.06.045.

87. Linssen GC, Rienstra M, Jaarsma T, et al. Clinical and prognostic effects of atrial fibrillation in heart failure patients with reduced and preserved left ventricular ejection fraction. Eur J Heart Fail 2011;13(10): 1111–20. http://dx.doi.org/10.1093/eurjhf/hfr066.

88. Rusinaru D, Leborgne L, Peltier M, et al. Effect of atrial fibrillation on long-term survival in patients hospitalised for heart failure with preserved ejection fraction. Eur J Heart Fail 2008;10(6):566–72. http://dx.doi.org/10.1016/j.ejheart.2008.04.002.

89. Alings M, Smit MD, Moes ML, et al. Routine versus aggressive upstream rhythm control for prevention of early atrial fibrillation in heart failure: background, aims and design of the RACE 3 study. Neth Heart J 2013. http://dx.doi.org/10.1007/s12471-013-0428-5.

90. Jones DG, Haldar SK, Hussain W, et al. A randomized trial to assess catheter ablation versus rate control in the management of persistent atrial fibrillation in heart failure. J Am Coll Cardiol 2013;61(18):1894–903. http://dx.doi.org/10.1016/j.jacc.2013.01.069.

91. Gheorghiade M, Vaduganathan M, Fonarow GC, et al. Anticoagulation in heart failure: current status and future direction. Heart Fail Rev 2012. http://dx.doi.org/10.1007/s10741-012-9343-x.

Atrial Fibrillation in Heart Failure in the Older Population

Patrick M. Heck, BM BCh[a],[*], Justin M.S. Lee, BM BCh[a],
Peter M. Kistler, MBBS, PhD[b],[c]

KEYWORDS

- Atrial fibrillation • Heart failure • Elderly • Ablation • Anticoagulation

KEY POINTS

- Atrial fibrillation (AF) and heart failure (HF) both have a higher incidence in the older patient and this is increasing.
- Older patients are more likely to have additional comorbidities that can make the management of AF and HF more complex.
- The risk of stroke secondary to AF in this population is high, making consideration of anticoagulation crucially important.
- Although data specifically targeting this patient group is scarce, it would appear that AF ablation can be undertaken safely, is as effective and superior to medical therapy.

INTRODUCTION

Atrial fibrillation (AF) is an important and often-underrecognized cause of cardiovascular morbidity and mortality. It is an arrhythmia that is commonly seen in the older patient, indeed the median age of patients with AF in early studies was 75 years.[1] Heart failure (HF) is also more frequently seen in the older patient with an approximate doubling of HF prevalence with each decade of life.[2] There is clear interaction between AF and HF, with evidence that HF can lead to AF and AF exacerbates HF. The prevalence of AF in individuals with HF is considerably greater than the general population and has been reported to be as high as 25%.[3] This increased prevalence appears related to the severity of the HF and ranges from 5% to 50% as the New York Heart Association (NYHA) classification of the patient increases from I to IV.[4] Taken together, these data make it apparent that AF and HF are frequently going to be encountered in the elderly patient. Elderly patients are more likely to have multiple comorbidities and polypharmacy, which complicate their management compared with their younger counterparts. This review focuses on the specific aspect of AF management in elderly (aged 70 years or more) patients with HF.

PHARMACOLOGIC MANAGEMENT

Older patients are often underrepresented in clinical trials. Pharmacokinetics are significantly altered in the elderly.[5] There is relatively lower muscle mass and higher body fat content, which alters the volume of distribution of drugs such as amiodarone. Hepatic drug metabolism is diminished, affecting drugs including propranolol,

None of the authors have any conflicts of interests to report.
Professor Peter M. Kistler is supported by a practitioner fellowship from the NHMRC. This research is supported in part by the Victorian Government's Operational Infrastructure Funding.
[a] Department of Cardiology, Papworth Hospital, Papworth Everard, Cambridge CB23 3RE, UK; [b] Department of Cardiology, Baker IDI, Melbourne, Australia; [c] Department of Cardiovascular Medicine, Alfred Heart Centre, Alfred Hospital, Baker IDI Heart and Diabetes Institute, University of Melbourne, Victoria 3004, Australia
* Corresponding author.
E-mail address: Patrick.heck@nhs.net

verapamil, and diltiazem. Renal dysfunction is also more common, reducing the elimination of drugs, including digoxin and sotalol. The older population has comorbidities, and polypharmacy can result in significant drug interactions.

Rate Versus Rhythm Control

The major decision in treatment of AF is whether to pursue a strategy to maintain sinus rhythm (SR) with potentially toxic antiarrhythmic drugs or to accept AF and target rate control; this is explored in detail in other articles in this issue. Current evidence indicates that in the absence of significant symptoms due to AF, clinical outcomes from rate control are equivalent to rhythm control.[6,7] Rhythm control should be favored in symptomatic patients. SR can be achieved with Class Ic or Class III antiarrhythmic drugs and/or electrical cardioversion. In the presence of structural heart disease Class Ic agents, such as flecainide, are generally avoided.[8,9] Rate control can be achieved with beta-blockers, calcium channel blockers or digoxin. Previously, guidelines have advocated the use of "strict" rate control[10] with resting heart rate less than 80 beats per minute, but recent evidence suggests that a more lenient target of less than 110 beats per minute could be adopted.[11]

The Atrial Fibrillation Follow-up Investigation of Rhythm Management (AFFIRM) study recruited more than 4000 patients with a mean age of 70 years, including 23% with a history of HF.[6] In the rhythm control arm, SR was maintained in 73% of patients at 3 years and 63% at 5 years and did not confer a survival advantage over rate control. Subgroup analysis did not identify a survival advantage according to left ventricular (LV) function.[12] However, in a post hoc "on-treatment" analysis, warfarin use and presence of SR were associated with a significant reduction in mortality, but the use of antiarrhythmic drugs was not.[13] This emphasizes the importance of anticoagulation and suggests that adverse effects of antiarrhythmic drugs may counteract the benefits of SR.

Similarly, the RAte Control versus Electrical cardioversion for atrial fibrillation (RACE) study randomized 522 patients (mean age 68 years) with persistent AF (median AF duration>300 days) to rate or rhythm control.[7] After a mean of 2.3 years, 39% of the rhythm-control group were in SR, compared with 10% of the rate-control group. Rate control was noninferior to rhythm control for the prevention of death and cardiovascular morbidity.

The Atrial Fibrillation and Congestive Heart Failure (AF-CHF) study randomized 1376 patients (mean age 67 years) to rate versus rhythm control in an HF population with NYHA class II to IV symptoms and LV ejection fraction (EF) less than 35%.[14] Once again, there was no significant difference between strategies in cardiovascular death, death from any cause, stroke, or worsening HF. Rhythm control was associated with an increase in hospitalization.

To date, clinical trials have used medical therapy in the rhythm control arm with few patients undergoing catheter ablation and this is explored in detail later. The benefits of rhythm control may be offset by the relative inefficacy and toxicity of current drugs. In the Carvedilol in Atrial Fibrillation Evaluation (CAFÉ) II trial of 61 patients comparing pharmacological rate versus rhythm control, NYHA class and 6-minute walk time (6MWT) distance were similar between patients assigned to rate or rhythm control, but those assigned to rhythm control had improved LV function, N-terminal pro-brain natriuretic peptide (NT-proBNP) concentration, and quality of life compared with those assigned to rate control.[15]

Pharmacologic Management

In the setting of significant structural heart disease, in particular HF, pharmacologic options for rhythm control of AF are almost exclusively limited to amiodarone according to European guidelines,[16] although US guidelines support the use of dofetilide as well.[17] A detailed review of pharmacological treatments in AF and HF is published elsewhere in this issue. This section will focus on the specific additional considerations in the elderly although there are limited data available specifically targeting this patient group.

Dofetilide is used infrequently because of the need for in-hospital initiation and the risks of proarrhythmia due to QT prolongation. In the Danish Investigations of Arrhythmia and Mortality ON Dofetilide (DIAMOND) study of dofetilide versus placebo in LV dysfunction post myocardial infarction, there was no effect on all-cause mortality.[20] Dofetilide was effective in converting AF and SR was maintained at 1 year in 79%.[21] Maintenance of SR was associated with significant reduction in mortality, whereas dofetilide therapy was associated with a significantly lower risk of congestive HF rehospitalization.

Dronedarone was developed as a modification of amiodarone in an attempt to maintain efficacy without toxicity and has shown some promise in studies.[22,23] In the ANDROMEDA study, dronedarone was trialed in patients with HF, with the study stopped early because of excess mortality in the dronedarone arm.[24] The current role of dronedarone is limited and is probably reserved for maintenance of SR in paroxysmal patients with AF with preserved systolic function.

Sotalol has a combined beta-blocker and class III effect. In the Sotalol Amiodarone Atrial Fibrillation Efficacy Trial (SAFE-T) study of patients with persistent AF, amiodarone and sotalol were equally efficacious in converting AF to SR, although amiodarone was superior for maintaining SR following electrical cardioversion.[18] Sotalol is renally excreted and at higher doses can lead to significant QT prolongation with risk of proarrhythmia in the elderly with HF. In addition, unlike other beta-blockers, such as bisoprolol and carvedilol, sotalol has no proven benefit in HF and so its use is not recommended in patients with AF and HF.[16,17]

Beta-blockers, in particular carvedilol, bisoprolol, and metoprolol, are recommended in current guidelines for treatment of HF because of their proven prognostic and symptomatic benefits.[19] In the Study of Effects of Nebivolol Intervention on Outcomes and Rehospitalization in Seniors (SENIORS) study, nebivolol, a beta-blocker with vasodilator properties, resulted in a reduction in the combined end point of death and hospital admissions in patients older than 70 years.[20] However, more recent data from the SENIORS study showed that nebivolol did not appear to confer clinical benefit in the AF subgroup, irrespective of ejection fraction.[21] In the Carvedilol Or Metoprolol European Trial (COMET)[22] study, although presence of AF was a poor prognostic factor, there was a relative benefit of carvedilol versus metoprolol in patients with AF and HF.

Digoxin is a second-line therapy for AF rate control and is also used in HF as a weak inotrope. Advanced age may predispose patients to an increased risk for digoxin toxicity because of decreased renal function, low body mass, and electrical conduction abnormalities. However, this was not observed in the Digitalis Investigation Group (DIG) trial, in which advanced age was not associated with an increased risk of digoxin toxicity.[23] These findings demonstrate that digoxin remains a useful agent in elderly patients with HF, although patients in this study were in SR. The combination of carvedilol and digoxin was better than either used alone in AF and HF, in terms of symptom control and ejection fraction in a small study by Khand and colleagues.[24]

Calcium channel blockers (eg, diltiazem and verapamil) are another option for rate control of AF when beta-blockers are contraindicated. A recent study compared the use of four different single dose drug regimens for rate control of AF in patients with a mean age of 71 years. This showed diltiazem 360 mg/d to be superior both in heart rate control and symptom improvement, although HF was an exclusion criteria for this study.[25]

THROMBOPROPHYLAXIS FOR AF IN THE OLDER PATIENT

Perhaps the most feared complication associated with AF is that of embolic stroke. Cardioembolic strokes tend to be more severe and are more likely to be fatal.[26] The risk of stroke attributable to AF increases markedly with age, such that in patients aged 80 to 89 years, AF accounts for more than 20% of their stroke risk, compared with only 1.5% in patients aged 50 to 59 years.[27] Using the recently validated risk-scoring tool for estimating stroke risk in AF, CHA_2DS_2-VASc (Congestive heart failure, Hypertension, Age >75, Diabetes, Stroke, Vascular disease, Age 65–75, Sex category), patients aged 75 years or more with HF (CHA_2DS_2-VASc of 3) have an annual risk of stroke or thromboembolism in excess of 5%.[28] Addressing thromboprophylaxis is fundamental to the management of any patient with AF.

Anticoagulation remains the cornerstone of treatment for the prevention of stroke in AF and this has been looked at in some detail earlier in this series. Oral anticoagulation (OAC) is recommended for anyone with a CHA_2DS_2-VASc score of 2 or higher and the improved safety profile afforded by the novel oral anticoagulants (NOACs) has led to the European Society of Cardiology extending this recommendation to those with a CHA_2DS_2-VASc score of 1 or higher. Generally, older patients with AF and HF require anticoagulation unless the bleeding risk is considered prohibitive.

Bleeding Risk in the Older Patient

OAC therapy in the elderly patient with AF and HF is not without potential risk of significant bleeding. Just as advancing age increases an individual's risk of stroke in AF and hence their potential gain from treatment with OAC, older patients are at higher risk of bleeding when taking OAC therapy.[29]

There are many potential barriers that can lead to the underprescription of OACs, but bleeding risk is the most frequently cited reason among elderly patients, with aspirin typically being used as an alternative. This is now a growing body of evidence to show that aspirin use in the elderly is not as benign as previously thought, with several studies reporting bleeding rates in the elderly taking aspirin equivalent to those receiving warfarin.[30–32] Concerns regarding bleeding risk, susceptibility to falls, patient avoidance of anticoagulation, and the requirement for interna- ilunal nnimalizml ially (INR) monilunnu have re sulted in a significant number of elderly patents not being anticoagulated and thus being inade- quately protected against stroke.[33,34]

Several bleeding risk scores have been intro- duced (Anticoagulation and Risk Factors in Atrial Fibrillation [ATRIA][35] and HAS-BLED[36] [hyperten- sion, abnormal renal/liver function, stroke, bleeding history or predisposition, labile INR, elderly, drugs/ alcohol concomitantly]) to provide physicians with the tools to objectively assess an individual's bleeding risk, enabling more informed discussions with the patient and family. In addition, 3 of the risk factors in the HAS-BLED scoring system are poten- tially reversible (*uncontrolled* hypertension, labile INRs, and drugs, such as aspirin or nonsteroidal anti-inflammatory drugs), thereby prompting the physician to minimize an individual's bleeding risk where possible.

The NOACs

The underuse of warfarin in the elderly with AF is multifactorial. In addition to the overestimation of bleeding risk in the older patient, another major deterrent is its fairly unappealing characteristics: narrow therapeutic range, variable dose response necessitating monitoring, and slow onset and offset of action. The NOACs have several distinct advantages in the older patient with AF. First, they have significantly fewer drug interactions than warfarin and older patients with HF are more likely to have comorbidities requiring the use of drugs that interfere with stable warfarin therapy.[37] The pharmacodynamics of the NOACs are more predictable and do not require moni- toring.[38] In addition, the reduced need for frequent monitoring will be especially advantageous in the elderly where mobility and access to anticoagula- tion services might be problematic.

At the time of writing this article, 3 new agents had received Food and Drug Administration approval for the use of stroke prevention in non- valvular AF: dabigatran etexilate, rivaroxaban, and apixaban. The data from trials leading to the approval of these drugs has been looked at in some detail elsewhere in this issue. In essence, the pivotal studies for each agent, in which they were compared with warfarin in nonvalvular AF, concluded *at least* noninferiority to warfarin in stroke prevention with a bleeding profile that was comparable or better.[39–41] There was a nonsignif- icant trend to increased extracranial hemorrhage in the elderly patients on higher dose (150 mg twice a day) dabigatran in the Randomized Evalu- ation of Long Term Anticoagulant Therapy (REL-Y)

study, perhaps favoring the 110 mg twice a day in this population.

The place of the NOACs in the management of AF in older patients remains to be firmly estab- lished. It is likely that a greater proportion of eligible patients with AF will now receive oral anti- coagulation therapy. Caution should be exercised when considering these agents in the very elderly, as these patients have been underrepresented in the NOAC trials, with the mean ages between 70 and 73 years. As with any new medication, ongoing surveillance on the safety and efficacy of NOACs in real-world medicine is critically important.

CATHETER ABLATION IN THE OLDER PATIENT

When discussing ablation for AF, it is important to make the distinction between ablation undertaken with the expectation of achieving SR and ablation of the atrioventricular node (AVN) combined with a pacemaker for optimizing rate control in AF. Abla- tion strategies in the nonelderly patient have been discussed elsewhere in this issue.

Catheter Ablation to Achieve SR

In appropriately selected patients with atrial fibril- lation catheter ablation of AF, with or without the use of antiarrhythmic drugs, is widely acknowl- edged as being superior to pharmacologic therapy alone in maintaining SR.[42,43] At present there are limited data that specifically address the issue of catheter ablation for the older patient with symp- tomatic AF and HF. A recent meta-analysis on the role of AF ablation in patients with HF concluded an overall improvement in symptoms and EF with catheter ablation,[44] however the mean age of patients in the studies analyzed ranged from 49 to 62 years. CABANA (catheter ablation vs antiarrhythmic drug therapy for AF) is a multicenter international randomized trial on catheter ablation for AF compared with medical therapy (without HF) targeting older patients or those with elevated stroke risk, with the primary end point of mortality. Unfortunately, the results are not yet available and we can only consider retrospective analyses and nonrandomized stu- dies to provide guidance (**Table 1**).[45–47,49–54]

There are 2 fundamental questions that need to be answered. First, is the ablation of AF in the older patient with HF effective? Second, is it safe? Neither question can be answered directly from the literature at present, but CASTLE-AF (Catheter Ablation vs Standard conventional Treatment in patients with LEft ventricular dysfunction and Atrial Fibrillation)[55] is an ongoing study aiming to

Table 1
Reported success rates for atrial fibrillation ablation in older patients

Study	No. of Patients	Age (y)	PAF (%)	Success Rate (%)	Follow-up (mo)
Bhargava et al,[45] 2004	103	>60	52	82	14.7
Bunch et al,[46] 2010	35	≥80	46	78	12
Corrado et al,[47] 2008	174	>75	55	95	20
Haegeli et al,[48] 2010	45	≥65	87	74	6
Hsieh et al,[49] 2005	37	>65	100	81	52
Kusumoto et al,[50] 2009	61	>75	34	82	12
Nademanee et al,[51] 2008	635	>65	40	81	27
Tan et al,[52] 2010	200	≥70	54	71	18
Traub et al,[53] 2009	15	≥70	100	60	12
Zado et al,[54] 2008	32	≥75	53	86	27

Abbreviation: PAF, paroxysmal atrial fibrillation.
 Data from Refs.[45–54]

address this question in patients with AF and HF without an age cutoff.

Although the number of patients in most studies is small and there is some heterogeneity in the reported success rates, catheter ablation of AF is associated with equivalent success rates to younger patients when undertaken in *highly selected* elderly patients.[56] In the series by Zado and colleagues,[54] the success rate was more than 85% in the group of patients older than 75; however, older patients were less likely to undergo a repeat ablation and more likely to remain on antiarrhythmic drugs, but only represented a small proportion of the study group overall. Similar findings on antiarrhythmic drug use after ablation were demonstrated in the series by Traub and colleagues[53] and Kusumoto and colleagues.[50]

Taken together, there are data to support the efficacy of AF ablation in nonelderly patients with HF and data to support the efficacy of AF ablation in the older patient without HF. However, we await the outcomes of large randomized studies, such as CABANA and CASTLE-AF[55] enrolling older patients with AF and structural heart disease before defining the role of catheter ablation in the older patient with AF and HF.

Safety is important in assessing the role of catheter ablation of AF in older patients with HF. In general terms, older patients are widely acknowledged to have higher complication rates for most medical or surgical interventions. Early data support this, with age older than 70 years shown to be associated with a fourfold increase in risk of major complications from AF ablation in a retrospective, single-center series reported by Spragg and colleagues.[57] This result was consistent with an earlier report by Oral and Morady[58] showing a

fourfold increase in risk of tamponade or stroke in patients older than 70 years.

However, with increasing experience and better tools to guide and deliver ablation, the procedure has become safer. More recent studies demonstrate equivalent safety in elderly compared with younger patients, although it must be acknowledged that these are *carefully selected* elderly patients.[46,47,50,53] Changes in ablation techniques combined with irrigated ablation, and refinement of periprocedural anticoagulation protocols are possibly responsible for the reduction in increased risk observed in earlier reports of ablation in the elderly.

Although there are no prospective, randomized trials to guide decision making in the elderly with AF and HF, catheter ablation appears to be effective and can be undertaken safely by experienced operators. This is reflected in the change in patient demographics reported in the most recent worldwide survey on AF reported by Cappato and colleagues.[59] Catheter ablation for AF is being undertaken in older patients and patients with worse LV function.[9,42]

Pacemaker Combined with AVN Ablation

The role of AVN ablation combined with permanent pacing is discussed in detail elsewhere.[60] AVN ablation provides effective rate control in drug-refractory AF, but must be preceded by pacemaker implantation.[61] Catheter "modification" of the AVN has also been described in an attempt to avoid pacemaker implantation, but the effects are not predictable, with potential complications, including polymorphic ventricular tachycardia or late atrioventricular block, and this is not recommended.[62,63] Brignole and colleagues[64] showed that a "pace and ablate" approach was superior to pharmacologic therapy in symptom control for AF. Significant improvement of LV function is seen in most patients following this procedure.[65] However, randomized trials support pulmonary vein isolation over AVN ablation in younger patients with AF and HF.[49,66]

AVN ablation and permanent pacing is often viewed as a more attractive therapy for the elderly.[67] However, there remains a paucity of randomized data comparing it to optimal medical therapy or catheter ablation of AF in elderly patients with AF and HF. Ablation of the AVN combined with permanent pacing does not prevent AF, and physicians must ensure appropriate anticoagulation is continued.

The choice of pacing system is important, especially in patients with HF. The clinician treating the patient with HF and uncontrolled AF with "pace and ablate" must consider whether it is appropriate to place a single-chamber pacemaker on the assumption that a tachycardia-mediated cardiomyopathy is present and will improve.[68] However, if there is a primary cardiomyopathy, chronic pacing of the right ventricle (RV) can be deleterious.[69–71] The Post AV Nodal Ablation Evaluation (PAVE) trial randomized patients (mean age 69 years and mean EF 46%) undergoing AVN ablation to receive either RV-only or biventricular pacing.[72] Biventricular pacing was shown to be superior to RV-only pacing, particularly in more severe LV function. Accordingly, major cardiology guidelines[42,73] advocate the implantation of a biventricular pacemaker to prevent deterioration in LV function when performing AVN ablation in a patient with AF and HF.[59,73]

AVN ablation is also recommended in guidelines to ensure complete biventricular capture in patients with HF and AF who already have a biventricular pacemaker implanted.[74,75] A recent meta-analysis by Ganesan and colleagues[76] reported that AVN ablation in patients with HF and biventricular pacemakers was associated with significant reductions in all-cause mortality and an improvement in NYHA functional class. The mean age of patients in this analysis ranged from 63 to 72 years.

SUMMARY

There are few randomized control trials that specifically assess the optimal management of AF in the older patient with HF. Studies are ongoing that will hopefully provide more evidence in this area.

Older patients with AF and HF are at significant risk for thromboembolic complications and should be anticoagulated unless the bleeding risk is considered prohibitive.

Rate control is equivalent to rhythm control in minimally symptomatic patients with AF. Rate control can be achieved medically, but often drugs are less well tolerated in the older patient and in these cases AVN ablation combined with biventricular pacing can be very effective.

Rhythm control for symptomatic benefit can be achieved pharmacologically or by catheter ablation, and there is growing evidence that catheter ablation of AF in older patients with HF is effective, superior to medical therapy alone, and can be delivered safely.

REFERENCES

1. Feinberg WM, Blackshear JL, Laupacis A, et al. Prevalence, age distribution, and gender of patients with atrial fibrillation. Analysis and implications. Arch Intern Med 1995;155(5):469–73.
2. Kannel WB, Belanger AJ. Epidemiology of heart failure. Am Heart J 1991;121(3 Pt 1):951–7.
3. Cleland JG, Swedberg K, Follath F, et al. The Euro-Heart Failure survey programme—a survey on the quality of care among patients with heart failure in Europe. Part 1: patient characteristics and diagnosis. Eur Heart J 2003;24(5):442–63.
4. Maisel WH, Stevenson LW. Atrial fibrillation in heart failure: epidemiology, pathophysiology, and rationale for therapy. Am J Cardiol 2003;91(6A):2D–8D.
5. Shi S, Klotz U. Age-related changes in pharmacokinetics. Curr Drug Metab 2011;12(7):601–10.
6. Wyse DG, Waldo AL, DiMarco JP, et al. A comparison of rate control and rhythm control in patients with atrial fibrillation. N Engl J Med 2002;347(23):1825–33.
7. Van Gelder IC, Hagens VE, Bosker HA, et al. A comparison of rate control and rhythm control in patients with recurrent persistent atrial fibrillation. N Engl J Med 2002;347(23):1834–40.
8. Echt DS, Liebson PR, Mitchell LB, et al. Mortality and morbidity in patients receiving encainide, flecainide, or placebo. The Cardiac Arrhythmia Suppression Trial. N Engl J Med 1991;324(12):781–8.
9. Akiyama T, Pawitan Y, Campbell WB, et al. Effects of advancing age on the efficacy and side effects of antiarrhythmic drugs in post-myocardial infarction patients with ventricular arrhythmias. The CAST Investigators. J Am Geriatr Soc 1992;40(7):666–72.
10. Fuster V, Ryden LE, Cannom DS, et al. ACC/AHA/ESC 2006 Guidelines for the Management of Patients with Atrial Fibrillation: a report of the American College of Cardiology/American Heart Association Task Force on Practice Guidelines and the European Society of Cardiology Committee

for Practice Guidelines (Writing Committee to Revise the 2001 Guidelines for the Management of Patients With Atrial Fibrillation): developed in collaboration with the European Heart Rhythm Association and the Heart Rhythm Society. Circulation 2006;114(7):e257–354.

11. Van Gelder IC, Groenveld HF, Crijns HJ, et al. Lenient versus strict rate control in patients with atrial fibrillation. N Engl J Med 2010;362(15): 1363–73.

12. Freudenberger RS, Wilson AC, Kostis JB. Comparison of rate versus rhythm control for atrial fibrillation in patients with left ventricular dysfunction (from the AFFIRM Study). Am J Cardiol 2007; 100(2):247–52.

13. Corley SD, Epstein AE, DiMarco JP, et al. Relationships between sinus rhythm, treatment, and survival in the Atrial Fibrillation Follow-Up Investigation of Rhythm Management (AFFIRM) Study. Circulation 2004;109(12):1509–13.

14. Roy D, Talajic M, Nattel S, et al. Rhythm control versus rate control for atrial fibrillation and heart failure. N Engl J Med 2008;358(25):2667–77.

15. Shelton RJ, Clark AL, Goode K, et al. A randomised, controlled study of rate versus rhythm control in patients with chronic atrial fibrillation and heart failure: (CAFE-II Study). Heart 2009; 95(11):924–30.

16. Camm AJ, Lip GY, De Caterina R, et al. 2012 focused update of the ESC Guidelines for the management of atrial fibrillation: an update of the 2010 ESC Guidelines for the management of atrial fibrillation. Developed with the special contribution of the European Heart Rhythm Association. Eur Heart J 2012;33(21):2719–47.

17. Wann LS, Curtis AB, Ellenbogen KA, et al. 2011 ACCF/AHA/HRS focused update on the management of patients with atrial fibrillation (update on dabigatran). A report of the American College of Cardiology Foundation/American Heart Association Task Force on Practice Guidelines. Heart Rhythm 2011;8(3):e1–8.

18. Singh BN, Singh SN, Reda DJ, et al. Amiodarone versus sotalol for atrial fibrillation. N Engl J Med 2005;352(18):1861–72.

19. Hunt SA, Abraham WT, Chin MH, et al. 2009 Focused update incorporated into the ACC/AHA 2005 Guidelines for the Diagnosis and Management of Heart Failure in Adults. A report of the American College of Cardiology Foundation/American Heart Association Task Force on Practice Guidelines developed in collaboration with the International Society for Heart and Lung Transplantation. J Am Coll Cardiol 2009;53(15):e1–90.

20. Flather MD, Shibata MC, Coats AJ, et al. Randomized trial to determine the effect of nebivolol on mortality and cardiovascular hospital admission in elderly patients with heart failure (SENIORS). Eur Heart J 2005;26(3):215–25.

21. Mulder BA, van Veldhuisen DJ, Crijns HJ, et al. Effect of nebivolol on outcome in elderly patients with heart failure and atrial fibrillation: insights from SENIORS. Eur J Heart Fail 2012;14(10): 1171–8.

22. Poole-Wilson PA, Swedberg K, Cleland JG, et al. Comparison of carvedilol and metoprolol on clinical outcomes in patients with chronic heart failure in the Carvedilol Or Metoprolol European Trial (COMET): randomised controlled trial. Lancet 2003;362(9377):7–13.

23. Ahmed A, Rich MW, Love TE, et al. Digoxin and reduction in mortality and hospitalization in heart failure: a comprehensive post hoc analysis of the DIG trial. Eur Heart J 2006;27(2):178–86.

24. Khand AU, Rankin AC, Martin W, et al. Carvedilol alone or in combination with digoxin for the management of atrial fibrillation in patients with heart failure? J Am Coll Cardiol 2003;42(11):1944–51.

25. Ulimoen SR, Enger S, Carlson J, et al. Comparison of four single-drug regimens on ventricular rate and arrhythmia-related symptoms in patients with permanent atrial fibrillation. Am J Cardiol 2013; 111(2):225–30.

26. Lin HJ, Wolf PA, Kelly-Hayes M, et al. Stroke severity in atrial fibrillation. The Framingham Study. Stroke 1996;27(10):1760–4.

27. Wolf PA, Abbott RD, Kannel WB. Atrial fibrillation as an independent risk factor for stroke: the Framingham Study. Stroke 1991;22(8):983–8.

28. Olesen JB, Lip GY, Hansen ML, et al. Validation of risk stratification schemes for predicting stroke and thromboembolism in patients with atrial fibrillation: nationwide cohort study. BMJ 2011;342:d124.

29. Fang MC, Go AS, Hylek EM, et al. Age and the risk of warfarin-associated hemorrhage: the anticoagulation and risk factors in atrial fibrillation study. J Am Geriatr Soc 2006;54(8):1231–6.

30. Rash A, Downes T, Portner R, et al. A randomised controlled trial of warfarin versus aspirin for stroke prevention in octogenarians with atrial fibrillation (WASPO). Age Ageing 2007;36(2):151–6.

31. Mant J, Hobbs FD, Fletcher K, et al. Warfarin versus aspirin for stroke prevention in an elderly community population with atrial fibrillation (the Birmingham Atrial Fibrillation Treatment of the Aged Study, BAFTA): a randomised controlled trial. Lancet 2007;370(9586):493–503.

32. Friberg L, Rosenqvist M, Lip GY. Evaluation of risk stratification schemes for ischaemic stroke and bleeding in 182 678 patients with atrial fibrillation: the Swedish Atrial Fibrillation cohort study. Eur Heart J 2012;33(12):1500–10.

33. Nieuwlaat R, Capucci A, Camm AJ, et al. Atrial fibrillation management: a prospective survey in

ESC member countries: the Euro Heart Survey on Atrial Fibrillation. Eur Heart J 2005;26(22):2422–34.

34. Man San Hing M, Laupacis A. Anticoagulant related bleeding in older persons with atrial fibrillation: physicians' fears often unfounded. Arch Intern Med 2003;163(13):1580–6.

35. Fang MC, Go AS, Chang Y, et al. A new risk scheme to predict warfarin-associated hemorrhage: the ATRIA (Anticoagulation and Risk Factors in Atrial Fibrillation) Study. J Am Coll Cardiol 2011; 58(4):395–401.

36. Pisters R, Lane DA, Nieuwlaat R, et al. A novel user-friendly score (HAS-BLED) to assess 1-year risk of major bleeding in patients with atrial fibrillation: the Euro Heart Survey. Chest 2010;138(5):1093–100.

37. Holbrook AM, Pereira JA, Labiris R, et al. Systematic overview of warfarin and its drug and food interactions. Arch Intern Med 2005;165(10): 1095–106.

38. De Caterina R, Husted S, Wallentin L, et al. New oral anticoagulants in atrial fibrillation and acute coronary syndromes: ESC Working Group on Thrombosis-Task Force on Anticoagulants in Heart Disease position paper. J Am Coll Cardiol 2012; 59(16):1413–25.

39. Connolly SJ, Ezekowitz MD, Yusuf S, et al. Dabigatran versus warfarin in patients with atrial fibrillation. N Engl J Med 2009;361(12):1139–51.

40. Granger CB, Alexander JH, McMurray JJ, et al. Apixaban versus warfarin in patients with atrial fibrillation. N Engl J Med 2011;365(11):981–92.

41. Patel MR, Mahaffey KW, Garg J, et al. Rivaroxaban versus warfarin in nonvalvular atrial fibrillation. N Engl J Med 2011;365(10):883–91.

42. Camm AJ, Lip GY, De Caterina R, et al. 2012 focused update of the ESC Guidelines for the management of atrial fibrillation: an update of the 2010 ESC Guidelines for the management of atrial fibrillation—developed with the special contribution of the European Heart Rhythm Association. Europace 2012;14(10):1385–413.

43. Wilber DJ, Pappone C, Neuzil P, et al. Comparison of antiarrhythmic drug therapy and radiofrequency catheter ablation in patients with paroxysmal atrial fibrillation: a randomized controlled trial. JAMA 2010;303(4):333–40.

44. Dagres N, Varounis C, Gaspar T, et al. Catheter ablation for atrial fibrillation in patients with left ventricular systolic dysfunction. A systematic review and meta-analysis. J Card Fail 2011;17(11):964–70.

45. Bhargava M, Marrouche NF, Martin DO, et al. Impact of age on the outcome of pulmonary vein isolation for atrial fibrillation using circular mapping technique and cooled-tip ablation catheter. J Cardiovasc Electrophysiol 2004;15(1):8–13.

46. Bunch TJ, Weiss JP, Crandall BG, et al. Long-term clinical efficacy and risk of catheter ablation for atrial fibrillation in octogenarians. Pacing Clin Electrophysiol 2010;33(2):146–52.

47. Corrado A, Patel D, Riedlbauchova L, et al. Efficacy, safety, and outcome of atrial fibrillation ablation in septuagenarians. J Cardiovasc Electrophysiol 2008;19(8):807–11.

48. Haegeli LM, Duru F, Lockwood EE, et al. Ablation of atrial fibrillation after the retirement age: considerations on safety and outcome. J Interv Card Electrophysiol 2010;28(3):193–7.

49. Hsieh MH, Tai CT, Lee SH, et al. Catheter ablation of atrial fibrillation versus atrioventricular junction ablation plus pacing therapy for elderly patients with medically refractory paroxysmal atrial fibrillation. J Cardiovasc Electrophysiol 2005;16(5):457–61.

50. Kusumoto F, Prussak K, Wiesinger M, et al. Radiofrequency catheter ablation of atrial fibrillation in older patients: outcomes and complications. J Interv Card Electrophysiol 2009;25(1):31–5.

51. Nademanee K, Schwab MC, Kosar EM, et al. Clinical outcomes of catheter substrate ablation for high-risk patients with atrial fibrillation. J Am Coll Cardiol 2008;51(8):843–9.

52. Tan HW, Wang XH, Shi HF, et al. Efficacy, safety and outcome of catheter ablation for atrial fibrillation in octogenarians. Int J Cardiol 2010;145(1): 147–8.

53. Traub D, Daubert JP, McNitt S, et al. Catheter ablation of atrial fibrillation in the elderly: where do we stand? Cardiol J 2009;16(2):113–20.

54. Zado E, Callans DJ, Riley M, et al. Long-term clinical efficacy and risk of catheter ablation for atrial fibrillation in the elderly. J Cardiovasc Electrophysiol 2008;19(6):621–6.

55. Marrouche NF, Brachmann J. Catheter ablation versus standard conventional treatment in patients with left ventricular dysfunction and atrial fibrillation (CASTLE-AF)—study design. Pacing Clin Electrophysiol 2009;32(8):987–94.

56. Yamada T, Kay GN. Catheter ablation of atrial fibrillation in the elderly. Pacing Clin Electrophysiol 2009;32(8):1085–91.

57. Spragg DD, Dalal D, Cheema A, et al. Complications of catheter ablation for atrial fibrillation: incidence and predictors. J Cardiovasc Electrophysiol 2008;19(6):627–31.

58. Oral H, Morady F. How to select patients for atrial fibrillation ablation. Heart Rhythm 2006;3(5):615–8.

59. Cappato R, Calkins H, Chen SA, et al. Updated worldwide survey on the methods, efficacy, and safety of catheter ablation for human atrial fibrillation. Circ Arrhythm Electrophysiol 2010;3(1):32–8.

60. Hoffmayer KS, Scheinman M. Current role of atrioventricular junction (AVJ) ablation. Pacing Clin Electrophysiol 2013;36(2):257–65.

61. Langberg JJ, Chin M, Schamp DJ, et al. Ablation of the atrioventricular junction with radiofrequency

energy using a new electrode catheter. Am J Cardiol 1991;67(2):142–7.

62. Menozzi C, Brignole M, Gianfranchi L, et al. Radiofrequency catheter ablation and modulation of atrioventricular conduction in patients with atrial fibrillation. Pacing Clin Electrophysiol 1994;17(11 Pt 2):2143–9.

63. Morady F, Hasse C, Strickberger SA, et al. Long-term follow-up after radiofrequency modification of the atrioventricular node in patients with atrial fibrillation. J Am Coll Cardiol 1997;29(1):113–21.

64. Brignole M, Menozzi C, Gianfranchi L, et al. Assessment of atrioventricular junction ablation and VVIR pacemaker versus pharmacological treatment in patients with heart failure and chronic atrial fibrillation: a randomized, controlled study. Circulation 1998;98(10):953–60.

65. Wood MA, Brown-Mahoney C, Kay GN, et al. Clinical outcomes after ablation and pacing therapy for atrial fibrillation: a meta-analysis. Circulation 2000; 101(10):1138–44.

66. Khan MN, Jais P, Cummings J, et al. Pulmonary-vein isolation for atrial fibrillation in patients with heart failure. N Engl J Med 2008;359(17):1778–85.

67. Hindricks G. The Multicentre European Radiofrequency Survey (MERFS): complications of radiofrequency catheter ablation of arrhythmias. The Multicentre European Radiofrequency Survey (MERFS) investigators of the Working Group on Arrhythmias of the European Society of Cardiology. Eur Heart J 1993;14(12):1644–53.

68. Lemery R, Brugada P, Cheriex E, et al. Reversibility of tachycardia-induced left ventricular dysfunction after closed-chest catheter ablation of the atrioventricular junction for intractable atrial fibrillation. Am J Cardiol 1987;60(16):1406–8.

69. Leong DP, Mitchell AM, Salna I, et al. Long-term mechanical consequences of permanent right ventricular pacing: effect of pacing site. J Cardiovasc Electrophysiol 2010;21(10):1120–6.

70. Sharma AD, Rizo-Patron C, Hallstrom AP, et al. Percent right ventricular pacing predicts outcomes in the DAVID trial. Heart Rhythm 2005;2(8):830–4.

71. Wilkoff BL, Cook JR, Epstein AE, et al. Dual-chamber pacing or ventricular backup pacing in patients with an implantable defibrillator: the Dual Chamber and VVI Implantable Defibrillator (DAVID) Trial. JAMA 2002;288(24):3115–23.

72. Doshi RN, Daoud EG, Fellows C, et al. Left ventricular-based cardiac stimulation post AV nodal ablation evaluation (the PAVE study). J Cardiovasc Electrophysiol 2005;16(11):1160–5.

73. Fuster V, Ryden LE, Cannom DS, et al. 2011 ACCF/AHA/HRS focused updates incorporated into the ACC/AHA/ESC 2006 Guidelines for the management of patients with atrial fibrillation: a report of the American College of Cardiology Foundation/American Heart Association Task Force on Practice Guidelines developed in partnership with the European Society of Cardiology and in collaboration with the European Heart Rhythm Association and the Heart Rhythm Society. J Am Coll Cardiol 2011;57(11):e101–98.

74. Dickstein K, Vardas PE, Auricchio A, et al. 2010 Focused Update of ESC Guidelines on device therapy in heart failure: an update of the 2008 ESC Guidelines for the diagnosis and treatment of acute and chronic heart failure and the 2007 ESC Guidelines for cardiac and resynchronization therapy. Developed with the special contribution of the Heart Failure Association and the European Heart Rhythm Association. Europace 2010;12(11):1526–36.

75. Epstein AE, Dimarco JP, Ellenbogen KA, et al. ACC/AHA/HRS 2008 guidelines for Device-Based Therapy of Cardiac Rhythm Abnormalities: executive summary. Heart Rhythm 2008;5(6):934–55.

76. Ganesan AN, Brooks AG, Roberts-Thomson KC, et al. Role of AV nodal ablation in cardiac resynchronization in patients with coexistent atrial fibrillation and heart failure. J Am Coll Cardiol 2012;59(8):719–26.

Case Selection for Cardiac Resynchronization in Atrial Fibrillation

John G.F. Cleland, MD, FRCP, FESC*,
Freidoon Keshavarzi, MD, MRCP, Pierpaolo Pellicori, MD,
Benjamin Dicken, MBBS, MRCP

KEYWORDS

- Cardiac resynchronization therapy • Atrial fibrillation • Atrioventricular resynchronization
- Biventricular capture • Heart failure

KEY POINTS

- Several guidelines make strong recommendations in favor of cardiac resynchronization therapy (CRT) for patients with atrial fibrillation (AF); however, avoiding implantation of CRT in patients with AF is more consistent with current evidence and reasonable clinical practice.
- Circumstances in which implantation of CRT into patients with AF should at least be considered include (1) those in whom a return to sinus rhythm is anticipated; (2) as a last resort in patients who lack better alternatives; and, perhaps, (3) patients with AF who otherwise are indicated for CRT and are about to receive either a standard pacemaker or an implantable defibrillator.
- Biventricular pacing cannot be effective unless AV conduction is suppressed.
- Failure of biventricular capture might explain the lack of benefit of CRT in AF; however, providing a possible explanation for failure does not constitute proof of efficacy. Further trials are required.

BACKGROUND

The prevalence of atrial fibrillation (AF) ranges from about 5% in patients with asymptomatic cardiac dysfunction to more than 50% of those with severe symptomatic heart failure.[1,2] In many patients, the onset of heart failure and AF coincide. Hypertension and coronary disease will often cause chronic cardiac dysfunction that progresses silently until symptoms are precipitated by an event such as the onset of AF or acute myocardial infarction.[3–5] In this sense, AF is the cause of heart failure, although rarely in isolation. Aggressive restoration of sinus rhythm may improve symptoms and quality of life in selected patients, although this has not yet been translated into an improvement in outcome.[6,7] The benefits of restoring sinus rhythm

in the one large trial that addressed this issue may have been offset by the adverse effects of amiodarone.[6]

The onset of AF in patients with preexisting heart failure indicates a poor prognosis.[8] Patients who develop heart failure as a consequence of AF (about 75% of those admitted when these two conditions coexist) have a better outcome than those who develop AF after the onset of heart failure.[9] Patients with chronic heart failure receiving contemporary therapy for heart failure, including beta-blockers, have a similar outcome, after adjusting for age and symptom severity, whether they are in persistent AF or in sinus rhythm, although patients with left bundle branch block might have a worse prognosis if in AF.[8,10,11]

Disclosures: Professor Cleland has received honoraria from Medtronic, Sorin and St Jude within the last 5 years for speaking at symposia and on advisory committees. Prof Cleland and Dr Dicken are investigators for the RESPOND study, funded by Sorin.
Department of Cardiology, Castle Hill Hospital, Hull York Medical School, University of Hull, Kingston-upon-Hull HU6 5JQ, UK
* Corresponding author.
E-mail address: j.g.cleland@hull.ac.uk

Heart Failure Clin 9 (2013) 461–474
http://dx.doi.org/10.1016/j.hfc.2013.07.001
1551-7136/13/$ – see front matter © 2013 Elsevier Inc. All rights reserved.

heartfailure.theclinics.com

Among patients with an implanted device that can record atrial arrhythmias, otherwise undetected paroxysmal AF may be present in more than 40% of patients[12–21]; when the burden is high (>3.8 hours per day), the risk of thromboembolic events, hospitalization for heart failure, and death increases substantially.[18] Studies in patients with less severe disease have also noted that only prolonged episodes of AF (>18 hours) seem to predict adverse outcomes.[22,23] Preimplant history is important both for predicting recurrent AF and the subsequent risk of embolic events.[18] About one-third of patients with a prior history of AF will develop a clinical overt recurrence in the following 1 to 2 years compared with about 10% without such a history (**Table 1**).[12–21] Device-detected episodes lasting more than 24 hours probably occur in only 5% to 10% of those without a history of AF but perhaps more than 20% of those with such a history (see **Table 1**). Clearly, AF is an important issue for many patients both before and after the implantation of a CRT device.

Pharmacologic treatment of heart failure can alter the risk of developing AF. Angiotensin-converting enzyme inhibitors, beta-blockers, and aldosterone antagonists have all been shown to reduce the incidence of AF in patients with heart failure and left ventricular systolic dysfunction (LVSD), whereas ivabradine, an agent that slows the rate of sinus node discharge, has been shown to increase the risk of AF.[1,2,24,25] The presence of AF may also alter the impact of treatment on the outcome. Patients with AF and LVSD do not seem to benefit from beta-1-selective blockers and may have a reduced response to carvedilol.[26] Drug therapy aimed at rhythm control for AF does not seem to improve the outcome of patients with heart failure and LVSD.[6] For patients in sinus rhythm, the optimal heart rate seems to be between 50 to 60 beats per minute (bpm); but for patients in AF, the optimal resting ventricular rate as observed in the clinic seems to be closer to 80 bpm.[27–29] The reason for this difference in optimal heart rate is unknown but could be related to excessive slowing of nocturnal ventricular rate with increased exposure to pause-dependent ventricular tachycardia.[29–31]

POTENTIAL MECHANISMS OF BENEFIT OF CARDIAC RESYNCHRONIZATION THERAPY

There is no doubt that cardiac resynchronization therapy (CRT) works, but exactly how it works remains elusive. It is likely that there are at least 4 major mechanisms in play, with the relative importance of each varying from one patient to the next and, perhaps, over time.

Studies attempting to predict the benefit from CRT have come up with remarkably little evidence to support any particular patient characteristic before implantation other than the QRS duration.[32] There are lots of observational studies purporting to show differences according to sex, cause of ventricular dysfunction, or QRS morphology; but these fail to disentangle factors reflecting the natural history of the disease from the effects of CRT. Identifying markers that predict the response to intervention rather than merely predictors of outcome in patients who have had the intervention requires randomized trials.[33] Further confusion has been caused by using improvements in LV function as a surrogate for response. It is true that patients with dilated cardiomyopathy have a greater improvement in LV function in response to CRT and a better prognosis compared with patients with ischemic heart disease (IHD). However, the change in prognosis wrought by CRT is similar or greater in patients with IHD.[32,34–36] So in population terms, if we want to improve the echocardiogram, we should implant CRT devices into patients with dilated cardiomyopathy; but if we want to prolong life, then we should choose to implant them into patients with LVSD caused by IHD.

Studies conducted at the time of CRT implantation provide some further insights into the likely mechanisms of benefit from CRT. The LV pacing site seems to be important. Pacing scarred regions should be avoided. Pacing regions exhibiting dyssynchrony that are far from the right ventricular (RV) pacing site seem successful.[37,38] The choice of LV pacing site can make a large difference to the effects of CRT on raising blood pressure, a candidate predictor of the longer-term benefits of CRT.[37,39]

Randomized controlled trials of device programming after implantation have been marred by the inclusion of all-comers, whether they have responded to the initial implantation or not and, therefore, provide little help in determining the importance of individualized programming among patients with a poor response to CRT.[40–44] Many patients respond to the standard factory CRT settings and may not benefit from reprogramming. Acute studies of programming suggest little effect of altering the inter-ventricular (VV) pacing interval on blood pressure or cardiac function in most patients but substantial differences with atrioventricular (AV) programming.[45,46] This finding implies that AV resynchronization might be more clinically important than VV resynchronization, as also suggested by a recent analysis of the MADIT-CRT (Multicenter Automatic Defibrillator Implantation with Cardiac Resynchronization Therapy) study.[47] If this is true, then CRT may deliver little or even no

Table 1
Studies investigating the incidence of AF in patients receiving CRT (where n >100)

Author, Pub Year	PAF if Reported	N =	Age (y)	IHD (%)	FU	Min Dur AF	AF: Device Diagnostics (%)	AF: Clinical n = (%)	Effect of AF on Clinical Outcome
Puglisi et al,[12] 2008	No	249	69	—	13 mo	>5 min (24 h)	42 (6)	—	Reduced activity
	Yes	161	—	—			47 (22)	—	
Borleffs et al,[13] 2009	No	223	—	—	32 mo	—	25	unknown	Less improvement
Caldwell et al,[14] 2009	No	101	66	60	—	30 s	27	—	Higher mortality if AF
	Yes	18	—		—		High	—	
Leclerq et al, 2010	No	82	70	28	6 mo	—	17	—	Less improvement
	Yes	38	—			—	29	—	
Marijon et al,[16] 2010	No	173	70	—	10 mo	—	28	—	Predicted clinical AF
Boriani et al,[17] 2011	—	1404	—	—	—	—	32	—	—
Shanmugam et al,[18] 2012	—	560	66	54	—	—	—	—	—
CARE-HF Control,[66] 2005	No	314	67	—	29 mo	—	Not applicable	30 (10)	Outcome worse in patients who developed AF who were assigned to either strategy; some attenuation of effect of CRT on M/M
	Yes	90						28 (31)	
CARE-HF CRT	No	330				>10 min (48 h)	93 (28)[a]	40 (12)	
	Yes	79					20 (25)[a]	26 (33)	
Padeletti et al,[20] 2008	No	323	68	49	12 mo	—	unknown	26 (8)	—
	Yes	71	—	—	—	—	unknown	25 (35)	—
MADIT-CRT 2011	—	1820	—	—	—	—	8	—	—
Santini et al,[21] 2011	—	—	—	—	13 mo	—	30	—	—

Abbreviations: Dur, duration; FU, follow-up; IHD, ischemic heart disease; MADIT-CRT, multicenter automatic defibrillator implantation with cardiac resynchronization therapy trial; Min, minimum; M/M, morbidity and mortality; PAF, paroxysmal atrial fibrillation; Pub, publication.
[a] This value does not include patients who were detected during clinical follow-up.
Data from Refs.[12–21,75]

benefit in the absence of atrial systole. However, the most striking marker of super response is the correction of mitral regurgitation.[34,48] The effects of CRT on mitral regurgitation are almost immediate,[34] and it is possible that it is the ventricular stimulation site that exerts the greater reduction in mitral regurgitation that is the optimal pacing site. Clearly, only patients who have mitral regurgitation can benefit from CRT by this mechanism.

To summarize, of the 4 likely main mechanisms of CRT benefit, 3 can be observed at the initial clinical assessment and are (1) correction of ventricular dyssynchrony; (2) correction of AV dyssynchrony including diastolic mitral regurgitation; and (3) reduction, when present, of mitral systolic regurgitation by resynchronizing papillary muscle contraction. These effects are then likely to lead to favorable LV remodeling, especially if the left ventricle is not heavily scarred. The fourth mechanism, the effects of CRT on arrhythmias, still requires longer-term verification and may be secondary to ventricular remodeling or caused by the prevention of pauses.

Patients with AF cannot benefit from AV resynchronization and can only benefit from VV resynchronization if ventricular capture occurs. This requires AV conduction to be slow or absent, which may be achieved by AV conduction system disease, by drugs, or (most reliably) by AV ablation. It is also possible that a more regular ventricular rhythm may improve cardiac performance as varying ventricular filling periods may lead to wide variations in filling pressures and autonomic feedback from one cardiac cycle to the next and long diastolic periods will lead to diastolic mitral regurgitation. The alternative to controlling ventricular rate is to try and restore sinus rhythm, either by pharmacologic or electrical cardioversion or by catheter ablation.[49,50]

CRT could affect the incidence of several arrhythmias. Reductions in atrial pressure should lead to a reduction in recurrent AF. Although some observational trials have suggested that CRT may reduce the AF burden according to the device diagnostics, randomized trials have been unable to show an effect on clinically relevant AF,[19,51] although longer-term follow-up suggests there may be delayed benefits perhaps consequent on late ventricular remodeling.[52] Possibly, the presence of a wire and the associated fibrotic reaction in the atrial wall is a stimulus to developing AF that negates the early hemodynamic benefits of CRT. However, it is likely, as with most treatments, that some patients benefit and some are harmed. With respect to the incidence of AF, harm and benefit seem to be in equilibrium.

CRT could also reduce the risk of ventricular arrhythmias. In the MADIT-CRT trial, implantation of CRT-defibrillator (D) rather than an implantable cardioverter defibrillator (ICD) was associated with a lower rate of ventricular arrhythmias requiring therapy, although there was no difference in mortality.[53] In CARE-HF (Cardiac Resynchronization-Heart Failure) trial, the implantation of a CRT pacemaker was associated with a reduction in sudden death compared with medical treatment alone.[36,53] The reduction in sudden death may have occurred only after the first year of follow-up, suggesting that ventricular remodeling may have played a role. However, it is possible that the greatest effect of CRT is in preventing pauses that represent a potentially significant direct cause of sudden death in advanced heart failure or a trigger for ventricular tachycardia.[31] This effect will only be observed in studies if the comparator group has no device. An important effect of CRT on prognosis may be its ability to prevent pauses without exacerbating dyssynchrony.

MANAGING AF IN PATIENTS WITH HEART FAILURE

Although there is no substantial study specifically investigating anticoagulants in patients with heart failure and AF, subgroup analyses and consensus generally support the use of anticoagulants.[54] Some observational trials have not supported this view.[55]

As noted earlier, the optimal ventricular rate in patients with heart failure and AF is uncertain and may be substantially higher than for patients in sinus rhythm.[29] Beta-blockers reduce the sympathetically driven component of heart rate, predominantly during the daytime and exercise; digoxin enhances the parasympathetic component, predominantly at rest and at night.[56] Beta-1-selective blockers seem less effective in improving the outcome of patients with heart failure if they are in AF rather than sinus rhythm.[9] The effects of digoxin on the outcome in patients with heart failure and AF remain unclear.[57]

Restoring sinus rhythm is intuitively appealing providing that treatment is not more toxic than the disease. The potential prognostic benefits of restoring the sinus rhythm with amiodarone or dronedarone seem to be neutralized by adverse effects of these drugs, although they might still improve the quality of life for some patients.[58–61] The benefits and risks of AV node or catheter ablation have not yet been adequately studied.[50] One small study suggested that pulmonary vein isolation was superior to biventricular pacing with AV node ablation in patients with heart failure and AF, again suggesting the importance of restoring atrial function and AV synchrony.[50] Another recent study in which 52 patients, most of whom did not have CRT devices, were randomly assigned to pharmacological ventricular rate control or pulmonary vein ablation, suggested that the latter strategy was associated with a greater improvement in quality of life and exercise capacity.[62] The rate and consequences of silent cerebral infarction after catheter ablation for AF are incompletely understood.[63] Unfortunately, a randomized trial of atrial overdrive pacing in patients with CRT failed to alter the incidence of AF.[20]

A further problem associated with AF in patients who receive a defibrillator in addition to CRT is an increased risk of inappropriate shocks, although contemporary conservative programming schemes with longer diagnostic delays (typically 20–30 beats) and widespread use of beta-blockers that reduce the risk of rapid ventricular response rates may have reduced this problem.[64,65]

CLINICAL EVIDENCE FOR CRT

Observational data are an unreliable guide to the benefits of therapy, especially when putative benefits, such as symptoms or ventricular function, have such a large subjective component.

When interpreting a clinical trial, it is important to consider what is being compared. Whether or not to implant a CRT device in patients on a background of pharmacologic therapy is one question (CARE-HF,[66] COMPANION [Comparison of Medical Therapy, Pacing, and Defibrillation in Heart Failure][67]); but whether or not to implant CRT or a backup pacemaker (MUSTIC [Multisite Stimulation in Cardiomyopathies],[68,69] MIRACLE [Multicenter InSync ICD Randomized Clinical Evaluation],[70] REVERSE [Resynchronization Reverses Remodelling in Systolic Left Ventricular Dysfunction trial][71]) or an ICD (MIRACLE-ICD,[72] MADIT-CRT,[73] REVERSE,[71] and RAFT [Resynchronization for Ambulatory Heart Failure Trial][74]) is quite another. The full potential range of CRT's benefit and harm can only be properly addressed in studies that have a device-free control group. Most studies comparing CRT with a control device programmed backup pacing at relatively low rates; this will have prevented profound bradycardia and its consequences. Studies comparing biventricular pacing and RV pacing after AV node ablation should be interpreted with caution. It is likely that AV node ablation with RV pacing is deleterious in patients with LVSD, although it may be innocuous in those without heart failure. This topic is discussed later. Better outcomes with biventricular pacing after

AV node ablation may indicate that it is less harmful than RV pacing but do not prove that it is better or safer than avoiding AV node ablation in the first place.

RANDOMIZED TRIALS OF CRT OR CRT-D COMPARED WITH NO DEVICE

The COMPANION study has not reported information on AF. In CARE-HF, patients assigned to CRT were slightly more likely to develop clinically overt AF.[19] This finding could reflect an increased rate of clinical detection of AF caused by the presence of the device, in addition to the obvious increase in detection of asymptomatic AF. Patients with new-onset AF did have a worse outcome, but this was largely explained by their intrinsically worse prognostic profile before the onset of AF. Prior history of AF, left atrial systolic volume, and plasma concentration of NT-proBNP predicted the development of AF.[19] The development of AF did not seem to detract from the benefits of CRT. Several explanations of these findings should be considered: CRT may have delivered benefits before AF developed; AF may have reverted spontaneously or with treatment; ventricular rate control may have been sufficient to ensure a high rate of ventricular capture; or it could be that simply preventing excessive bradycardia in these patients may be beneficial. In other words, CARE-HF does not provide robust evidence that CRT is effective in patients with AF.

RANDOMIZED TRIALS OF CRT COMPARED WITH BACKUP PACING WITHOUT AV NODE ABLATION

The MIRACLE studies have not reported information on AF. MADIT-CRT showed no overall difference between CRT-D and ICD on device-related occurrence of atrial arrhythmias, although the analysis suggested that patients who developed a marked reduction in left atrial volume had a lower incidence of atrial arrhythmias and a markedly better prognosis.[75] In this sense, the left atrium seems to be a good barometer of LV and overall cardiac performance. The RAFT study failed to show a difference between treatments in patients with AF despite a powerful reduction in morbidity and mortality in patients in sinus rhythm (**Fig. 1**).[76] However, only one patient received AV node ablation, and insufficient ventricular rate control probably prevented a high rate of biventricular capture. RAFT did suggest trends to improved quality of life and reductions in heart failure hospitalization among patients with AF.[76]

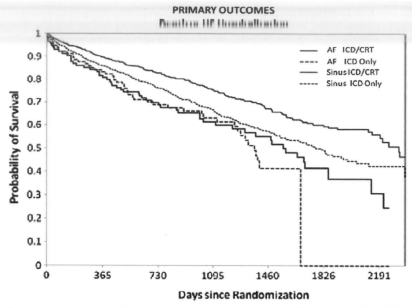

Fig. 1. Effects of cardiac resynchronization on the primary outcome of death or heart failure (HF) hospitalization. (*From* Healey JS, Hohnloser SH, Exner DV, et al, RAFT Investigators. Cardiac resynchronization therapy in patients with permanent atrial fibrillation: results from the Resynchronization for Ambulatory Heart Failure Trial (RAFT). Circ Heart Fail 2012;5(5):568; with permission.)

RANDOMIZED TRIALS COMPARING AV NODE ABLATION AND PACING WITH MEDICAL THERAPY

Although some advocate routine AV node ablation to ensure high rates of ventricular capture, others suggest that AV node ablation is only required in a minority of patients.[77–79]

There are no relevant randomized trials among patients with heart failure and a low LV ejection fraction (LVEF). A meta-analysis of trials including 314 patients mostly with a normal ejection fraction has been conducted.[80] Symptoms generally improved with AV node ablation, but there was insufficient information to identify whether the procedure increased or reduced risks. In a subgroup with a mean ejection fraction of 44%, a 4% improvement in ejection fraction was observed. Many experts advise an increased ventricular pacing rate after AV node ablation to reduce the risk of sudden death.[80,81]

RANDOMIZED TRIALS OF CRT COMPARED WITH BACKUP PACING WITH ROUTINE AV NODE ABLATION

Five trials (**Table 2**), including 637 patients, have compared RV backup pacing with CRT, although only one, MUSTIC-AF, was conducted exclusively in patients with heart failure and a LVEF of 35% or less.[82] Overall, these trials suggested a favorable

trend on mortality (risk ratio 0.75, 95% confidence interval [CI] 0.43–1.30; $P = .30$), a substantial reduction in hospitalization for heart failure (risk ratio 0.38, 95% CI 0.17–0.85; $P = .02$), and improvement in LVEF by about 2% but no benefit on quality of life or walking distance.[82,83] The results of MUSTIC-AF are consistent with the pooled data.[69] The largest of these studies was the PAVE (Post AV Nodal Ablation Evaluation) study, which enrolled 252 patients with a mean LVEF of 46%.[84] By 6 months, patients assigned to CRT improved their 6-minute walk test more than those assigned to RV pacing. LVEF was unchanged with CRT but decreased with RV pacing. The deterioration in LV function with RV pacing may have accounted for the significantly worse survival of those assigned to RV pacing.

Two small, randomized, crossover trials have compared LV pacing with CRT in patients with AF. One trial of 13 patients suggested that cardiac function and symptom improvement might be superior with CRT compared with LV pacing.[85] The other trial of 56 patients suggested little incremental benefit of either LV pacing or CRT compared with RV pacing on symptoms or walking distance; but both LV pacing and CRT improved LVEF, LV volumes, and mitral regurgitation by similar amounts.[86]

Other studies, such as RD-HF,[87] Homburg Biventricular Pacing Evaluation,[88] and BLOCK-HF (Biventricular Pacing for Atrio-ventricular Block

Table 2
Randomized trials of CRT compared with backup pacing with routine AV node ablation

Comparison	Reference	N with AF	Comparison	Outcome
CRT vs no device			No relevant trials	
CRT vs backup pacing without AVNA	RAFT	229	ICD vs CRT-D	No benefit
RCTs of AVNA	AVERT-AF[90]	180	ICD vs CRT-D + AVNA	Ongoing
	CAAN-HF	550	CRT-D vs CRT-D + AVNA	Ongoing (ClinicalTrials.gov: NCT01522898)
	RAFT-AF	1000	Rhythm control (drugs ± CA) vs rate control (drugs ± AVNA and pacing)	ClinicalTrials.gov: NCT01420393
RCTs of device after routine AVNA	Meta-analysis[82]		RVP (± ICD) vs CRT-D	Favorable trend on mortality. Significant reduction in hospitalizations for heart failure.

Abbreviations: AVNA, atrioventricular node ablation; CA, catheter ablation; CAAN-HF, cardiac resynchronization therapy and AV nodal ablation trial in atrial fibrillation; RCTs, randomized controlled trials; RVP, right ventricular pacing.

and Systolic Dysfunction in Heart Failure),[89] have compared RV pacing with CRT in patients with high-grade AV block who may or may not have been in AF. These studies have also suggested a benefit, but it remains unclear whether the presence of AF influenced the response to CRT or whether, in the absence of atrial systole, differences merely reflect the avoidance of RV-only pacing rather than an intrinsic benefit from CRT.

In summary, these trials strongly suggest that CRT is superior to RV pacing; but this may be because CRT prevents the adverse effects of RV pacing rather than an intrinsic benefit of CRT in patients with AF.

RANDOMIZED TRIALS OF AV NODE ABLATION

No randomized study has specifically compared medical management without AV node ablation with CRT and AV node ablation as necessary to ensure high rates of biventricular capture, and yet this is what guidelines generally advocate. For patients with AF who have received a CRT device, no randomized study has compared medical management with AV node ablation; but such a study is now underway (see **Table 2** CAAN-HF [Cardiac Resynchronization Therapy and AV Nodal Ablation Trial in Atrial Fibrillation]) (ClinicalTrials.gov: NCT01522898). A randomized study, the AVERT-AF trial (Atrio-VEntricular Junction Ablation Followed by Resynchronization Therapy in patients with CHF and AF) is testing the hypothesis

that AV node ablation followed by CRT improves symptoms and exercise capacity compared with pharmacologic rate control and an ICD in patients with chronic AF and depressed ejection fraction, regardless of ventricular rate or QRS duration.[90] This study, which should now be complete, will not address the issue of whether patients with a prolonged QRS duration who are in AF should receive CRT or, indeed, any device at all.

OBSERVATIONAL STUDIES

Observational studies provide important information on prognosis and outcome with therapy and to that extent provide insights into met and unmet needs.[33] Cohort studies are a poor substitute for randomized trials but can help create hypotheses.

One of the earliest reports of CRT for AF was a study in which patients who had severe heart failure consequent on AV node ablation and RV pacing. Patients improved with an upgrade to CRT.[91] The extent to which this was caused by better care or correcting problems caused by RV pacing is not clear.

In a meta-analysis of 5 observational studies including 1164 patients, of whom 367 had AF (207 of whom had AV node ablation), mortality and improvement in symptoms after CRT were similar regardless of cardiac rhythm, although patients with AF may have fared less well in terms of exercise capacity and quality of life.[92] In a meta-analysis of 6 observational studies including 768 with AF, the 339 patients who had an AV node ablation to ensure ventricular capture with CRT had a substantially better prognosis than those who did not (risk ratio 0.42, 95% CI 0.26–0.68) and a greater improvement in New York Heart Association functional class (risk ratio −0.52, 95% CI −0.87 to −0.17).[93] This is illustrated by the largest of these reports from Gasparini and colleagues (**Figs. 2** and **3**).[94,95] However, higher-risk patients may have been less likely to receive AV node ablation and more likely to receive medications with adverse effects on outcome; therefore, these results may be biased. Reducing a ventricular rate to less than about 80 bpm is associated with a worse outcome in patients with heart failure and AF, perhaps because of exacerbation of nocturnal pauses that provoke lethal arrhythmias.[29]

If biventricular pacing is an important mechanism for the effect of CRT, then ensuring ventricular capture will be important. Two substantial observational studies[94–96] have suggested that for patients with AF, very high rates of capture (in excess of 95%) according to the device diagnostic algorithms, which might only be achieved by AV node ablation, are associated with dramatically better outcomes (**Fig. 4**). It is not immediately clear why such high rates of capture are required for CRT to be effective. One explanation is that the device diagnostics are only the tip of the iceberg reflecting a much more serious loss of ventricular capture rate. In some patients, a 5% to 10% loss

of capture according to device diagnostics may be associated with more than 40% loss of capture when analyzed by Holter monitoring.[97]

SPECIFIC CASE SELECTION
Scenario 1: Patients are Expected to Return to Sinus Rhythm

A substantial proportion of younger patients who have a short history both of heart failure and of AF should return to sinus rhythm after implantation of CRT, especially if echocardiography shows that the left atrium is not grossly dilated. Such patients should be selected for CRT as though they were in sinus rhythm. Cardioversion may be considered at the time of implantation provided that patients are anticoagulated. Patients who fail initial attempts at cardioversion should have a further attempt after a few months once the LV lead has been shown to be in a stable position. Short-term use of amiodarone may increase the chance of a return of sinus rhythm.

Scenario 2: Patients are Indicated for an ICD and, Apart From AF, are Indicated for CRT

Devices are expensive, and all procedures carry a risk. Implanting the right device at the first attempt reduces patient morbidity and costs. Although the RAFT trial provides the largest body of evidence that upgrading an ICD to CRT-D has no effect on prognosis, there are several arguments against

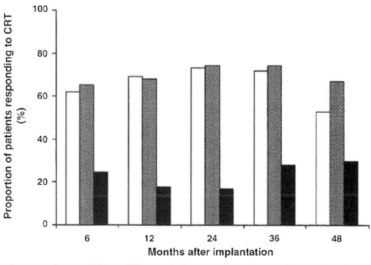

Fig. 2. Percentage of responders to CRT at different follow-up times in an observational study is presented. The open bars refer to sinus rhythm patients; the ruled bars relate to AF with AV junction ablation; and, finally, the solid bars refer to AF without AV junction ablation. There was a significantly higher proportion of responders in patients with sinus rhythm or AF with AF junction ablation compared with patients with AF without AF junction ablation. (*From* Gasparini M, Auricchio A, Regoli F, et al. Four-year efficacy of cardiac resynchronization therapy on exercise tolerance and disease progression: the importance of performing atrioventricular junction ablation in patients with atrial fibrillation. J Am Coll Cardiol 2006;48(4):741; with permission.)

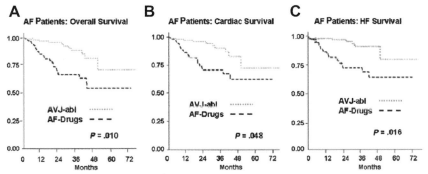

Fig. 3. Pharmacologic therapy for rate control in 125 patients and AV node ablation done in 118. Comparison of Kaplan-Meier estimates of overall (A), cardiac (B), and heart failure (C) survival between patients with AF who underwent AV junction ablation (AVJ-abl) and patients with AF treated only with negative chronotropic drugs. P values shown derived from the adjusted hazards ratio analysis stratified according to the corresponding cause of death. (*From* Gasparini M, Auricchio A, Metra M, et al. Long-term survival in patients undergoing cardiac resynchronization therapy: the importance of performing atrio-ventricular junction ablation in patients with permanent atrial fibrillation. Eur Heart J 2008;29(13):1648; with permission.)

ICD as the preferred option in patients otherwise indicated for CRT. RAFT did suggest some improvement in symptoms and reduction in heart failure hospitalization among patients with AF.[76] Only one patient had AV node ablation in RAFT. It is possible that the benefits would have been greater had a more aggressive strategy to ensure biventricular capture been adopted, although clearly this is speculation. If an ICD is implanted but subsequently an upgrade to CRT-D is considered appropriate, this creates a dilemma. Should the potential benefits of an early upgrade be foregone to incur the risk and costs of a potential second procedure? Ultimately, implanting a CRT-D device with selective AV node ablation depending on the progression of symptoms may be the best strategy. On current evidence, any patient with substantial LVSD who is in AF and who is going to receive a device and who is otherwise indicated for CRT should have a CRT device rather than RV pacing or an ICD.

Scenario 3: Patients have AF, Severe Heart Failure Recalcitrant to Best Drug Therapy, and are Otherwise Indicated for CRT

These patients have a limited number of options: LV assist device or a heart transplant. Under these circumstances, in the absence of the possibility of participating in a randomized controlled trial, it seems reasonable to consider CRT if the other alternatives are considered unattractive.

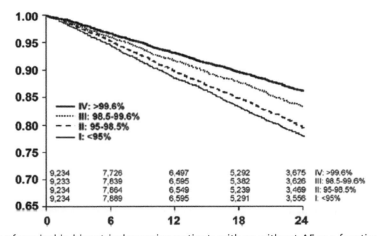

Fig. 4. Probability of survival in biventricular pacing patients with or without AF as a function of percentage of biventricular pacing capture. Patients with biventricular pacing greater than 99.6% experienced a 24% reduction in mortality compared with the other groups (hazard ration 0.76, P<.001). (*Adapted from* Hayes DL, Boehmer JP, Day JD, et al. Cardiac resynchronization therapy and the relationship of percent biventricular pacing to symptoms and survival. Heart Rhythm 2011;8:1469–75; with permission.)

Scenario 4: Patients have AF and Mild to Moderate Heart Failure on Pharmacologic Therapy but are Otherwise Indicated for CRT but have no Mandate for or are Unwilling to Have an ICD

These patients should not have CRT based on current evidence. CRT might be superior to AV node ablation and RV pacing, but then what is the evidence in support of the latter strategy? Ideally, they should be enrolled in a randomized controlled trial comparing CRT (or CRT-D) with no device in patients who would be indicated for a CRT if they were in sinus rhythm (LVEF <40%, QRS duration >140 ms).[32] Unfortunately, no trial fits these criteria that the authors are aware of.

REFERENCES

1. Khand A, Rankin AC, Kaye GC, et al. Systematic review of the management of atrial fibrillation in patients with heart failure. Eur Heart J 2000;21: 614–32.
2. Khand A, Cleland JG, Deedwania P. Prevention of and medical therapy for atrial arrhythmias in heart failure. Heart Fail Rev 2002;7:267–83.
3. Shelton RJ, Clark AL, Kaye GC, et al. The atrial fibrillation paradox of heart failure. Congest Heart Fail 2010;16(1):3–9.
4. Khand AU, Shaw M, Gemmel I, et al. Do discharge codes underestimate hospitalisation due to heart failure? Validation study of hospital discharge coding for heart failure. Eur J Heart Fail 2005; 7(5):792–7.
5. Khand AU, Gemmell I, Rankin AC, et al. Clinical events leading to the progression of heart failure: insights from a national database of hospital discharges. Eur Heart J 2001;22:153–64.
6. Roy D, Talajic M, Nattel S, et al. Rhythm control versus rate control for atrial fibrillation and heart failure. N Engl J Med 2008;358(25):2667–77.
7. Shelton RJ, Clark AL, Goode KM, et al. A randomized controlled study of rate versus rhythm control in patients with chronic atrial fibrillation and heart failure: (CAFE-II Study). Heart 2009; 95(11):924–30.
8. Swedberg K, Olsson LG, Charlesworth A, et al. Prognostic relevance of atrial fibrillation in patients with chronic heart failure on long-term treatment with beta-blockers: results from COMET. Eur Heart J 2005;26:1303–8.
9. Smit MD, Moes ML, Maass AH, et al. The importance of whether atrial fibrillation or heart failure develops first. Eur J Heart Fail 2012;14(9): 1030–40.
10. Baldasseroni S, De BL, Fresco C, et al. Cumulative effect of complete left bundle-branch block and chronic atrial fibrillation on 1-year mortality and hospitalization in patients with congestive heart failure. A report from the Italian network on congestive heart failure (in-CHF database). Eur Heart J 2002; 23(21):1692–8.
11. Mamas MA, Caldwell JC, Chacko S, et al. A meta-analysis of the prognostic significance of atrial fibrillation in chronic heart failure. Eur J Heart Fail 2009;11(7):676–83.
12. Puglisi A, Gasparini M, Lunati M, et al. Persistent atrial fibrillation worsens heart rate variability, activity and heart rate, as shown by a continuous monitoring by implantable biventricular pacemakers in heart failure patients. J Cardiovasc Electrophysiol 2008;19(7):693–701.
13. Borleffs CJ, Ypenburg C, van Bommel RJ, et al. Clinical importance of new-onset atrial fibrillation after cardiac resynchronization therapy. Heart Rhythm 2009;6(3):305–10.
14. Caldwell JC, Contractor H, Petkar S, et al. Atrial fibrillation is under-recognized in chronic heart failure: insights from a heart failure cohort treated with cardiac resynchronization therapy. Europace 2009; 11(10):1295–300.
15. Leclercq C, Padeletti L, Cihak R, et al. Incidence of paroxysmal atrial tachycardias in patients treated with cardiac resynchronization therapy and continuously monitored by device diagnostics. Europace 2010;12(1):71–7.
16. Marijon E, Jacob S, Mouton E, et al. Frequency of atrial tachyarrhythmias in patients treated by cardiac resynchronization (from the Prospective, Multicenter Mona Lisa Study). Am J Cardiol 2010; 106(5):688–93.
17. Boriani G, Gasparini M, Landolina M, et al. Incidence and clinical relevance of uncontrolled ventricular rate during atrial fibrillation in heart failure patients treated with cardiac resynchronization therapy. Eur J Heart Fail 2011;13(8):868–76.
18. Shanmugam N, Boerdlein A, Proff J, et al. Detection of atrial high-rate events by continuous home monitoring: clinical significance in the heart failure-cardiac resynchronization therapy population. Europace 2012;14(2):230–7.
19. Hoppe UC, Casares JM, Eiskjaer H, et al. Effect of cardiac resynchronization on the incidence of atrial fibrillation in patients with severe heart failure. Circulation 2006;114(1):18–25.
20. Padeletti L, Muto C, Maounis T, et al. Atrial fibrillation in recipients of cardiac resynchronization therapy device: 1-year results of the randomized MASCOT trial. Am Heart J 2008;156(3):520–6.
21. Santini M, Gasparini M, Landolina M, et al. Device-detected atrial tachyarrhythmias predict adverse outcome in real-world patients with implantable biventricular defibrillators. J Am Coll Cardiol 2011; 57(2):167–72.

22. Healey JS, Connolly SJ, Gold MR, et al. Subclinical atrial fibrillation and the risk of stroke. N Engl J Med 2012;366(2):120–9.

23. Capucci A, Santini M, Padeletti L, et al. Monitored atrial fibrillation duration predicts arterial embolic events in patients suffering from bradycardia and atrial fibrillation implanted with antitachycardia pacemakers. J Am Coll Cardiol 2005;46(10): 1913–20.

24. Swedberg K, Komajda M, Bohm M, et al, on behalf of the SHIFT Investigators. Ivabradine and outcomes in chronic heart failure (SHIFT): a randomised controlled study. Lancet 2010;376: 875–85.

25. Swedberg K, Zannad F, McMurray JJ, et al. Eplerenone and atrial fibrillation in mild systolic heart failure: results from the EMPHASIS-HF (Eplerenone in Mild Patients Hospitalization And Survival Study in Heart Failure) study. J Am Coll Cardiol 2012;59(18): 1598–603.

26. Rienstra M, Damman K, Mulder BA, et al. Beta-blockers and outcome in heart failure and atrial fibrillation; a meta-analysis. J Am Coll Cardiol HF 2013;1(1):21–8.

27. Bohm M, Borer J, Ford I, et al. Heart rate at baseline influences the effect of ivabradine on cardiovascular outcomes in chronic heart failure: analysis from the SHIFT study. Clin Res Cardiol 2013;102(1):11–22.

28. Cullington D, Goode KM, Clark AL, et al. Heart rate achieved or beta-blocker dose in patients with chronic heart failure: which is the better target? Eur J Heart Fail 2012;14(7):737–47.

29. Cullington D, Goode KM, Cleland JG, et al. Is heart rate important for patients with heart failure in atrial fibrillation? 2013.

30. Gronefeld GC, Israel CW, Padmanabhan V, et al. Ventricular rate stabilization for the prevention of pause dependent ventricular tachyarrhythmias: results from a prospective study in 309 ICD recipients. Pacing Clin Electrophysiol 2002;25(12): 1708–14.

31. Aizawa Y, Sato A, Watanabe H, et al. Dynamicity of the J-wave in idiopathic ventricular fibrillation with a special reference to pause-dependent augmentation of the J-wave. J Am Coll Cardiol 2012;59(22): 1948–53.

32. Cleland JG, Abraham WT, Linde C, et al. An individual patient meta-analysis of five randomized trials assessing the effects of cardiac resynchronization therapy on morbidity and mortality in patients with symptomatic heart failure. Eur Heart J 2013. [E-pub ahead of print].

33. Cleland JG, Tavazzi L, Daubert JC, et al. Cardiac resynchronization therapy. Are modern myths preventing appropriate use? J Am Coll Cardiol 2009; 53(7):608–11.

34. Ghio S, Freemantle N, Scelsi L, et al. Long term left ventricular reverse remodelling with cardiac resynchronization therapy. Results from the CARE-HF trial. Eur J Heart Fail 2009;11(5):480–8.

35. Cleland JG, Freemantle N, Erdmann E, et al. Long-term mortality with cardiac resynchronization therapy in the Cardiac Resynchronization-Heart Failure (CARE-HF) trial. Eur J Heart Fail 2012; 14(6):628–34.

36. Cleland JG, Daubert JC, Erdmann E, et al, on behalf of the CARE-HF Study Investigators. Longer-term effects of cardiac resynchronization therapy on mortality in heart failure (the Cardiac Resynchronization - Heart Failure (CARE-HF) trial extension phase). Eur Heart J 2006;27(16): 1928–32.

37. Cowburn PJ, Leclercq C. How to improve outcomes with cardiac resynchronisation therapy: importance of lead positioning. Heart Fail Rev 2012;17(6):781–9.

38. Khan FZ, Virdee MS, Palmer CR, et al. Targeted left ventricular lead placement to guide cardiac resynchronization therapy: the TARGET study: a randomized, controlled trial. J Am Coll Cardiol 2012; 59(17):1509–18.

39. Richardson M, Freemantle N, Calvert MJ, et al. Predictors and treatment response with cardiac resynchronisation therapy in patients with heart failure characterised by dyssynchrony: a predefined analysis from the CARE-HF Trial. Eur Heart J 2007;28(15):1827–34.

40. Ellenbogen KA, Gold MR, Meyer TE, et al. Primary results from the SmartDelay determined AV optimization: a comparison to other delay methods used in cardiac resynchronization therapy (SMART-AV) trial: a randomized trial comparing empirical, echocardiography-guided and algorithmic atrioventricular delay programming in cardiac resynchronization therapy. Circulation 2010;122:2660–8.

41. Boriani G, Biffi M, Muller CP, et al. A prospective randomized evaluation of VV delay optimization in CRT-D recipients: echocardiographic observations from the RHYTHM II ICD study. Pacing Clin Electrophysiol 2009;32(Suppl 1):S120–5.

42. Rao RK, Kumar UN, Schafer J, et al. Reduced ventricular volumes and improved systolic function with cardiac resynchronization therapy: a randomized trial comparing simultaneous biventricular pacing, sequential biventricular pacing, and left ventricular pacing. Circulation 2007;115:2136–44.

43. Abraham WT, Leon AR, St John Sutton MG, et al. Randomized controlled trial comparing simultaneous versus optimized sequential interventricular stimulation during cardiac resynchronization therapy. Am Heart J 2012;164(5):735–41.

44. Ritter P, Delnoy PP, Padeletti L, et al. A randomized pilot study of optimization of cardiac

resynchronization therapy in sinus rhythm patients using a peak endocardial acceleration sensor vs standard methods. Europace 2012;14(9):1324–33.

45. Whinnett ZI, Davies JE, Willson K, et al. Haemodynamic effects of changes in atrioventricular and interventricular delay in cardiac resynchronisation therapy show a consistent pattern: analysis of shape, magnitude and relative importance of atrioventricular and interventricular delay. Heart 2006; 92(11):1628–34.

46. Whinnett ZI, Francis DP, Denis A, et al. Comparison of different invasive hemodynamic methods for AV delay optimization in patients with cardiac resynchronization therapy: implications for clinical trial design and clinical practice. Int J Cardiol 2013. [Epub ahead of print].

47. Brenyo A, Kutyifa V, Moss AJ, et al. Atrioventricular delay programming and the benefit of cardiac resynchronization therapy in MADIT-CRT. Heart Rhythm 2013;10(8):1136–43.

48. Cleland JG, Freemantle N, Ghio S, et al. Predicting the long-term effects of cardiac resynchronisation therapy on mortality from baseline variables and the early response: a report from CARE-HF (Cardiac Resynchronisation in Heart Failure). J Am Coll Cardiol 2008;52:438–45.

49. Hsu LF, Jais P, Sanders P, et al. Catheter ablation for atrial fibrillation in congestive heart failure. N Engl J Med 2004;351(23):2373–83.

50. Khan MN, Jais P, Cummings J, et al. Pulmonary-vein isolation for atrial fibrillation in patients with heart failure. N Engl J Med 2008;359(17):1778–85.

51. Kies P, Leclercq C, Bleeker GB, et al. Cardiac resynchronisation therapy in chronic atrial fibrillation: impact on left atrial size and reversal to sinus rhythm. Heart 2006;92(4):490–4.

52. Hugl B, Bruns HJ, Unterberg-Buchwald C, et al. Atrial fibrillation burden during the post-implant period after CRT using device-based diagnostics. J Cardiovasc Electrophysiol 2006;17(8):813–7.

53. Ouellet G, Huang DT, Moss AJ, et al. Effect of cardiac resynchronization therapy on the risk of first and recurrent ventricular tachyarrhythmic events in MADIT-CRT. J Am Coll Cardiol 2012;60(18):1809–16.

54. McMurray JJ, Adamopoulos S, Anker SD, et al. ESC guidelines for the diagnosis and treatment of acute and chronic heart failure 2012: the task force for the diagnosis and treatment of acute and chronic heart failure 2012 of the European Society of Cardiology. Developed in collaboration with the Heart Failure Association (HFA) of the ESC. Eur J Heart Fail 2012;14(8):803–69.

55. Carson PE, Johnson GR, Dunkman WB, et al. The influence of atrial fibrillation on prognosis in mild to moderate heart failure: the V-HeFT studies. Circulation 1993;87:VI102–10.

56. Khand AU, Rankin AC, Martin W, et al. Carvedilol alone or in combination with digoxin for the management of atrial fibrillation in patients with heart failure. J Am Coll Cardiol 2003;42:1944–51.

57. Gheorghiade M, Fonarow GC, Van Veldhuisen DJ, et al. Lack of evidence of increased mortality among patients with atrial fibrillation taking digoxin: findings from post hoc propensity-matched analysis of the AFFIRM trial. Eur Heart J 2013;34(20):1489–97.

58. Chatterjee S, Ghosh J, Lichstein E, et al. Meta-analysis of cardiovascular outcomes with dronedarone in patients with atrial fibrillation or heart failure. Am J Cardiol 2012;110(4):607–13.

59. Connolly SJ, Camm AJ, Halperin JL, et al. Dronedarone in high-risk permanent atrial fibrillation. N Engl J Med 2011;365(24):2268–76.

60. Torp-Pedersen C, Metra M, Spark P, et al, for the COMET Investigators. The safety of amiodarone in patients with heart failure. J Card Fail 2007;13(5):340–5.

61. Kober L, Torp-Pedersen C, McMurray JJ, et al. Increased mortality after dronedarone therapy for severe heart failure. N Engl J Med 2008;358(25):2678–87.

62. Jones DG, Haldar SK, Hussain W, et al. A randomized trial to assess catheter ablation versus rate control in the management of persistent atrial fibrillation in heart failure. J Am Coll Cardiol 2013;61(18):1894–903.

63. Gaita F, Caponi D, Pianelli M, et al. Radiofrequency catheter ablation of atrial fibrillation: a cause of silent thromboembolism? Magnetic resonance imaging assessment of cerebral thromboembolism in patients undergoing ablation of atrial fibrillation. Circulation 2010;122(17):1667–73.

64. Daubert JP, Zareba W, Cannom DS, et al. Inappropriate implantable cardioverter-defibrillator shocks in MADIT II: frequency, mechanisms, predictors, and survival impact. J Am Coll Cardiol 2008; 51(14):1357–65.

65. Cleland JG, Buga L. Defibrillators - a shocking therapy for cardiomyopathy? Nat Rev Cardiol 2010; 7(2):69–70.

66. Cleland JG, Daubert JC, Erdmann E, et al, for the Cardiac Resynchronisation - Heart Failure (CARE-HF) Study Investigators. The effect of cardiac resynchronization on morbidity and mortality in heart failure. N Engl J Med 2005;352(15):1539–49.

67. Bristow MR, Saxon LA, Boehmer J, et al, for the Comparison of Medical Therapy, Pacing, and Defibrillation in Heart Failure (COMPANION) Investigators. Cardiac-resynchronization therapy with or without an implantable defibrillator in advanced chronic heart failure. N Engl J Med 2004;350:2140–50.

68. Cazeau S, Leclerc C, Lavergne T, et al, Multisite Stimulation in Cardiomyopathies (MUSTIC) Study Investigators. Effects of multisite biventricular pacing in patients with heart failure and intraventricular conduction delay. N Engl J Med 2001; 344:873–80.

69. Leclercq C, Walker S, Linde C, et al. Comparative effects of permanent biventricular and right-univentricular pacing in heart failure patients with chronic atrial fibrillation. Eur Heart J 2002;23: 1780–7.

70. Abraham WT, Fisher WG, Smith AL, et al, for the MIRACLE Study Group. Cardiac resynchronisation in chronic heart failure. N Engl J Med 2002;346(24): 1845–53.

71. Daubert JC, Gold MR, Abraham WT, et al, on behalf of the REVERSE Study Group. Prevention of disease progression by cardiac resynchronization therapy in patients with asymptomatic or mildly symptomatic left ventricular dysfunction. J Am Coll Cardiol 2009;54:1837–46.

72. Young J, Abraham WT, Smith AL, et al, Multicenter InSync ICD Randomized Clinical Evaluation (MIRACLE ICD) Trial Investigators. Combined cardiac resynchronisation and implantable cardioversion defibrillation in advanced chronic heart failure. The MIRACLE ICD trial. JAMA 2003;289: 2685–94.

73. Moss AJ, Hall WJ, Cannom DS, et al. Cardiac-resynchronization therapy for the prevention of heart-failure events. N Engl J Med 2009;361(14): 1329–38.

74. Tang AS, Wells GA, Talajic M, et al. Cardiac-resynchronization therapy for mild-to-moderate heart failure. N Engl J Med 2010;363(25):2385–95.

75. Brenyo A, Link MS, Barsheshet A, et al. Cardiac resynchronization therapy reduces left atrial volume and the risk of atrial tachyarrhythmias in MADIT-CRT (Multicenter Automatic Defibrillator Implantation Trial with Cardiac Resynchronization Therapy). J Am Coll Cardiol 2011;58(16):1682–9.

76. Healey JS, Hohnloser SH, Exner DV, et al. Cardiac resynchronization therapy in patients with permanent atrial fibrillation: results from the Resynchronization for Ambulatory Heart Failure Trial (RAFT). Circ Heart Fail 2012;5(5):566–70.

77. Tolosana JM, Arnau AM, Madrid AH, et al. Cardiac resynchronization therapy in patients with permanent atrial fibrillation. Is it mandatory to ablate the atrioventricular junction to obtain a good response? Eur J Heart Fail 2012;14(6):635–41.

78. Khadjooi K, Foley PW, Chalil S, et al. Long-term effects of cardiac resynchronisation therapy in patients with atrial fibrillation. Heart 2008;94(7): 879–83.

79. Schutte F, Ludorff G, Grove R, et al. Atrioventricular node ablation is not a prerequisite for cardiac resynchronization therapy in patients with chronic atrial fibrillation. Cardiol J 2009;16(3):246–9.

80. Chatterjee NA, Upadhyay GA, Ellenbogen KA, et al. Atrioventricular nodal ablation in atrial fibrillation: a meta-analysis and systematic review. Circ Arrhythm Electrophysiol 2012;5(1):68–76.

81. Geelen P, Brugada J, Andries E, et al. Ventricular fibrillation and sudden death after radiofrequency catheter ablation of the atrioventricular junction. Pacing Clin Electrophysiol 1997; 20(2 Pt 1):343–8.

82. Stavrakis S, Garabelli P, Reynolds DW. Cardiac resynchronization therapy after atrioventricular junction ablation for symptomatic atrial fibrillation: a meta-analysis. Europace 2012;14:1490–7.

83. Chatterjee NA, Upadhyay GA, Ellenbogen KA, et al. Atrioventricular nodal ablation in atrial fibrillation: a meta-analysis of biventricular vs. right ventricular pacing mode. Eur J Heart Fail 2012;14(6): 661–7.

84. Doshi RN, Daoud EG, Fellows C, et al, for the PAVE Study Group. Left ventricular-based cardiac stimulation Post AV Nodal Ablation Evaluation (The PAVE Study). J Cardiovasc Electrophysiol 2005; 16:1160–5.

85. Garrigue S, Bordachar P, Reuter S, et al. Comparison of permanent left ventricular and biventricular pacing in patients with heart failure and chronic atrial fibrillation: prospective haemodynamic study. Heart 2002;87(6):529–34.

86. Brignole M, Gammage M, Puggioni E, et al. Comparative assessment of right, left, and biventricular pacing in patients with permanent atrial fibrillation. Eur Heart J 2005;26(7):712–22.

87. Leclercq C, Cazeau S, Lellouche D, et al. Upgrading from single chamber right ventricular to biventricular pacing in permanently paced patients with worsening heart failure: The RD-CHF Study. Pacing Clin Electrophysiol 2007;30(Suppl 1):S23–30.

88. Kindermann M, Hennen B, Jung J, et al. Biventricular versus conventional right ventricular stimulation for patients with standard pacing indication and left ventricular dysfunction: the Homburg Biventricular Pacing Evaluation (HOBIPACE). J Am Coll Cardiol 2006;47(10):1927–37.

89. Curtis AB, Worley SJ, Adamson PB, et al. Biventricular pacing for atrioventricular block and systolic dysfunction. N Engl J Med 2013;368(17):1585–93.

90. Hamdan MH, Freedman RA, Gilbert EM, et al. Atrioventricular junction ablation followed by resynchronization therapy in patients with congestive heart failure and atrial fibrillation (AVERT-AF) study design. Pacing Clin Electrophysiol 2006;29(10): 1081–8.

91. Leon AR, Greenberg JM, Kanuru N, et al. Cardiac resynchronization in patients with congestive heart failure and chronic atrial fibrillation: effect of

upgrading to biventricular pacing after chronic right ventricular pacing. J Am Coll Cardiol 2002; 39:1258–63.

92. Upadhyay GA, Choudhry NK, Auricchio A, et al. Cardiac resynchronization in patients with atrial fibrillation: a meta-analysis of prospective cohort studies. J Am Coll Cardiol 2008;52(15): 1239–46.

93. Ganesan AN, Brooks AG, Roberts-Thomson KC, et al. Role of AV nodal ablation in cardiac resynchronization in patients with coexistent atrial fibrillation and heart failure: a systematic review. J Am Coll Cardiol 2012;59(8):719–26.

94. Gasparini M, Auricchio A, Metra M, et al. Long-term survival in patients undergoing cardiac resynchronization therapy: the importance of performing atrio-ventricular junction ablation in patients with permanent atrial fibrillation. Eur Heart J 2008; 29(13):1644–52.

95. Gasparini M, Auricchio A, Regoli F, et al. Four-year efficacy of cardiac resynchronization therapy on exercise tolerance and disease progression: the importance of performing atrioventricular junction ablation in patients with atrial fibrillation. J Am Coll Cardiol 2006;48(4):734–43.

96. Hayes DL, Boehmer JP, Day JD, et al. Cardiac resynchronization therapy and the relationship of percent biventricular pacing to symptoms and survival. Heart Rhythm 2011;8(9):1469–75.

97. Kamath GS, Cotiga D, Koneru JN, et al. The utility of 12-lead Holter monitoring in patients with permanent atrial fibrillation for the identification of nonresponders after cardiac resynchronization therapy. J Am Coll Cardiol 2009;53(12):1050–5.

Cardiac Resynchronization Therapy Mechanisms in Atrial Fibrillation

Zachary I. Whinnett, BMedSci, BMBS, MRCP, PhD*,
Darrel P. Francis, FRCP, MD

KEYWORDS

- Biventricular pacing • Cardiac resynchronization therapy • Atrial fibrillation

KEY POINTS

- The process of comparing multiple settings is the acid test of the resynchronization hypothesis, largely unacknowledged by the clinical and scientific community.
- Lack of a visible prominent effect of interventricular (VV) adjustment on hemodynamics is proof that either the resynchronization concept is plain wrong or the measurement protocol was designed to be so vulnerable to error that it cannot detect this important effect.
- The hazard of VV delay optimization lies in the widespread failure to perceive natural biologic variability, which is often mistaken for failure of the operator to make measurements correctly. Measurement variability causes false optima to appear with VV delay adjustment and makes the size of the optimization benefit become exaggerated.
- Using sensitive (narrow-error-bar) methods, VV delay optimization produces relatively small increments in hemodynamic effects over and above programming a nominal setting of VV 0 ms.

INTRODUCTION

It has been commonly assumed that the mechanism through which biventricular pacemakers (BVPs) improve cardiac function is by resynchronization of ventricular activation, which is why it is commonly referred to as cardiac resynchronization therapy (CRT). Resynchronization means restoration of simultaneity, which can only mean of the ventricles (because the atria are never supposed to contract simultaneously with the ventricles). The mental picture conjured by that term and conveyed when speaking to nonspecialists is almost always that of ventricular walls contracting incoordinately under native conduction and then brought back into correct mutual timing by the pacemaker. The visual impact and cognitive catchiness of the concept is overwhelming.

Under this hypothesis, patients with atrial fibrillation (AF) should be in as strong a position to benefit from BVP as those in sinus rhythm, because both groups are equally liable to ventricular dyssynchrony.

In routine clinical practice, BVPs are frequently implanted into patients who are in permanent AF (23% in a large European survey[1]).

After implantation of a BVP in a patient with AF, there are 2 main targets for optimizing therapy. First, measures can be taken to ensure high percentages of ventricular pacing that allow adequate

Funding Sources: The authors would like to acknowledge support from the British Heart Foundation DF (FS/10/38/28268).
International Centre for Circulatory Health, National Heart and Lung Institute, Imperial College London, 59-61 North Wharf Road, London W2 1LA, UK
* Corresponding author.
E-mail address: z.whinnett@imperial.ac.uk

Heart Failure Clin 9 (2013) 475–488
http://dx.doi.org/10.1016/j.hfc.2013.07.005
1551-7136/13/$ – see front matter

delivery of therapy. Second, the relative timing of stimulation of the 2 pacing leads can be adjusted (VV delay). If the mechanism through which BVP delivers its beneficial effect is predominantly ventricular resynchronization, then adjusting VV delay would be expected to produce large changes in cardiac function.

This article examines how to assess the reliability of potential techniques for performing optimization and explores whether the effort required for optimization is likely worthwhile.

CRT IN PATIENTS WITH ATRIAL FIBRILLATION

Would a patient with AF and left bundle branch block (LBBB) stand to benefit from BVP? Even a devotee of the resynchronization concept accepts that the presence of AF might impair the ability of BVP to give benefit. The variable intrinsic atrioventricular (AV) conduction might cause some beats to not have BV capture by the pacemaker and, therefore, incomplete delivery of biventricular pacing.

Therefore, it is not possible to simply assume that the benefit observed in patients with sinus rhythm also applies to patients in AF.

The evidence base for BVP in patients with AF has been predominantly derived from observational case series.[2–10] These data suggest that the benefits seem attenuated compared with patients in sinus rhythm.[11,12]

Only small numbers of patients with permanent AF have been included in the landmark randomized studies to assess the impact of CRT on clinical outcome measures. It is difficult to understand why these randomized trials—outwardly designated trials of cardiac resynchronization—were not designed to cover a full spread of patients with heart failure and LBBB. Until new studies are carried out, guidance is based on interpretation of the data that did arise.[13,14]

In a predefined substudy of the RAFT (Resynchronization–Defibrillation for Ambulatory Heart Failure Trial), patients with permanent AF, New York Heart Association class II or III heart failure, left ventricular (LV) ejection fraction less than or equal to 30%, and QRS duration greater than or equal to 120 ms were randomized to receive BVP or no BVP, with all patients receiving a defibrillator; 229 patients were randomized. The principal result of the study is that the event rate was low in both arms and, therefore, the CI for the primary outcome of death or heart failure hospitalization between those assigned to CRT–implantable cardioverter defibrillator (ICD) and those assigned ICD was wide,[15] ranging from 0.65 to 1.41. The point estimate was 0.96 ($P = .82$), but the CI includes an

effect as strong as seen in CARE-HF (Cardiac Resynchronization Heart Failure) trial, for instance.

The MUSTIC-AF (Multisite Stimulation in Cardiomyopathy Atrial Fibrillation) trial, which deliberately focused on AF and addressed symptoms, did find evidence of symptomatic advantage of BVP over pure right ventricular (RV) pacing[13] but it should be borne in mind that RV pacing on its own was found harmful in the DAVID (Dual Chamber and VVI Implantable Defibrillator) trial,[16] so the favorable outcome in the BVP arm should not be assumed due to a salutary effect of BVP: it may simply be a neutral alternative to harmful RV pacing.

The absence of conclusive evidence of benefit from randomized studies to support the use of CRT in patients with AF may be explained by the following:

1. Insufficient numbers of patients entered into randomized studies

Many more sinus rhythm patients than AF patients have been entered into randomized studies. Therefore, even if BVP is equally effective in both groups, the AF studies are likely to be underpowered.

2. Lack of consistent biventricular capture through lack of AV node ablation

In AF, native RR interval varies because of variable arrival of atrial wavefronts and possibly also variable AV node conduction. This means that a regular programmed ventricular pacing rate may fail to capture every beat consistently, because of intermittent breakthrough of native conduction.[17] If there is reduced delivery of therapy, perhaps in the 60% to 75% range, then a study approximately 2.5 times as large as those performed in sinus rhythm is required. In reality, AF studies have been smaller than their sinus rhythm counterparts.

3. The effect may be smaller in AF

Even if ventricular resynchronization is the primary driver of the benefit of CRT in sinus rhythm, there may be a contribution from coordination of atrial versus ventricular contraction (this is not resynchronization but might be called euchronization).[18] The beneficial effect of BVP in AF might, therefore, be smaller than in sinus rhythm.

OPTIMIZING DELIVERY OF BIVENTRICULAR PACING

In order to ensure high percentages of ventricular pacing, hence, the opportunity for adequate delivery of therapy, it is important to ensure that native conduction does not unfavorably compete with BVP, so that ventricular resynchronization is successfully delivered.

High percentages of ventricular pacing may be achieved pharmacologically by adequate uptitration of medication to control ventricular rate. Relying on the percent biventricular pacing data stored in the pacemaker to determine this may be misleading, because these rates may include fusion and pseudofusion between pacing from the device and intrinsic atrioventricular conduction.[19]

AV node ablation can deliver a more powerful guarantee of the effectiveness of adequate rate control. Some operators are anxious about the potential adverse consequences of converting a patient with stable status, who is nonpacemaker dependent, into a patient who is totally dependent on the pacemaker for survival.

Although observational studies report strong symptomatic responses to ablation plus BVP[3,6–9,20] there are 2 limitations. First, these procedures are by their nature only likely to be carried out by groups with a strong belief in the rationale and, therefore, any outcome markers that require human judgment should not be assumed free of innocent bias. Second, they have all covered only the short term. Adverse consequences that take longer to materialize, such as the undesirable sequelae of total pacing dependency, may not have manifested at the time the studies were evaluated.

The net clinical effect of biventricular pacing in AF is difficult to guess from the clinical outcome data that exist to date. The randomized experience is small, and the nonrandomized experience (like all observational data) is open to an unquantifiable degree of natural observer bias.

What is needed are reliable experimental data, which may take the form of physiologic measurements with and without BVP, with careful attention to bias-resistance and reliability of the data within individual patients. Alternatively, they may take the form of outcome trials with event endpoints, although, for the reasons described previously, these have to be much larger than their sinus rhythm predecessors to achieve the same degree of statistical power.

OPTIMIZATION OF INTERVENTRICULAR DELAY

The typical nominal VV delay is close to 0 ms (ie, virtually simultaneous onset of stimulation). Adjusting the VV delay is expected to change the degree of ventricular resynchronization. There are theoretic reasons why it may be necessary to adjust the VV delay in order to obtain maximal improvements in ventricular resynchronization. For example, if the LV lead is positioned in an area of slow conduction, there may be a significant time delay before the pacing stimulus spreads to activate the left ventricle. In this case, it may be rational to program the LV lead to pace before the RV lead in order to allow a greater bulk of the ventricular myocardium to be activated approximately synchronously.

Several different methods have been proposed to guide the process of assessing the impact of adjusting the VV delay. Because supporting evidence on the long-term benefit of BVP optimization from large clinical trials is lacking, guidelines provide little scientifically supported guidance on how to program VV delay in AF.[21]

The lack of supporting evidence for optimization may be because there is no or little incremental benefit to be obtained from optimizing VV delay over and above the nominal delay. Alternatively, it may be that there are advantageous VV delays, but the methods used for optimization were unreliable and did not identify them correctly.

In order to establish which of these explanations is most likely, there must be a mechanism for assessing the reliability of an optimization method. Before proceeding to clinical outcome studies, simple steps can be taken to determine whether an optimization method has a high likelihood of delivering reliable results. A rigorously conducted large-scale clinical outcome study assessing an optimization method that does not reliably identify the true optimal VV delay will not find a beneficial effect for VV optimization. It will not be possible to determine whether the lack of benefit is because VV optimization is not important or whether it is simply due to the failure of the optimization method tested.

IS A PROPOSED OPTIMIZATION METHOD SUFFICIENTLY RELIABLE TO DELIVER CLINICALLY USEFUL RESULTS?

It is unwise to proceed directly to a clinical trial with an optimization scheme before establishing its reliability; this can be done cheaply. This article sets out a series of steps that can be used to assess any optimization method, beginning with simple tests that can be done in a few minutes in 1 or 2 patients.

Step 1: Does the Proposed Optimization Scheme Identify a Singular Optimal Value?

An optimization scheme must select a single VV delay (or a narrow range of VV delays) if it is to make any meaningful claim of being an optimization scheme at all.

For example, a scheme that selects a broad range, such as "anywhere from LV first by 80 ms to RV first by 80 ms," is so vague as to be little better than completely uninformative. Taken to its extreme, a scheme could declare all possible VV delays to be optimal: there is no reason to consider this an optimization scheme.

Ideally, a scheme should provide the optimum to the level of precision to which a device can be programmed. For devices that can only be programmed to the nearest 10-ms step, there is no need to know the optimum to any greater degree of precision than this. Despite being easy to determine, the majority of optimization schemes do not report a degree of precision for the value determined as the optimum.

Aside from a too-wide range of proposed optimality, the second undesirable pattern is the dual-peaked optimum. How can LV first by 20 ms and RV first by 40 ms be equally optimal, with intervening settings worse? Uncritical acceptance of dual-peaked optima allows virtually any pattern to be taken as a valid set of optimization measurements. There is little physiologic justification for dual peaks. At the least, a dual-peaked pattern should be the subject of blinded verification from separate data by an independent observer, and, if confirmed, patients should undergo detailed assessment of the physiologic process underlying the phenomenon, which might turn out to be a landmark finding in fundamental mechanisms.

The ability to identify a singular region on the VV delay spectrum as optimal is the most basic requirement for an optimization scheme. It takes only a handful of patients to test singularity of most of the proposed methods. For example, to assess whether optimization performed using left ventricular outflow tract (LVOT) velocity-time integral (VTI) measurements identify a singular region would only require about 7 minutes per patient (3 beats per VV delay, across 7 VV delays, allowing 20 seconds per VTI measurement). Readers are encouraged to test this.

Step 2: Is It Reproducible?

Once a scheme has demonstrated adequate singularity, it can then go forward for the slightly more time-consuming test of reproducibility. If a test is not singular, there is no point assessing it for reproducibility. The reason for this is as follows. A scheme that is not singular either provides too broad a territory of supposed optimality or provides multiple disconnected regions of optimality. In either case, if a second test is carried out, whether the second result is consistent with the

first in the first case is always judged successful or in the second case is impossible to judge.

For example, if the scheme addresses a spectrum of possibilities from "LV first by 120 ms" to "RV first by 80 ms" and declares that "LV first by 80 ms to RV first by 40 ms" are all optimal, then a second test that declares the optimum is "LV first by 40 ms to RV first by 80 ms" is judged a match—even though in both cases they cover half the range.

In another example, if the first test declares the optimum to be "LV first by 120 ms or RV first by 40 ms" and the second test declares it "LV first by 40 ms or RV first by 80 ms," they may at first be considered almost concordant (due to the near match of RV 40 ms and RV 80 ms) but on further reflection it becomes clear that almost any finding on the second test would be considered a perfect or near match.

So singularity is a vital prerequisite, but how exactly should reproducibility itself be judged?

1. Independent data sets acquired separately

The key to reproducibility is the identification of equivalence or near-equivalence of VV delay optimum by independent observers who acquire separate data blinded to each other's findings. It is grossly inadequate to ask 2 observers to examine the same acquired set of data (it makes no more sense than asking 2 observers to look at the same reading displayed on a blood pressure machine and call it reproducibility).

The enemy of optimization is biologic variability that is continually producing fluctuations in any measured variable. In this environment, there is great opportunity for differences between observations at different VV delays to be the result of these natural biologic fluctuations and not the VV delay itself. For this reason, the 2 operators should acquire separate data. If under these circumstances they obtain the same optimum, then the scheme is sufficiently robust to overcome this noise.

2. Blinding

In clinical practice, most workers have an inherent recognition that the techniques they use are less good than claimed, although they rarely voice this concern. The principal hallmark of the presence of this gestalt knowledge is the behavior of peeking at previous results before making a new measurement. This happens in assessment of LV function and of valvular function[22] and is even condoned in guidelines.

When practitioners conduct peeking, to ensure that values make physiologic sense in the context, they are recognizing that the noise in the measurement is so great that they have to select between the various measurements, using some external knowledge in order to achieve an expected pattern. In such an environment, once they conduct one optimization, they tend to tune the results of the second to match the results of the first.

A simple solution to this is to ask 2 independent operators to conduct entirely separate optimizations on the same patient immediately successively without the 2 operators communicating or viewing each other's data. Alternatively, the process could be automated so that the human tendency to manipulate the interpretation of one set of data to match that of the other is avoided.

Again, although this process of testing reproducibility takes a little forethought to understand why it is necessary, its actual execution is easy and quick.

3. Willingness to publish unpleasant results

Individuals testing reproducibility should be willing to publish the findings even if they do not fit their prejudice or a department's liking. It should not be assumed that findings that discord with prejudice are incorrect. Instead, it may be the failure of previous workers to report findings that may have resulted in the present worker having a wrong prejudice. In any case, a biologic observation is a biologic observation and not an assay of the staff member, so no shame should be accrued from realizing that a scheme is not reproducible.

4. Calculate and display the relevant variable, not an irrelevant one

When the data of the 2 optimizations are collected in a handful of patients, the relevant calculation is the SD of difference between the optimal VV delays. This is carried out by listing the VV delay selected by operator 1 in the first column, the VV delay selected by operator 2 in the second column, and the difference in the third column. The difference should be signed (ie, if operator 2 picked a more positive VV delay in a particular patient, it would be marked as a positive difference; meanwhile if that operator picked a more negative VV delay in another patient, it would be marked as a negative difference).

On average (unless an operator is biased toward reporting a higher or lower value consistently), the mean of those differences tends to be distributed at approximately 0. The relevant question is how wide that distribution is, which can be conveniently calculated as the SD of those differences. There are several variables that there is no point in calculating.

Whether operator 1 and operator 2 are significantly different

It is of no use to calculate whether operator 2 reports a significantly higher optimum or not than operator 1. This is only of interest if there was a concern that one operator had a consistent tendency to pick higher or lower values. If they were both selecting purely randomly, without making any biologic measurement, they would have no difference in their mean optima (because they are drawn from identical distribution) even though such an optimization process would be completely useless.

What proportion of patients is within the 95% Bland-Altman CI bands?

There is essentially no point reporting this because the CI bands are designed to capture approximately 95% of the cases on a parametric basis. Deviations from 95% occur by chance due to the shapes of the distribution and give no useful information on the reliability of the technique.

Difference in LVOT VTI or other measurement between settings

The question is how widely the repeat VV optima are distributed, not the measured consequences on the VTI or other physiologic variables. Although it might be intuitively attractive for a clinician to report whether operator 1 and operator 2 generated similar physiologic consequences, selecting settings entirely at random, even with physiology that is strongly dependent on VV delay, results in a near-0 difference between the 2 operators. Again this is because the physiologic responses are drawn from the same distribution, not because the VV delays are equal.

Step 3: Is the Value Identified as Optimal Biologically Plausible?

For any scheme that passes both singularity and reproducibility criteria, it is time to test its physiologic plausibility. For example, a scheme that always defines the optimum VV delay in women as RV first by 60 ms and in men as LV first by 80 ms would meet criteria of singularity and reproducibility, because each patient is always allocated a consistent value, but would not be biologically plausible.

There are several aspects to biologic plausibility. A scheme that for most patients picked RV first by a high degree (eg, 60 ms or 80 ms) would suffer from the apprehension that it is delivering largely RV pacing, which, as is known from trials, such as DAVID, is likely harmful.[16]

Plotting the distribution of optima obtained may give clues to plausibility. It would be expected, from induction from the concept behind BVP, that VV optima most commonly are in the vicinity of VV 0 ms or slightly left first. It would be expected that RV first or very extreme LV first would be identified as optimal in only a minority of patients.

This 3-step process (singularity, reproducibility, and plausibility) can be checked inexpensively and can be conducted for multiple variables in the same study without loss of power. The authors have conducted such a study for markers that are electrical (QRS duration), flow based (LVOT VTI), and pressure based (noninvasive beat-by-beat blood pressure) to show how it could work in this screening process.[23]

Step 4: Does the Optimization Method Result in Improvements in Cardiac Function?

Singular, reproducible, and plausible optimization schemes are still not yet necessarily ready for large-scale trailing.

Optima based on intracardiac measurements need not necessarily agree with each other or produce overall improvements in cardiac function, because there are many potential variables, and maximization of one may be at the expense of another. Outside the heart, however, what generates pressure is what generates flow, so these 2 variables tend to be affected in the same direction by any change in VV delay timing. All other peripherally measured variables are downstream consequences of pressure and/or flow and, therefore, are likely to be affected concordantly. It is implausible for a peripheral variable to have a VV delay optimum that is substantially different from the optimum for pressure and flow.

Optimization should be expected to deliver an increment in cardiac function. The size of the increment can be determined in relation to the status at a reference VV delay, such as 0 ms. For example, if a VV delay of LV first 60 ms is identified as optimal, it can be compared with VV 0 ms in order to determine the magnitude of the increment in blood pressure or flow that is gained by programming the optimized setting. It is important to ensure that if using a measure of cardiac function to both identify the optimal delay and assess the impact of programming the optimal delay, that separate measurements are used to identify the optimal VV delay from those used to determine the hemodynamic impact. Otherwise, there is likely to be a positive bias, which results in an overestimation of the magnitude of improvement in cardiac function.[24] Therefore, one set of measurements should be made to identify the optimal delay and separate measurements made to compare this optimal delay with the reference.

Step 5: Choosing an Optimization Scheme

After these stages, only methods that identify a singular optimum, are reproducible, and are plausible are left. They have good agreement with measures of cardiac function. It is likely that optimization methods demonstrating these properties will show clustering with regard to the VV delay identified as optimal. These schemes will therefore show good agreement with each other with regard to the VV delay determined as optimal. Each scheme would be already validated against all the others in that cluster. With all schemes in the cluster reporting similar optima, any one of the schemes could be chosen for clinical use, perhaps based on cost or local convenience.

No endpoint trials need be carried out before this stage. At this stage, if 2 different measures of cardiac function consistently identify different optima, to assist in choosing between the schemes it may be helpful to conduct a clinical trial. **Box 1** shows the process for identifying a reliable scheme for optimization of VV delay.

HAZARDS OF JUDGING A BOOK BY ITS COVER OR AN ARTICLE BY ITS TITLE

Several different methods have been proposed to guide VV delay optimization. Although little recognized, it is not sufficient to settle on a parameter and measure it at each setting, choosing the setting with the best value, because the measurements may vary spontaneously with time due to natural biologic fluctuation. If thought is not applied, these biologic fluctuations may be mistaken for the effect of VV delay; thereby, a random VV delay setting may unknowingly become selected.

The protocol used to acquire data needs careful planning so that enough steps are taken to minimize the effects of biologic variability. If these steps have not been taken, then the findings may be incorrect. If the planning has not been carried out, then the investigators will not have realized

---

Box 1
Process for identifying a reliable scheme for optimization of VV delay

Step 1: Does the proposed optimization scheme identify a singular optimal value?

Step 2: Is it reproducible?

Step 3: Is the value identified as optimal biologically plausible?

Step 4: Does the optimization method result in improvements in cardiac function?

Step 5: Choosing an optimization scheme

that they need to take these steps. If signal has been overwhelmed by noise, a study's investigators are unlikely to report it (they may not even know). The only sign of this that a reader can realistically expect to see is the absence of evidence of meticulous quantification of natural biologic variability by the investigators.

It is tempting to classify articles on optimization by their choice of variable measured for optimization (eg, VTI of Doppler, pulse pressure, or LV dP/dt_{max}). But the crucial distinction is not the choice of variable but the choice to measure the variable sufficiently precisely to make the optimization singular, reproducible, and plausible.[25] For each variable there is noise. By measuring (not guessing) the magnitude of the noise, it is possible to calculate how many replicate measurements are required for an optimization of any desired degree of precision.[26,27]

If the steps taken to minimize the effect of noise have not been carefully planned, then even measures that have the potential to be excellent candidates as a means for guiding optimization may fail.

dP/dt_{max}, for example, has strong theoretic grounds for being a good marker of cardiac function. Many different protocols have been used for acquiring invasive dP/dt_{max} to guide AV delay optimization. Some investigators have simply used a single 30-second recording and not compared this to a reference setting[28] whereas others have compared single measurements of calculation of the relative change in dP/dt_{max} with a reference setting[29] and others have used multiple measurements of the relative change.[30–32] Reproducibility is poor if only single measurements are made and is much improved by making multiple measurements.[25]

The foregoing makes it clear that it is insufficient to choose a marker that has strong a priori validity, and insufficient to simply measure it invasively. It is essential that carefully preplanned steps are taken to minimize the effect of noise that occurs due to background spontaneous variations that occur even in dP/dt_{max} measurements.

It is not only the parameter proposed as an optimization marker but also the way in which it is recorded (ie, precisely what noise reduction steps are included and quantitatively how these were decided on) that determines whether it can be a reliable method to guide optimization.

EXAMPLES OF VARIABLES THAT CAN BE MEASURED FOR OPTIMIZATION

A wide variety of variables can be proposed for optimization, including electrical, pressure-based, and flow-based.

LVOT VTI

The intuitively most attractive variable to maximize while optimizing VV delay is cardiac output.[33–35] At a fixed heart rate, this is equivalent to maximizing stroke volume. For a constant outflow tract diameter, this is also equivalent to maximizing stroke distance or VTI. Typically this is recorded noninvasively using Doppler echocardiography, although it can be recorded invasively using a flow wire.[36] At each pacemaker setting, a sample of pulsed wave Doppler traces is acquired from the LVOT, while keeping the probe position constant between settings. It is often recommended to average the VTIs of 3 beats, although articles describing the technique commonly show the process carried out on a single beat per setting. Increments of 20 ms in the VV delay are commonly recommended. The VV delay setting that yields the highest VTI is selected as the optimum.

The authors' group has assessed noninvasive outflow tract VTI as a tool for VV delay optimization in AF.[23] Six consecutive beats of LVOT flow were acquired (**Fig. 1**). The average of the 6 beats was taken as the value for that setting. The authors assessed singularity, reproducibility, and plausibility of the data.

Singularity
The number of optimizations in which there is a single peak of clearly maximum VTI (judged from the raw points, not the curve) is few. Applying curve fitting increases the proportion but there are still many of the 40 optimizations in which the curves are noncurved or inverted. Each inverted curve is noise rather than physiologically meaningful, but what may not be obvious is that it has a counterpart that is correctly oriented but also noise, because it is the nature of random noise to be equal in each direction. Therefore, the number of curves that are biologic meaningful may be as few as 50% or less of those acquired.

Reproducibility
In **Fig. 1**, it can be seen that only 9 of the 20 patients tested have a pair of curves that are both correctly oriented. In the remaining 11, it is not possible to establish reproducibility. In the 9, most have fairly good agreement between the optima indicated by the 2 curves. This is an example of the phenomenon explained earlier: in the absence of strong singularity, there is little point in addressing reproducibility of the optimum. The SD of difference was 34 ms.

Biologic Plausibility
There is no point addressing biologic plausibility because singularity is poor as is reproducibility.

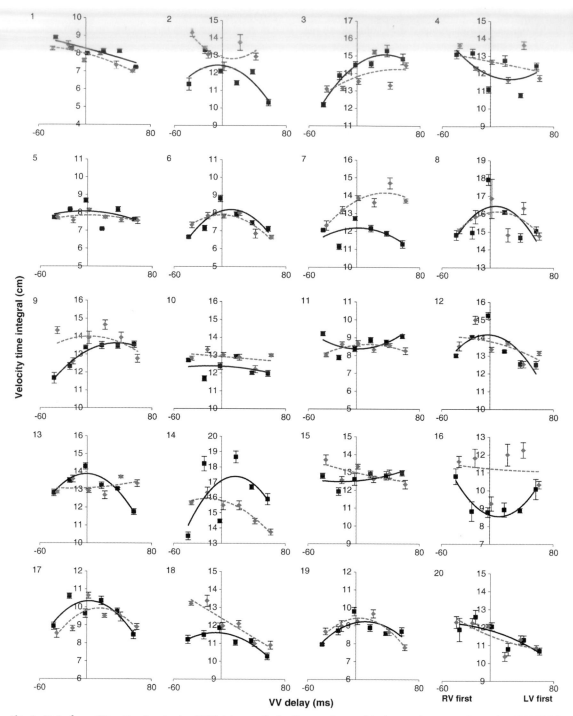

Fig. 1. Data from 20 patients who had VV delay optimization performed twice on the same day, using LVOT VTI. Data for the first optimization is displayed in black and the second in gray. A parabola was fitted and the peak of the parabola was considered to represent the optimal VV delay (optimum = largest VTI). (*From* Kyriacou A, Li Kam Wa ME, Pabari PA, et al. A systematic approach to designing reliable VV optimization methodology: assessment of internal validity of echocardiographic, electrocardiographic and haemodynamic optimization of cardiac resynchronization therapy. Int J Cardiol 2012 Mar 26. [Epub ahead of print]; with permission.)

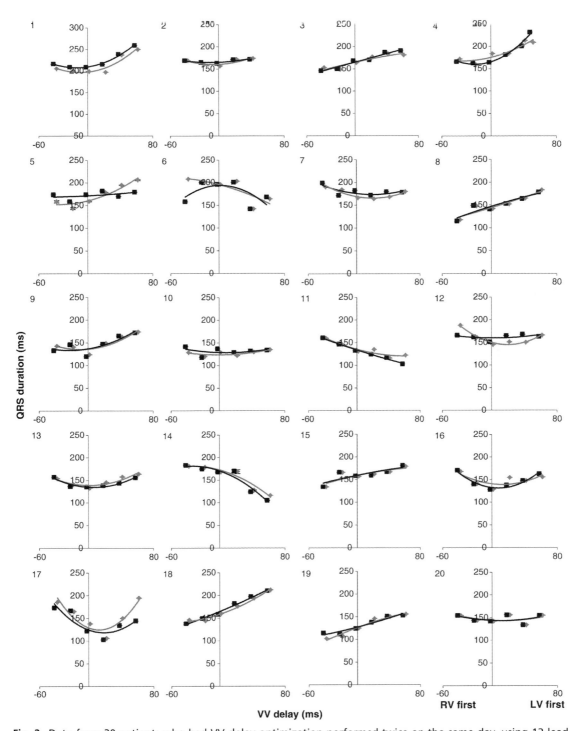

Fig. 2. Data from 20 patients who had VV delay optimization performed twice on the same day, using 12-lead ECG QRS width. Data for the first optimization is displayed in black and the second optimization is displayed in gray. A parabola was fitted for optimization session and the trough of the parabola was considered to represent the optimal VV delay (optimum = narrowest QRS). (*From* Kyriacou A, Li Kam Wa ME, Pabari PA, et al. A systematic approach to designing reliable VV optimization methodology: assessment of internal validity of echocardiographic, electrocardiographic and haemodynamic optimization of cardiac resynchronization therapy. Int J Cardiol 2012 Mar 26. [Epub ahead of print]; with permission.)

This analysis does not show that measurement of flow is doomed to be ineffective for VV optimization. It only shows that the protocol carried out, measuring 6 beats, cannot reliably identify a singular or reproducible optimum. It is entirely possible that an approach that averaged more beats might vanquish the noise sufficiently to make the approach feasible. This does not seem, however, to have yet been tested. Efforts to optimize VV delay by LVOT VTI have often claimed to use 3 beats per setting, and lectures have sometimes shown examples using only 1 beat per setting. It is hard to understand how such attempts could be anything other than futile.

QRS Minimization

With wide QRS a prime criterion for implantation of CRT, it is intellectually attractive to aim to adjust VV delay in a manner to restore QRS width to as close as possible to a normal narrow duration.

Whether competitive narrowing of QRS is a physiologically ideal target is not known, but the authors' experiments may have cast some light.

Singularity

QRS duration can easily be measured precisely, as readily seen from the error bars in **Fig. 2** too narrow to see in many cases (just visible for the gray). In almost every case, there is a clear optimum (ie, VV delay which minimizes QRS duration).

Reproducibility

The replicate data sets are closely concordant, as evidenced by the almost overlapping curves in many cases.

Biologic Plausibility

The concern for QRS duration is that some of the VV delays identified as apparently optimal, in terms of QRS minimization, are not VV delays that spring to mind as physiologically desirable. For example, in patients 3, 5, 8, 15, 18, and 19, the VV delay consistently selected as optimal by both replicate VV optimization processes was RV first by 60 ms. If 30% of cases require such extreme RV preactivation for optimality, then some of the understanding of the mechanism of CRT and cardiac function must be incorrect. **Fig. 3** shows plot of the distribution of VV delays identified as optimal using QRS minimization.

Pressure

The authors' group has conducted a series of experiments over the past 10 years on the potential for using blood pressure, which can be measured beat-to-beat noninvasively, as a marker for optimization of BVPs.[30–32] Pressure has the advantage over flow in that it can be acquired automatically with no human intervention required, which makes it more convenient than echo Doppler.

Singularity

Most of the 40 optimizations shown in **Fig. 4** identified a clear optimum VV delay.

Reproducibility

The test-retest variability of the optimum by this BP protocol was an SD of differences of 10.2 ms.

Plausibility

Eighteen of the 20 patients showed on both optimization sessions an optimum that was in the central region that biologically might appear most plausible. No post hoc data editing took place.

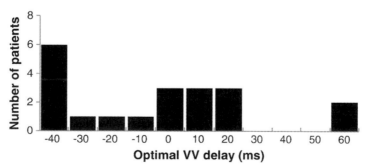

Fig. 3. Plot of the distribution of VV delays identified as optimal using QRS minimization. A high proportion of optima with significant (−40 ms) RV pre-excitation was identified as optimal. (*From* Kyriacou A, Li Kam Wa ME, Pabari PA, et al. A systematic approach to designing reliable VV optimization methodology: assessment of internal validity of echocardiographic, electrocardiographic and haemodynamic optimization of cardiac resynchronization therapy. Int J Cardiol 2012 Mar 26. [Epub ahead of print]; with permission.)

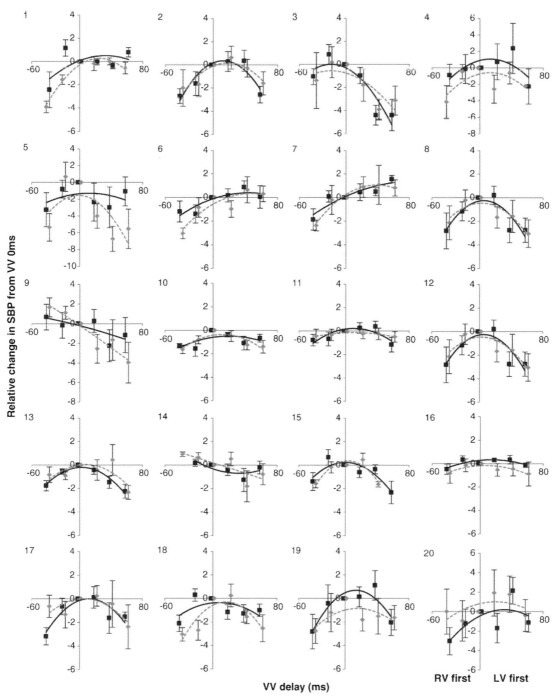

Fig. 4. Data from 20 patients who had VV delay optimization performed twice on the same day, using noninvasive systolic blood pressure (SBP). In order to minimize noise, each tested VV delay was compared with the reference VV delay of 0 ms and the relative change in systolic blood pressure was calculated by subtracting the mean SBP of the 10 beats immediately after the transition from the 10 beats immediately before the transition. A mean of 8 replicate measurements was used. Data for the first optimization is displayed in black and the second optimization is displayed in gray. A parabola was fitted in all optimization sessions and the peak of the parabola was considered to represent the optimal VV delay (optimum = highest relative SBP). (*From* Kyriacou A, Li Kam Wa ME, Pabari PA, et al. A systematic approach to designing reliable VV optimization methodology: assessment of internal validity of echocardiographic, electrocardiographic and haemodynamic optimization of cardiac resynchronization therapy. Int J Cardiol 2012 Mar 26. [Epub ahead of print]; with permission.)

IS TIME SPENT OPTIMIZING VV DELAY RATHER THAN SIMPLY PROGRAMMING SIMULTANEOUS RV AND LV PACING LIKELY TO DELIVER CLINICAL USEFUL IMPROVEMENTS IN CARDIAC FUNCTION?

Although many clinicians consider it not worthwhile to optimize VV delay, the articles that report the results of VV optimization characteristically indicate large increments in physiologic variables measured. How can these be reconciled?

There is a serious trap into which it is easily possible to fall when optimizing VV delay by maximizing a physiologic variable. Consider an extreme case where the biologic variable measured has no relation to VV delay at all and only shows random biologic variability. If N settings are tested, 1 of which is the 0 VV delay that is the reference state, then because of natural variability, there is always 1 VV delay whose measurement is highest. On average, in 1 out of N cases, this is VV 0; in the remaining (N-1)/N cases, it is some other delay. Thus, as more settings are tested, the greater the chance that a non-0 setting will be selected as optimal.

But the problem has even worse ramifications. Clinicians mindful of the need for clinical audit might attempt to calculate the average benefit in the variable achieved by VV optimization. Because, in each case, they would use the increment from VV 0 ms to the optimal VV delay, and in each case that increment would be positive (except in the 1/N cases, in which it is 0 because the VV 0-ms setting happened by chance to give the highest measurement), the increment would be a list of exclusively positive numbers (with a few 0s). Necessarily, such a list would be statistically significantly larger than 0.

Therefore, in any statistical test, the optimization process would seem to have statistically significantly increased the measurement, such as of LVOT VTI, even though in reality the optimization was no more than selecting a VV delay setting at random. In real life, VV delay may be making a contribution, but the size of it is unknown unless special steps are taken to eradicate the noise component.

Therefore, estimating the increment achieved by VV optimization must not be carried out using data that have wide error bars. Using a high degree of replication, such as can be achieved with pressure, and curve fitting to minimize the effect of noise,[27] it is possible to visualize the effect of adjusting VV delay and gauge the likely magnitude of contribution of moving VV delay away from 0 ms.

From the authors' AF study of VV optimization, it seems that in most cases the optimum VV delay gives systolic blood pressure less than 1 mm Hg higher than would be achieved by VV 0-ms pacing. Because blood pressure is approximately 100 mm Hg, the authors interpret this as an increment in cardiac output or stroke volume of less than 1%. To put this into context, simply switching on CRT (in sinus rhythm) to optimal AV delay (in patients in SR) increases blood pressure by approximately 6%. Thus, the amount gained by most patients from VV optimization is less than one-sixth the effect of CRT itself.

SUMMARY

VV delay optimization is a fascinating and potentially hazardous pursuit. The fascination lies in that the process of comparing multiple settings is the acid test of the resynchronization hypothesis, largely unacknowledged by the clinical and scientific community. Lack of a visible prominent effect of VV adjustment on hemodynamics is proof that either the resynchronization concept is plain wrong, or the measurement protocol design is so vulnerable to error that it cannot detect this important effect. The hazard lies in the widespread failure to perceive natural biologic variability, which is often mistaken for failure of the operator to make measurements correctly. Measurement variability causes false optima to appear with VV delay adjustment and makes the size of the optimization benefit become exaggerated.

Using sensitive (narrow-error-bar) methods, VV delay optimization produces small increments in hemodynamic effects over and above programming a nominal setting of VV 0 ms.

REFERENCES

1. Dickstein K, Bogale N, Priori S, et al. The European cardiac resynchronization therapy survey. Eur Heart J 2009;30:2450–60.
2. Molhoek SG, Bax JJ, Bleeker GB, et al. Comparison of response to cardiac resynchronization therapy in patients with sinus rhythm versus chronic atrial fibrillation. Am J Cardiol 2004;94:1506–9.
3. Gasparini M, Auricchio A, Regoli F, et al. Four-year efficacy of cardiac resynchronization therapy on exercise tolerance and disease progression. The importance of performing atrioventricular junction ablation in patients with atrial fibrillation. J Am Coll Cardiol 2006;48:734–43.
4. Kies P, Leclercq C, Bleeker GB, et al. Cardiac resynchronisation therapy in chronic atrial fibrillation: impact on left atrial size and reversal to sinus rhythm. Heart 2006;92:490–4.
5. Delnoy PP, Ottervanger JP, Luttikhuis HO, et al. Comparison of usefulness of cardiac resynchronization therapy in patients with atrial fibrillation and

heart failure versus patients with sinus rhythm and heart failure. Am J Cardiol 2007;99:1252–7.

6. Ferreira AM, Adragao P, Cavaco DM, et al. Benefit of cardiac resynchronization therapy in atrial fibrillation patients vs patients in sinus rhythm: the role of atrioventricular junction ablation. Europace 2008;10: 809–15.

7. Gasparini M, Auricchio A, Metra M, et al. Long term survival in patients undergoing cardiac resynchronization therapy: the importance of performing atrio-ventricular junction ablation in patients with permanent atrial fibrillation. Eur Heart J 2008;29: 1644–52.

8. Tolosana JM, Hernandez Madrid A, Brugada J, et al. Comparison of benefits and mortality in cardiac resynchronization therapy in patients with atrial fibrillation versus patients in sinus rhythm. Am J Cardiol 2008;102:444–9.

9. Dong K, Shen WK, Powell BD, et al. Atrioventricular nodal ablation predicts survival benefit in patients with atrial fibrillation receiving cardiac resynchronization therapy. Heart Rhythm 2010;7:1240–5.

10. Khadjooi K, Foley PW, Chalil S, et al. Long-term effects of cardiac resynchronisation therapy in patients with atrial fibrillation. Heart 2008;94:879–83.

11. Wilton SB, Leung AA, Ghali WA, et al. Outcomes of cardiac resynchronization therapy in patients with versus those without atrial fibrillation: a systematic review and meta-analysis. Heart Rhythm 2011;8: 1088–94. http://dx.doi.org/10.1016/j.hrthm.2011.02. 014.

12. Wilton SB, Kavanagh KM, Aggarwal SG, et al. Association of rate-controlled persistent atrial fibrillation with clinical outcome and ventricular remodelling in recipients of cardiac resynchronization therapy. Can J Cardiol 2011;27(6):787–93. http://dx.doi.org/ 10.1016/j.cjca.2011.06.004.

13. Leclercq C, Walker S, Linde C, et al. Comparative effects of permanent biventricular and right-univentricular pacing in heart failure patients with chronic atrial fibrillation. Eur Heart J 2002;23(22): 1780–7.

14. Linde C, Leclercq C, Rex S, et al. Long-term benefits of biventricular pacing in congestive heart failure: results from the MUltisite STimulation in cardiomyopathy (MUSTIC) study. J Am Coll Cardiol 2002;40: 111–8.

15. Healey JS, Hohnloser SH, Exner DV, et al, RAFT Investigators. Cardiac resynchronization therapy in patients with permanent atrial fibrillation: results from the Resynchronization for Ambulatory Heart Failure Trial (RAFT). Circ Heart Fail 2012; 5:566–70.

16. Wilkoff BL, Cook JR, Epstein AE, et al, Dual Chamber and VVI Implantable Defibrillator Trial Investigators. Dual-chamber pacing or ventricular backup pacing in patients with an implantable defibrillator: the Dual Chamber and VVI Implantable Defibrillator (DAVID) Trial. JAMA 2002;288: 3115–23.

17. Mullens W, Grimm RA, Verga T, et al. Insights from a cardiac resynchronization optimization clinic as part of a heart failure disease management program. J Am Coll Cardiol 2009;53:765–73.

18. Kyriacou A, Pabari P, Francis D. Cardiac resynchronization therapy is certainly cardiac therapy, but how much resynchronization and how much atrioventricular delay optimization? Heart Fail Rev 2012; 17:727–36.

19. Kamath GS, Cotiga D, Koneru JN, et al. The utility of 12-lead Holter monitoring in patients with permanent atrial fibrillation for the identification of nonresponders after cardiac resynchronization therapy. J Am Coll Cardiol 2009;53:1050–5.

20. Ganesan AN, Brooks AG, Roberts-Thomson KC, et al. Role of AV nodal ablation in cardiac resynchronization in patients with coexistent atrial fibrillation and heart failure a systematic review. J Am Coll Cardiol 2012;59(8):719–26.

21. Daubert JC, Saxon L, Adamson PB, et al, European Heart Rhythm Association, European Society of Cardiology, Heart Rhythm Society, Heart Failure Society of America, American Society of Echocardiography, American Heart Association, European Association of Echocardiography, Heart Failure Association. 2012 EHRA/HRS expert consensus statement on cardiac resynchronization therapy in heart failure: implant and follow-up recommendations and management. Heart Rhythm 2012;9(9):1524–76.

22. Finegold JA, Manisty CH, Cecaro F, et al. Choosing between velocity-time-integral ratio and peak velocity ratio for calculation of the dimensionless index (or aortic valve area) in serial follow-up of aortic stenosis. Int J Cardiol 2012. [Epub ahead of print].

23. Kyriacou A, Li Kam Wa ME, Pabari PA, et al. A systematic approach to designing reliable VV optimization methodology: assessment of internal validity of echocardiographic, electrocardiographic and haemodynamic optimization of cardiac resynchronization therapy. Int J Cardiol 2012. [Epub ahead of print].

24. Pabari PA, Willson K, Stegemann B, et al. When is an optimization not an optimization? Evaluation of clinical implications of information content (signal-to-noise ratio) in optimization of cardiac resynchronization therapy, and how to measure and maximize it. Heart Fail Rev 2011;16:277–90.

25. Whinnett ZI, Francis DP, Denis A, et al. Comparison of different invasive hemodynamic methods for AV delay optimization in patients with cardiac resynchronization therapy: implications for clinical trial design and clinical practice. Int J Cardiol 2013. http://dx.doi.org/10.1016/j.ijcard.2013.01.216.

26. Francis DP. How to reliably deliver narrow individual-patient error bars for optimization of pacemaker AV or VV delay using a "pick-the-highest" strategy with haemodynamic measurements. Int J Cardiol 2013;163:221–5. http://dx.doi.org/10.1016/j.ijcard.2012.03.128.

27. Francis DP. Precision of a Parabolic Optimum Calculated from Noisy Biological Data, and Implications for Quantitative Optimization of Biventricular Pacemakers (Cardiac Resynchronization Therapy). Applied Mathematics 2011;2:1497–506.

28. Perego GB, Chianca R, Facchini M, et al. Simultaneous vs sequential biventricular pacing in dilated cardiomyopathy: an acute hemodynamic study. Eur J Heart Fail 2003;5:305–13.

29. Bogaard MD, Doevendans PA, Leenders GE, et al. Can optimization of pacing settings compensate for a non-optimal left ventricular pacing site? Europace 2010;12:1262–9.

30. Whinnett ZI, Davies JE, Willson K, et al. Haemodynamic effects of changes in AV and VV delay in cardiac resynchronisation therapy show a consistent pattern: analysis of shape, magnitude and relative importance of AV and VV delay. Heart 2006;92:1628–34.

31. Whinnett ZI, Briscoe C, Davies JE, et al. The atrioventricular delay of cardiac resynchronization can be optimized hemodynamically during exercise and predicted from resting measurements. Heart Rhythm 2008;5:378–86.

32. Whinnett ZI, Nott G, Davies JE, et al. Efficiency, reproducibility and agreement of five different hemodynamic measures for optimization of cardiac resynchronization therapy. Int J Cardiol 2008;129:216–26.

33. Waggoner AD, de las Fuentes L, Davila-Roman VG. Doppler echocardiographic methods for optimization of the atrioventricular delay during cardiac resynchronization therapy. Echocardiography 2008;25(9):1047–55.

34. Boriani G, Muller CP, Seidl KH, et al. Randomized comparison of simultaneous biventricular stimulation versus optimized interventricular delay in cardiac resynchronization therapy. The Resynchronization for the Hemodynamic Treatment for Heart Failure Management II implantable cardioverter defibrillator (RHYTHM II ICD) study. Am Heart J 2006;151:1050–8.

35. Leon AR, Abraham WT, Brozena S, et al. Cardiac resynchronization with sequential biventricular pacing for the treatment of moderate-to-severe heart failure. J Am Coll Cardiol 2005;46:2298–304.

36. Kyriacou A, Whinnett ZI, Sen S, et al. Improvement in coronary blood flow velocity with acute biventricular pacing is predominantly due to an increase in a diastolic backward-travelling decompression (suction) wave. Circulation 2012;126:1334–44.

The Role of Ablation of the Atrioventricular Junction in Patients with Heart Failure and Atrial Fibrillation

Eszter M. Vegh, MD[a], Nitesh Sood, MD[b],
Jagmeet P. Singh, MD, PhD, DPhil[a],*

KEYWORDS

- AV junction ablation • Cardiac resynchronization therapy • Therapy refractory atrial fibrillation

KEY POINTS

- Ablation of the atrioventricular junction (AVJ) is a technically easy procedure that is safe and has a high success rate as an intervention for effective ventricular rate control in patients in symptomatic atrial fibrillation.
- AVJ ablation has been reported to improve quality of life, left ventricular ejection fraction, and exercise duration in patients with symptomatic atrial fibrillation and minimize the incidence of inappropriate shocks.
- Because right ventricular pacing after AVJ ablation may result in a decrease in left ventricular function and worsening of heart failure symptoms, there is increasing evidence to support the effectiveness of cardiac resynchronization therapy in atrial fibrillation populations.
- After receiving resynchronization therapy, AVJ ablation increases the proportion of biventricular pacing and thereby improves the response to cardiac resynchronization therapy in this cohort of patients.

INTRODUCTION

Heart failure (HF) and atrial fibrillation (AF) are at epidemic proportions in the modern world. HF affects more than 5 million Americans and is one of the leading causes of morbidity and mortality.[1] Similarly, more than 2 million people in the United States and a similar number in Europe have AF, with an increasing prevalence in the aging population. Based on Framingham follow-up data, the current lifetime risks for development of AF are 1 in 4 for men and women 40 years of age and older.[2]

AF is a common precipitating factor for HF decompensation in patients with both preserved and depressed left ventricular ejection fraction (LVEF).[3,4] AF also portends an adverse long-term prognosis in such patients.[5] Moreover, the incidence of AF increases with an increasing severity of HF: the incidence being 4% in patients with New York Heart Association (NYHA) functional class I,[3] 10% to 27% in NYHA II to III,[6] and increasing to 50% in patients with NYHA class IV HF.[7] AF has also been associated with an increased incidence of both appropriate and inappropriate implantable cardioverter defibrillator (ICD) shocks, both of which have been associated with HF decompensation and mortality in patients with cardiomyopathy.[8,9]

Rate and rhythm control strategies have both been shown to ameliorate symptoms of AF in

Disclosures: EMV and NS have no disclosures. JPS: Lectures, consulting and research grants from Biotronik, Boston Scientific, Medtronic, Sorin Group, and St. Jude Medical.
[a] Cardiac Arrhythmia Service, Massachusetts General Hospital, Harvard Medical School, 55 Fruit Street, Boston, MA 02114, USA; [b] Division of Cardiology, Lahey Clinic, Tufts University, 41 Burlington Mall Road, Burlington, MA 01805, USA
* Corresponding author.
E-mail address: jsingh@partners.org

Heart Failure Clin 9 (2013) 489–499
http://dx.doi.org/10.1016/j.hfc.2013.07.003
1551-7136/13/$ – see front matter © 2013 Elsevier Inc. All rights reserved.

eligible symptoms. Although a strategy of rhythm control has been reported to improve ejection fraction and quality of life in some series,[10] there is no conclusive evidence to suggest that rate control is inferior to rhythm control in patients with HF and irreversible systolic dysfunction.[11–13] This is particularly relevant to some older populations with AF and HF, who may not be suitable for aggressive treatment with antiarrhythmic drugs or catheter ablation.

The strategy of "Ablate and Pace" using atrioventricular junction (AVJ) ablation is an accepted but underused treatment option for patients with symptomatic, drug refractory AF. It is supported by a substantial amount of literature accumulated over a period of greater than 30 years and has recently proved to be an effective strategy to ensure optimal biventricular pacing in patients with AF and cardiomyopathy, undergoing cardiac resynchronization therapy.[14–17]

HISTORY OF AVJ ABLATION

AVJ ablation was first performed in 1981 in a patient suffering from recurrent episodes of drug refractory, symptomatic AF.[18] Scheinman[19] published a report of 5 cases of AVJ ablation in 1982. An electrode catheter was positioned via a transvenous approach at the site of largest His bundle potential. A series of direct current (DC) defibrillation shocks (300–500 J) were delivered until atrioventricular (AV) block was achieved. Four of the 5 patients continued to have AV block, whereas one patient died suddenly at 5.5 weeks after the procedure.[19] Soon after, Gallagher and colleagues[20] reported their results with DC shock-induced AVJ ablation in a series of 9 patients. After being established in canine experiments, radiofrequency ablation gathered ground in the late 1980s, and soon superseded DC shock ablation for the AVJ.[21]

ABLATION OF AVJ: DIFFERENT TECHNIQUES

The goal of AVJ ablation is to achieve conduction block in the compact AV node ideally with a stable junctional escape rhythm after ablation. The actual ablation procedure is technically simple with a low risk of complications as well as a high early and long-term success rate (>98%).[22]

Right-sided Approach

The right-sided method is nearly always attempted first and accounts for most cases. Catheters are typically introduced via a transvenous femoral approach into the right atrium. After mapping a His bundle potential in the right ventricular septal region, the ablation catheter is withdrawn slowly toward the right atrium with a clockwise torque. At the optimal location for ablation, a larger atrial than ventricular electrogram and a His bundle potential should be recorded. Ablation at the proximal part of the conduction apparatus (ie, toward the atrium) is preferred to allow for a junctional rather than a ventricular escape rhythm. Radiofrequency energy is delivered usually for 30 to 60 seconds at temperatures typically of 55 to 70°C at a maximum of 60 W. Early nodal acceleration during ablation suggests an effective ablation lesion (**Fig. 1**).

Left-sided Approach

A highly calcified AV node and/or edema after an unsuccessful right-sided ablation attempt may necessitate a left-sided approach to AVJ ablation. The ablation catheter is introduced through the femoral artery or transseptally to the left side of the ventricular membranous septum. Anatomically this lies immediately inferior to the right fibrous trigone and the junction of the right and the noncoronary cusps of the aortic valve. The penetrating bundle of His enters the left ventricular (LV) outflow tract in this region and is not protected by the central fibrous body. Sousa and colleagues[23] first described this method using 20 to 36 W of energy for 15 to 30 seconds. Later, Marshall and colleagues reported no major complications with high energy, temperature, and duration, similar to a right-sided ablation. Nevertheless, vascular complications, the risks associated with transseptal puncture, and the need for peri-procedural anticoagulation increase the theoretical risk associated with this left-sided approach.

Modification of the Slow Pathway

AF has been associated with AV node remodeling and preferential conduction over the slow AV nodal pathway.[24] Thus, modification of the slow pathway has been explored as an alternative strategy for rate control in patients with drug refractory, symptomatic AF. A few small, single-center studies have reported similar reductions in ventricular rate,[25] but this technique is not routinely used due to a higher resumption of conduction.

Approach from Superior Veins

Some operators have explored ablation of the AV node through access from the cephalic/axillary/subclavian venous system at the time of pacemaker implant.[26] This approach has been reported to reduce both the procedure and the fluoroscopy times, with similar procedural efficacy.[26] This approach may also reduce potential femoral vascular complications and is an alternative for patients with

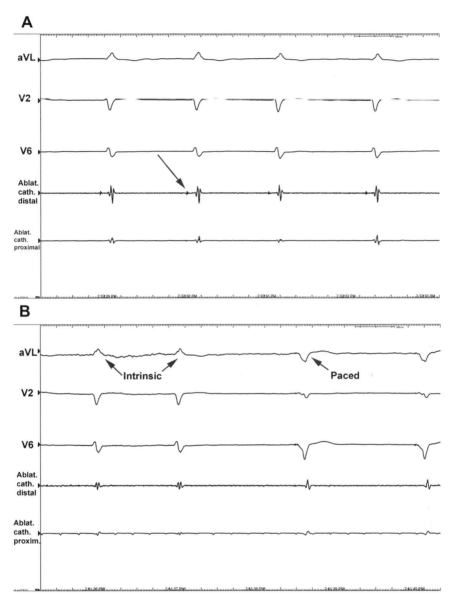

Fig. 1. Electrocardiographic representation of AVN ablation. (*A*) Registered potentials: the arrow points to the His signal. (*B*) The patient attained complete AV block after 3 seconds of ablation. The alteration of QRS morphology indicates the modified activation sequence.

an inferior vena cava filter (which does not provide an absolute contraindication), obstruction, or other issues that limit access from the inferior veins.

BENEFITS OF AVJ ABLATION

Ablation of the AVJ leads to several clinical benefits, although through mechanisms that are not completely understood. Presumably the most important component is prevention of tachycardia-mediated cardiomyopathy. In experimental models, chronic rapid ventricular pacing has been demonstrated to induce biventricular failure. Myocardial energy

depletion, ischemia, cellular, and extracellular remodeling and abnormalities of calcium regulation were observed and considered plausible mechanisms. End-stage HF status was reached within 3 to 5 weeks of right ventricular (RV) pacing in dogs; however, the process was reversible in the first 1 to 2 weeks.[27] A second mechanism for the benefit of AVJ ablation is via the regularization of R-R intervals. Clinically, lone AF has been shown to cause LV dysfunction and idiopathic cardiomyopathy, which is reversible after AVJ ablation.[28–30] Clark and colleagues[31] assessed invasive hemodynamics pre- and post-AVJ ablation comparing irregular

R-R intervals during AF to RV paced rhythm with the preablation mean rate. Irregular R-R intervals (representing altering durations between two ventricular beats) demonstrated a significantly decreased cardiac output (4.4 ± 1.6 vs 5.2 ± 2.4 L/min, $P<.01$), increased pulmonary capillary wedge pressure (17 ± 7 vs 14 ± 6 mm Hg, $P<.002$), and increased right atrial pressure (10 ± 6 vs 8 ± 4 mm Hg, $P<.05$) when compared with the paced group at preablation mean heart rate.

Pharmacologic rate control is the first line of treatment of rate control in AF. However, after an unsuccessful trial of medical treatment, AVJ ablation is a reasonable next option.[32] In the Ablate and Pace Trial, 156 highly symptomatic persistent and paroxysmal AF patients were treated with AVJ ablation. At the 12 months follow-up, the authors reported an improved quality of life but no statistically significant change in LVEF and exercise capacity compared with baseline. Notably, the authors reported 23 deaths (5 classified as sudden cardiac death, SCD; 14.7%) in 156 patients included in this study.[28] Subsequently, Ozcan and colleagues[29] reported long-term survival after AVJ ablation. Patients with AF undergoing AVJ ablation were compared with age-matched and sex-matched control subjects free of AF and consecutive AF patients receiving only pharmacologic therapy. A total of 250 patients were followed for a mean period of 3.5 years. The authors observed a similar survival in AVJ-ablated patients as in the general population and AF patients treated with pharmacologic rate control. However, mortality in subjects treated with AVJ ablation was significantly elevated in patients with underlying heart disease. A meta-analysis published by the authors' group examined the safety, efficacy, and effectiveness of AVJ ablation versus pharmacologic treatment of rate control in AF. The authors' analyses showed that, compared with subjects receiving pharmacotherapy, those receiving AVJ ablation obtained a statistically significant improvement in quality-of-life indices and LVEF, and a modest but statistically nonsignificant improvement in functional status and echocardiographic variables. Periprocedural complications were relatively rare, with the incidence of death being 0.27%, malignant arrhythmia 0.57%, that the authors considered too low to draw any safety conclusions. No significant differences were found between all-cause mortality in AVJ ablation versus medical therapy for rate control of AF.[22]

PACING AFTER AVJ ABLATION
Deleterious Effects of RV Pacing

Multiple studies have reported increased numbers of HF hospitalizations and enhanced mortality associated with high percentage of RV pacing (>40%).[33–35] Long-term follow-up of the MADIT II study reported increased mortality in ICD patients with a high percentage of RV pacing.[36] RV pacing has been shown to result in abnormal activation sequence leading to both electrical and mechanical interventricular dyssynchrony.[37,38] RV pacing has also been associated with worsening diastolic dysfunction and increased levels of inflammatory markers.[39,40]

Evidence for Biventricular Versus RV Pacing in Patients with Preserved Systolic Function (LVEF >45%)

RV pacing after AVJ ablation may result in a decrease in LVEF and worsening of HF symptoms.[15,41] Recent studies have evaluated the potential benefit of a universal biventricular pacing approach after AVJ ablation. The PAVE Study Group randomized patients to either CRT-P (cardiac resynchronization therapy-pacemaker) or RV pacing after AVJ ablation (n = 101 vs 81). Patients treated with CRT-P had a significant improvement in 6-minute walk distance (82.9 ± 94.7 m vs 61.2 ± 90.0 m, $P = .04$), and higher ejection fraction (46 ± 13% vs 41 ± 13%, $P = .03$) 6 months after ablation when compared with the RV paced group. This improvement in 6-minute walk time was higher in patients with more advanced HF (LVEF ≤45% and NYHA II/III symptoms).[41]

Brignole and colleagues[15] recently published the results of a similar study, whereby they hypothesized a superiority of CRT (n = 97) versus RV (n = 89) pacing in reducing HF events in patients with permanent AF undergoing AVJ ablation. During their median follow-up of 20 months, there was a decreased incidence of a composite endpoint of HF hospitalization, worsening symptoms, and mortality in the CRT group. In multivariable analyses, CRT remained the single independent predictor of a lack of HF events. This effect was seen in patients irrespective of ejection fraction. Recent 2-year data from the Pacing to Prevent Cardiac Enlargement trial, that compared biventricular to right ventricular pacing in patients with normal ejection fraction and sinus bradycardia, echoed similar effects on the prevention of deleterious LV remodeling in patients receiving biventricular compared to RV pacing.[42]

Biventricular Versus RV Pacing in Patients with Depressed Systolic Function

Current guidelines recommend biventricular pacing in patients with irreversible cardiomyopathy with LVEF ≤35% undergoing AVJ ablation for AF or who otherwise meet criteria for CRT-D.[32]

Patients with tachycardia-mediated cardiomyopathy with an LVEF ≤35% should be initially implanted with RV pacing lead only.[43]

CLINICAL IMPLICATIONS AND AVJ ABLATION AS A TREATMENT MODALITY: CURRENT GUIDELINES

Current guidelines recommend single-chamber pacemaker implant for patients with normal LV function or reversible LV dysfunction undergoing AVJ ablation for AF.[32] Biventricular defibrillator/pacemaker is indicated in patients with irreversible cardiomyopathy and LVEF of ≤35%. A LV lead upgrade is indicated in patients with LVEF greater than 35% at implant who subsequently develop RV pacing-induced cardiomyopathy and/or HF.

Class II A (Level of Evidence: B)

It is reasonable to use ablation of AV node or accessory pathway to control heart rate when pharmacologic therapy is insufficient or associated with side effects.

Class II B (Level of Evidence: C)

When rate cannot be controlled by pharmacologic therapy or tachycardia-induced cardiomyopathy is suspected, catheter-driven AV node ablation may be considered in patients with AF to control heart rate.

Class III

Catheter ablation of AV node should not be used in AF to control heart rate without a prior trial of medications.

AVJ ABLATION AS A TREATMENT MODALITY
Preserved LVEF Greater than 45%

Symptomatic
AF is a common precipitant of hospitalization in patients with HF with preserved ejection fraction. Loss of atrial systole and irregular R-R intervals are the most likely mechanisms. Patients with AF and HF with preserved ejection fraction tend to be older and mostly not candidates for aggressive rhythm control strategy with anti-arrhythmic drugs or catheter ablation.[31,44] AVJ ablation may be an effective treatment in this patient group after a trial of pharmacologic therapy.

Asymptomatic
Many studies have shown that rate control is equivalent to rhythm control in asymptomatic patients with permanent AF and preserved ejection fraction. Moreover, a recent randomized trial (RACE II) suggested that lenient heart rate control

(<110 bpm) may be an optimal strategy for patients with ejection fraction greater than 40%.[45] Thus, patients with asymptomatic permanent AF with preserved ejection fraction may be treated conservatively without aggressive measures. The exercise treadmill test may help with assessing symptoms because, for instance, individuals with rapid ventricular rates during exercise associated with symptoms and/or reduced functional capacity are not truly "asymptomatic." Holter monitors can be used to verify adequate heart rate control over 24 to 48 hours. An "Ablate and Pace" strategy may be appropriate for patients with suboptimal functional capacity, exercise-induced rapid ventricular rates associated with symptoms, inadequate heart rate control (>110 bpm), or those unable to tolerate pharmacologic treatment. In current practice, younger patients with symptomatic AF are often considered better candidates for a trial of anti-arrhythmic therapy or catheter ablation of AF.

Patients with Systolic Dysfunction

Symptomatic
Patients with either tachycardia-mediated cardiomyopathy or symptomatic AF and LV dysfunction should be managed aggressively. In such patients, associated comorbidities such as renal and liver dysfunction frequently limit the use of antiarrhythmic medications. Dofetilide and amiodarone may be safe in patients with LV dysfunction but require close monitoring.[46,47] Class IC drugs are contraindicated in patients with structural heart disease.[48] Sotalol should be used with caution especially in severely depressed LV dysfunction and advanced NYHA class.[49] Notably, dronedarone was recently reported to be associated with increase risk of mortality in patients with LV dysfunction and HF.[50]

A prospective randomized study compared AVJ ablation and biventricular pacing to catheter ablation for patients with AF and LV dysfunction. This study included patients with drug refractory AF, LVEF less than 40% that were at least NYHA class II/III. Patients with normal sinus rhythm after catheter ablation demonstrated a greater improvement in ejection fraction (35% vs 28%), 6-minute walk distance (340 m vs 297 m), and quality-of-life indices. The success rate for pulmonary vein isolation in this study was 88% with anti-arrhythmic drugs and 71% without anti-arrhythmic drugs at 6 months.[51] However, other studies reported variable results with catheter ablation for AF in patients with LV dysfunction.[52-54] Notably, the lack of a standardized ablative approach, frequent need for repeat procedures, and lack of robust data demonstrating benefit makes catheter ablation less attractive as a first-line approach to patients with AF and LV dysfunction. Catheter ablation for AF may be more likely to benefit selected groups of patients, such as those with tachycardia-related cardiomyopathy and paroxysmal or early persistent AF; this is currently being investigated in a prospective trial (CASTLE-HF).[55] Until further data are available, AVJ ablation and biventricular pacing remain a viable and beneficial approach in the treatment of symptomatic drug/ablation refractory AF in patients with LV dysfunction.

Asymptomatic

Even in asymptomatic patients, AF is associated with worse prognosis (CHARM).[56] Pharmacologic rate versus rhythm control was tested in a prospective randomized trial in patients with paroxysmal and persistent AF and HF with an LVEF less than 35% (AF-CHF). The rhythm control strategy with amiodarone and electrical cardioversion showed no benefit, and conversely, reported increased hospitalizations during follow-up.[13] The authors recommend Holter monitor and exercise treadmill test to ascertain symptoms and adequate heart rate control. A trial of sinus rhythm after cardioversion may also be attempted in such patients, to ascertain differences in functional status between sinus rhythm and AF. Truly asymptomatic patients with adequate heart rate control have not been reported to benefit from aggressive rhythm control or by a strategy of AVJ ablation and biventricular pacing. It is essential to evaluate the often subtle symptoms carefully that may arise from AF in patients with irreversible systolic dysfunction and HF. Of note, a lenient rate control strategy has not been extensively evaluated in the HF and cardiomyopathy populations, because patients with ejection fraction less than 40% were excluded from the RACE II trial.[45] Indeed, one study showed an increase in HF hospitalizations in patients with cardiomyopathy and AF whose average ventricular rate was greater than 90 bpm in a 1-month period.[57] Thus, ventricular rate–related symptoms should be carefully assessed in the reduced ejection fraction group.

Prevention of Appropriate ICD Shocks

Many studies have shown that AF is associated with a higher incidence of appropriate shocks in patients with an ICD.[58] This finding has been reported in patients with persistent AF, whereas episodes of paroxysmal AF have also been shown to precede appropriate ICD shocks in 20% of patients.[59] Studies suggest that exacerbations in HF, with electrophysiological abnormalities, mechano-electrical feedback from hemodynamic compromise, rate-related ischemia, ventricular arrhythmias associated with use of anti-arrhythmic drugs, and sympatho-excitation from heart rate irregularity are possible contributing mechanisms for this association.[58–60] These patients frequently have added comorbidities like renal dysfunction, diabetes, and hypertension, hence limiting the choices and dosages of pharmacologic rate control.

Prevention of Inappropriate ICD Shocks

Subanalyses of 2 major primary prevention trials (MADIT-II and SCD-HeFT) have reported an association between inappropriate shocks with increased mortality during follow-up.[8,9] AF remains the most prominent cause of inappropriate ICD shocks.[60–62] A large population-based cohort study of the LATITUDE database demonstrated that this increase in mortality was only seen in patients who received inappropriate shocks for AF.[63] Patients who received inappropriate shocks for other reasons (eg, sensing problems, supraventricular tachyarrhythmias) lacked a similar increase in mortality.[59,63] Hence, it may very well be that the additive effect of AF and shocks is responsible for this association.

Accordingly, patients that receive either appropriate or inappropriate ICD shocks secondary to AF should be aggressively considered for AVJ ablation or rhythm control strategy for management of AF.

Treating Ineffective Biventricular Pacing

Biventricular pacing has been demonstrated to reduce composite endpoint of mortality and HF in patients with cardiomyopathy and AF.[17,64–66] However, this requires a high percentage of biventricular pacing to optimize the response to CRT.[67] AF in patients with native conduction decreases true biventricular capture. The combined effects of AF and decreased percentage of biventricular pacing are additive in increasing mortality.[68,69] The presence of biventricular fusion (hybrid between paced and intrinsic QRS morphologies) and pseudofusion (pacing artifact delivered but intrinsic QRS morphology not altered) can artificially elevate the apparent percentage of biventricular pacing, yet without the benefits of true cardiac resynchronization.[70] Although the cutoff for percentage of biventricular pacing in reducing mortality was recently described in a large cohort of patients (>98.7%),[67] a similar cutoff for patients with AF and biventricular fusion has not been reported.

AVJ ablation has been reported to improve survival and functional status in patients with AF implanted with cardiac resynchronization therapy.[15,17,71] Ganesan and colleagues[14] reported a review and meta-analysis of clinical studies examining the impact of AVJ ablation in CRT-AF patients. This study included 6 trials and compared CRT-AF patients with and without AVJ ablation. Patients without AVJ ablation had higher all-cause (RR 0.42) and cardiovascular (RR 0.44) mortality. Heterogeneity in assessment of functional status precluded definite conclusion for this outcome.[14] Gasparini and colleagues[17] also found a significant increase in the LVEF of patients with CRT and AF with versus without AVJ ablation (37.1 vs 23.7% at 1 year, 39.5 vs 25.0% at 4-year follow-up).

Accordingly, patients with CRT and AF who are deemed to be nonresponders should undergo a careful assessment of true biventricular pacing, which may include a 24- to 48-hour Holter monitor to assess the percentage of paced beats that may truly be fused with intrinsic (dyssynchronous) activation. Patients who fail to respond clinically to resynchronization therapy with a suboptimal percentage of biventricular pacing should be treated aggressively to increase this percentage. Pharmacologic approaches with AV nodal blocking agents is the first-line treatment. Adverse effects of these medications are common in patients with advanced cardiomyopathy and HF. Lack of effective AV node blockade or adverse effects of pharmacologic agents should prompt consideration for AVJ ablation in these patients.

COMPLICATIONS OF AVJ ABLATION

Iatrogenic pacemaker dependency is likely to be a primary hesitation in recommending AVJ ablation more universally for rate control in patients with AF. Indeed, pacemaker dysfunction or loss of capture from lead dislodgment or fracture could be fatal in such patients. However, in a recent meta-analysis of AVJ ablation in AF, the authors' group found the incidence of lead failure as low as 0.23%.[22] Ganesan and colleagues[14] also did not report any major complications secondary to pacemaker dysfunction in their recent meta-analysis.

As an invasive procedure, AVJ carries inherent risks of femoral vascular complications, such as bleeding, hematoma, fistula, and venous thrombosis. Rare complications include intracardiac shunt, cardiac perforation, pericardial tamponade, tricuspid valve regurgitation, infection, and even death. The incidence of complications is approximately 3%, but with major complications is less than 2%.[72] According to the NASPE Prospective

Voluntary Registry only 5 significant complications were reported during AVJ ablation of 646 patients, whereby the overall success rate was 97.4%.[73]

Sudden cardiac death after AVJ ablation was described in early studies and also in major trials.[19] The Ablate and Pace Trial reported 11 cases of death, and underlying structural heart disease was found to be a major predisposing factor.[28] Ozcan and colleagues[29] reported 4 likely and 3 possible procedure-related SCD cases in 334 AVJ ablation procedures. They found that risk of death was highest in the first 2 days after ablation. Diabetes, NYHA ≥2, ventricular arrhythmias present preprocedure, mitral or aortic stenosis, aortic regurgitation, and chronic obstructive pulmonary disease were independent predictors of mortality.

Ventricular tachyarrhythmias and SCD may contribute to mortality after AVJ ablation and are assumed to be triggered by bradycardia and pause-dependent polymorphic ventricular tachycardia.[74] To prevent this phenomenon, Geelen and colleagues[75] compared a postablation lower rate limit for pacing to 90 bpm (n = 235) for the first 1 to 3 months postablation compared with a group of patients (n = 100) with a lower rate limit ≤70 bpm. Notably, they found less SCD (0 vs 6 cases) in the higher base rate group despite no significant differences in baseline characteristics between groups. Postablation ventricular fibrillation was observed only during slow ventricular pacing or escape rhythm. Thus, current practice is to set an elevated pacing rate for some months after AVJ ablation, then reduce the rate over time.

It is important to remember clearly that AVJ-ablated patients demand constant ventricular pacing, leading to early battery depletion demanding more frequent generator replacement with its attendant complications.

AVJ ablation does not address AF per se, and patients still require oral anticoagulation according to their risk for stroke as codified in the CHA_2DS_2-VASc score.

LV–right atrial shunt is an extremely rare complication of AVJ ablation. During ablation, the catheter is positioned toward the apex of the triangle of Koch, directly above the septal leaflet of tricuspid valve. This leaflet is 5 to 10 mm more apically located than the mitral valve and above it the superior AV portion of the membranous septum can be found. This membranous septum can be perforated due to radiofrequency ablation in this area.[76] Can and colleagues[77] reported a patient with such an LV-RA shunt and a 76-mm Hg gradient at 5 months with mild to moderate RV dilatation. Nevertheless, this patient remained stable with NYHA I and II HF during follow-up with conservative management.

Of note, AVERT-AF (Atrio-Ventricular Junction Ablation Followed By Resynchronization Therapy In patients with CHF and AF) is a prospective, randomized, multicenter trial examining AVJ ablation versus pharmacologic rate control in CRT-AF population with respect to functional status, quality of life, and survival. The AVERT-AF is designed to test exercise capacity and functional status, as primary endpoints in patients with chronic AF and depressed ejection fraction, regardless of rate or QRS duration. The results are expected soon.[78]

SUMMARY

AVJ ablation is a technically straightforward and relatively safe procedure, with a high success as an intervention to achieve effective ventricular rate control in patients in symptomatic AF. It has been reported to improve quality of life, LVEF, and exercise duration in these patients. There is increasing evidence that supports its effectiveness in the CRT-AF population to improve response to resynchronization. It is important to remember, however, that patients after AVJ ablation become pacemaker-dependent and still require appropriate antithrombotic therapy to prevent stroke.

REFERENCES

1. Roger VL, Go AS, Lloyd-Jones DM, et al. Executive summary: heart disease and stroke statistics–2012 update: a report from the American Heart Association. Circulation 2012;125:188–97.

2. Lloyd-Jones DM, Wang TJ, Leip EP, et al. Lifetime risk for development of atrial fibrillation: the Framingham Heart Study. Circulation 2004;110: 1042–6.

3. Maisel WH, Stevenson LW. Atrial fibrillation in heart failure: epidemiology, pathophysiology, and rationale for therapy. Am J Cardiol 2003;91:8.

4. Rosenberg MA, Manning WJ. Diastolic dysfunction and risk of atrial fibrillation: a mechanistic appraisal. Circulation 2012;126:2353–62.

5. Dries DL, Exner DV, Gersh BJ, et al. Atrial fibrillation is associated with an increased risk for mortality and heart failure progression in patients with asymptomatic and symptomatic left ventricular systolic dysfunction: a retrospective analysis of the SOLVD trials. Studies of Left Ventricular Dysfunction. J Am Coll Cardiol 1998;32:695–703.

6. Pedersen OD, Bagger H, Keller N, et al. Efficacy of dofetilide in the treatment of atrial fibrillation-flutter in patients with reduced left ventricular function: a Danish investigations of arrhythmia and mortality on dofetilide (diamond) substudy. Circulation 2001;104:292–6.

7. Effects of enalapril on mortality in severe congestive heart failure. Results of the Cooperative North Scandinavian Enalapril Survival Study (CONSENSUS). The CONSENSUS Trial Study Group. N Engl J Med 1987;316:1429–35.

8. Daubert JP, Zareba W, Cannom DS, et al. Inappropriate implantable cardioverter-defibrillator shocks in MADIT II: frequency, mechanisms, predictors, and survival impact. J Am Coll Cardiol 2008;51: 1357–65.

9. Poole JE, Johnson GW, Hellkamp AS, et al. Prognostic importance of defibrillator shocks in patients with heart failure. N Engl J Med 2008;359:1009–17.

10. Hagens VE, Crijns HJ, Van Veldhuisen DJ, et al. Rate control versus rhythm control for patients with persistent atrial fibrillation with mild to moderate heart failure: results from the RAte Control versus Electrical cardioversion (RACE) study. Am Heart J 2005;149:1106–11.

11. Bolliger CT, Guckel C, Engel H, et al. Prediction of functional reserves after lung resection: comparison between quantitative computed tomography, scintigraphy, and anatomy. Respiration 2002;69:482–9.

12. Van Gelder IC, Hagens VE, Bosker HA, et al. A comparison of rate control and rhythm control in patients with recurrent persistent atrial fibrillation. N Engl J Med 2002;347:1834–40.

13. Roy D, Talajic M, Nattel S, et al. Rhythm control versus rate control for atrial fibrillation and heart failure. N Engl J Med 2008;358:2667–77.

14. Ganesan AN, Brooks AG, Roberts-Thomson KC, et al. Role of AV nodal ablation in cardiac resynchronization in patients with coexistent atrial fibrillation and heart failure a systematic review. J Am Coll Cardiol 2012;59:719–26.

15. Brignole M, Botto G, Mont L, et al. Cardiac resynchronization therapy in patients undergoing atrioventricular junction ablation for permanent atrial fibrillation: a randomized trial. Eur Heart J 2011;32:2420–9.

16. Dong K, Shen WK, Powell BD, et al. Atrioventricular nodal ablation predicts survival benefit in patients with atrial fibrillation receiving cardiac resynchronization therapy. Heart Rhythm 2010;7:1240–5.

17. Gasparini M, Auricchio A, Metra M, et al. Long-term survival in patients undergoing cardiac resynchronization therapy: the importance of performing atrio-ventricular junction ablation in patients with permanent atrial fibrillation. Eur Heart J 2008;29: 1644–52.

18. Scheinman MA. Reflections on the first catheter ablation of the atrioventricular junction. Pacing Clin Electrophysiol 2003;26:2315–6.

19. Scheinman MM, Morady F, Hess DS, et al. Catheter-induced ablation of the atrioventricular junction to control refractory supraventricular arrhythmias. JAMA 1982;248:851–5.

20. Gallagher JJ, Svenson RH, Kasell JH, et al. Catheter technique for closed-chest ablation of the atrioventricular conduction system. N Engl J Med 1982;306:194–200.

21. Olgin JE, Scheinman MM. Comparison of high energy direct current and radiofrequency catheter ablation of the atrioventricular junction. J Am Coll Cardiol 1993;21:557–64.

22. Chatterjee NA, Upadhyay GA, Ellenbogen KA, et al. Atrioventricular nodal ablation in atrial fibrillation: a meta-analysis and systematic review. Circ Arrhythm Electrophysiol 2012;5:68–76.

23. Sousa J, el-Atassi R, Rosenheck S, et al. Radiofrequency catheter ablation of the atrioventricular junction from the left ventricle. Circulation 1991; 84:567–71.

24. Zhang Y, Mazgalev TN. Atrioventricular node functional remodeling induced by atrial fibrillation. Heart Rhythm 2012;9:1419–25.

25. Williamson BD, Man KC, Daoud E, et al. Radiofrequency catheter modification of atrioventricular conduction to control the ventricular rate during atrial fibrillation. N Engl J Med 1994;331:910–7.

26. Kalaga R, Kahr R, Migeed M, et al. Comparison of single and double vein approaches for His bundle ablation and pacemaker placement for symptomatic rapid atrial fibrillation. J Interv Card Electrophysiol 2009;24:113–7.

27. Shinbane JS, Wood MA, Jensen DN, et al. Tachycardia-induced cardiomyopathy: a review of animal models and clinical studies. J Am Coll Cardiol 1997;29:709–15.

28. Kay GN, Ellenbogen KA, Giudici M, et al. The Ablate and Pace Trial: a prospective study of catheter ablation of the AV conduction system and permanent pacemaker implantation for treatment of atrial fibrillation. APT Investigators. J Interv Card Electrophysiol 1998;2:121–35.

29. Ozcan C, Jahangir A, Friedman PA, et al. Long-term survival after ablation of the atrioventricular node and implantation of a permanent pacemaker in patients with atrial fibrillation. N Engl J Med 2001; 344:1043–51.

30. Wood MA, Brown-Mahoney C, Kay GN, et al. Clinical outcomes after ablation and pacing therapy for atrial fibrillation: a meta-analysis. Circulation 2000; 101:1138–44.

31. Clark DM, Plumb VJ, Epstein AE, et al. Hemodynamic effects of an irregular sequence of ventricular cycle lengths during atrial fibrillation. J Am Coll Cardiol 1997;30:1039–45.

32. Fuster V, Ryden LE, Cannom DS, et al. 2011 ACCF/AHA/HRS focused updates incorporated into the ACC/AHA/ESC 2006 Guidelines for the management of patients with atrial fibrillation: a report of the American College of Cardiology Foundation/American Heart Association Task Force on Practice Guidelines developed in partnership with the European Society of Cardiology and in collaboration with the European Heart Rhythm Association and the Heart Rhythm Society. J Am Coll Cardiol 2011;57:101–98.

33. Wilkoff BL, Cook JR, Epstein AE, et al. Dual-chamber pacing or ventricular backup pacing in patients with an implantable defibrillator: the Dual Chamber and VVI Implantable Defibrillator (DAVID) Trial. JAMA 2002;288:3115–23.

34. Brignole M, Gammage M, Puggioni E, et al. Comparative assessment of right, left, and biventricular pacing in patients with permanent atrial fibrillation. Eur Heart J 2005;26:712–22.

35. Sweeney MO, Ellenbogen KA, Tang AS, et al. Atrial pacing or ventricular backup-only pacing in implantable cardioverter-defibrillator patients. Heart Rhythm 2010;7:1552–60.

36. Barsheshet A, Wang PJ, Moss AJ, et al. Reverse remodeling and the risk of ventricular tachyarrhythmias in the MADIT-CRT (Multicenter Automatic Defibrillator Implantation Trial-Cardiac Resynchronization Therapy). J Am Coll Cardiol 2011;57:2416–23.

37. Bank AJ, Kaufman CL, Burns KV, et al. Intramural dyssynchrony and response to cardiac resynchronization therapy in patients with and without previous right ventricular pacing. Eur J Heart Fail 2010; 12:1317–24.

38. Bank AJ, Schwartzman DS, Burns KV, et al. Intramural dyssynchrony from acute right ventricular apical pacing in human subjects with normal left ventricular function. J Cardiovasc Transl Res 2010;3:321–9.

39. Rubaj A, Rucinski P, Oleszczak K, et al. Inflammatory activation following interruption of long-term cardiac resynchronization therapy. Heart Vessels 2012. http://dx.doi.org/10.1007/s00380-012-0285-y.

40. Fang F, Zhang Q, Chan JY, et al. Deleterious effect of right ventricular apical pacing on left ventricular diastolic function and the impact of pre-existing diastolic disease. Eur Heart J 2011;32:1891–9.

41. Doshi RN, Daoud EG, Fellows C, et al. Left ventricular-based cardiac stimulation post AV nodal ablation evaluation (the PAVE study). J Cardiovasc Electrophysiol 2005;16:1160–5.

42. Chan JY, Fang F, Zhang Q, et al. Biventricular pacing is superior to right ventricular pacing in bradycardia patients with preserved systolic function: 2-year results of the PACE trial. Eur Heart J 2011; 32:2533–40.

43. Tracy CM, Epstein AE, Darbar D, et al. 2012 ACCF/AHA/HRS Focused Update of the 2008 Guidelines for Device-Based Therapy of Cardiac Rhythm Abnormalities: a Report of the American College of Cardiology Foundation/American Heart Association Task Force on Practice Guidelines. J Am Coll Cardiol 2012;60:1297–313.

44. Linderer T, Chatterjee K, Parmley WW, et al. Influence of atrial systole on the Frank-Starling relation and the end-diastolic pressure-diameter relation of the left ventricle. Circulation 1983;67:1045–53.

45. Van Gelder IC, Groenveld HF, Crijns HJ, et al. Lenient versus strict rate control in patients with atrial fibrillation. N Engl J Med 2010;362:1363–73.

46. Torp-Pedersen C, Moller M, Bloch-Thomsen PE, et al. Dofetilide in patients with congestive heart failure and left ventricular dysfunction. Danish Investigations of Arrhythmia and Mortality on Dofetilide Study Group. N Engl J Med 1999;341:857–65.

47. Effect of prophylactic amiodarone on mortality after acute myocardial infarction and in congestive heart failure: meta-analysis of individual data from 6500 patients in randomised trials. Amiodarone Trials Meta-Analysis Investigators. Lancet 1997;350: 1417–24.

48. Echt DS, Liebson PR, Mitchell LB, et al. Mortality and morbidity in patients receiving encainide, flecainide, or placebo. The Cardiac Arrhythmia Suppression Trial. N Engl J Med 1991;324:781–8.

49. Waldo AL, Camm AJ, deRuyter H, et al. Effect of d-sotalol on mortality in patients with left ventricular dysfunction after recent and remote myocardial infarction. The SWORD Investigators. Survival With Oral d-Sotalol. Lancet 1996;348:7–12.

50. Kober L, Torp-Pedersen C, McMurray JJ, et al. Increased mortality after dronedarone therapy for severe heart failure. N Engl J Med 2008;358: 2678–87.

51. Khan MN, Jais P, Cummings J, et al. Pulmonary-vein isolation for atrial fibrillation in patients with heart failure. N Engl J Med 2008;359:1778–85.

52. Efremidis M, Sideris A, Xydonas S, et al. Ablation of atrial fibrillation in patients with heart failure: reversal of atrial and ventricular remodelling. Hellenic J Cardiol 2008;49:19–25.

53. MacDonald MR, Connelly DT, Hawkins NM, et al. Radiofrequency ablation for persistent atrial fibrillation in patients with advanced heart failure and severe left ventricular systolic dysfunction: a randomised controlled trial. Heart 2011;97:740–7.

54. Dagres N, Varounis C, Gaspar T, et al. Catheter ablation for atrial fibrillation in patients with left ventricular systolic dysfunction. A systematic review and meta-analysis. J Card Fail 2011;17:964–70.

55. Marrouche NF, Brachmann J, CASTLE-AF Steering Committee. Catheter ablation versus standard conventional treatment in patients with left ventricular dysfunction and atrial fibrillation (CASTLE-AF) - study design. Pacing Clin Electrophysiol 2009;32:987–94.

56. Olsson LG, Swedberg K, Ducharme A, et al. Atrial fibrillation and risk of clinical events in chronic heart failure with and without left ventricular systolic dysfunction: results from the Candesartan in Heart failure-Assessment of Reduction in Mortality and morbidity (CHARM) program. J Am Coll Cardiol 2006;47:1997–2004.

57. Sarkar S, Koehler J, Crossley GH, et al. Burden of atrial fibrillation and poor rate control detected by continuous monitoring and the risk for heart failure hospitalization. Am Heart J 2012;164:616–24.

58. Fischer A, Ousdigian KT, Johnson JW, et al. The impact of atrial fibrillation with rapid ventricular rates and device programming on shocks in 106,513 ICD and CRT-D patients. Heart Rhythm 2012;9:24–31.

59. Kleemann T, Hochadel M, Strauss M, et al. Comparison between atrial fibrillation-triggered implantable cardioverter-defibrillator (ICD) shocks and inappropriate shocks caused by lead failure: different impact on prognosis in clinical practice. J Cardiovasc Electrophysiol 2012;23:735–40.

60. van Rees JB, Borleffs CJ, de Bie MK, et al. Inappropriate implantable cardioverter-defibrillator shocks: incidence, predictors, and impact on mortality. J Am Coll Cardiol 2011;57:556–62.

61. Saxon LA, Hayes DL, Gilliam FR, et al. Long-term outcome after ICD and CRT implantation and influence of remote device follow-up: the ALTITUDE survival study. Circulation 2010;122:2359–67.

62. Stempniewicz P, Cheng A, Connolly A, et al. Appropriate and inappropriate electrical therapies delivered by an implantable cardioverter-defibrillator: effect on intracardiac electrogram. J Cardiovasc Electrophysiol 2011;22:554–60.

63. Powell BD, Asirvatham SJ, Perschbacher DL, et al. Noise, Artifact, and Oversensing Related Inappropriate ICD Shock Evaluation: ALTITUDE NOISE Study. Pacing Clin Electrophysiol 2012;35(7): 863–9.

64. Khadjooi K, Foley PW, Chalil S, et al. Long-term effects of cardiac resynchronisation therapy in patients with atrial fibrillation. Heart 2008;94:879–83.

65. Gasparini M, Auricchio A, Regoli F, et al. Four-year efficacy of cardiac resynchronization therapy on exercise tolerance and disease progression: the importance of performing atrioventricular junction ablation in patients with atrial fibrillation. J Am Coll Cardiol 2006;48:734–43.

66. Hoppe UC, Casares JM, Eiskjaer H, et al. Effect of cardiac resynchronization on the incidence of atrial fibrillation in patients with severe heart failure. Circulation 2006;114:18–25.

67. Hayes DL, Boehmer JP, Day JD, et al. Cardiac resynchronization therapy and the relationship of percent biventricular pacing to symptoms and survival. Heart Rhythm 2011;8:1469–75.

68. Gasparini M, Cappelleri A. Atrial arrhythmias after cardiac resynchronization therapy: an inverse correlation with achieving 100% biventricular pacing and cardiac resynchronization therapy effectiveness. Europace 2010;12:9–10.

69. Gasparini M, Steinberg JS, Arshad A, et al. Resumption of sinus rhythm in patients with heart failure and permanent atrial fibrillation undergoing cardiac resynchronization therapy: a longitudinal observational study. Eur Heart J 2010;31: 976–83.

70. Kamath GS, Cotiga D, Koneru JN, et al. The utility of 12-lead Holter monitoring in patients with permanent atrial fibrillation for the identification of nonresponders after cardiac resynchronization therapy. J Am Coll Cardiol 2009;53:1050–5.

71. Upadhyay GA, Choudhry NK, Auricchio A, et al. Cardiac resynchronization in patients with atrial fibrillation: a meta-analysis of prospective cohort studies. J Am Coll Cardiol 2008;52:1239–46.

72. Hoffmayer KS, Scheinman M. Current role of atrioventricular junction (AVJ) ablation. Pacing Clin Electrophysiol 2013;36:257–65.

73. Scheinman MM, Huang S. The 1998 NASPE prospective catheter ablation registry. Pacing Clin Electrophysiol 2000;23:1020–8.

74. Brandt RR, Shen WK. Bradycardia-induced polymorphic ventricular tachycardia after atrioventricular junction ablation for sinus tachycardia-induced cardiomyopathy. J Cardiovasc Electrophysiol 1995; 6:630–3.

75. Geelen P, Brugada J, Andries E, et al. Ventricular fibrillation and sudden death after radiofrequency catheter ablation of the atrioventricular junction. Pacing Clin Electrophysiol 1997;20:343–8.

76. Sharma AK, Chander R, Singh JP. AV nodal ablation-induced Gerbode defect (LV-RA Shunt). J Cardiovasc Electrophysiol 2011;22:1288–9.

77. Can I, Krueger K, Chandrashekar Y, et al. Images in cardiovascular medicine. Gerbode-type defect induced by catheter ablation of the atrioventricular node. Circulation 2009;119:553–6.

78. Hamdan MH, Freedman RA, Gilbert EM, et al. Atrioventricular junction ablation followed by resynchronization therapy in patients with congestive heart failure and atrial fibrillation (AVERT-AF) study design. Pacing Clin Electrophysiol 2006;29:1081–8.

Ablation of Atrial Tachycardia and Atrial Flutter in Heart Failure

Ayotunde Bamimore, MB, ChB,
Paul Mounsey, BSc, BM BCh, PhD, MRCP*

KEYWORDS

• Tachyarrhythmia • Heart failure • Atrial flutter • Atrial tachycardia • Ablation

KEY POINTS

• Atrial tachycardia (AT) and atrial flutter (AFL) are common tachyarrhythmias in the heart failure population.
• They commonly lead to, exacerbate, and increase the morbidity and mortality associated with heart failure and, thereby, warrant urgent and early definitive therapy in the form of catheter ablation.
• Catheter ablation requires careful patient stabilization and extensive preprocedural planning, particularly with regards to anesthesia, strategy, catheter choice, mapping system, and fluid balance, to increase efficacy and limit adverse effects.
• Heart failure may limit the success of catheter ablation with higher reported recurrence rates and, in selected patients, a hybrid epicardial-endocardial ablation can be considered.

Atrial tachyarrhythmias are common in patients with heart failure and vice versa.[1] Several publications highlight the development of heart failure in patients with poorly controlled atrial tachyarrhythmias as well as the development of atrial arrhythmias in heart failure patients previously known to be in sinus rhythm. The structural, electrophysiologic, and neuroendocrine changes that occur in one facilitate the development of the other, thereby setting up a vicious cycle, such that atrial tachyarrhythmias beget heart failure and heart failure begets atrial tachyarrhythmias. This statement, however true, is an oversimplification of a complex relationship.

Atrial tachyarrhythmias are those tachycardias that are initiated or sustained by the atria and do not require the atrioventricular (AV) node or ventricles for perpetuation. They may be regular or irregular. The irregular atrial arrhythmias are atrial fibrillation (AF) and multifocal AT whereas regular atrial tachyarrhythmias were previously classified as AT and AFL. This outdated classification of regular atrial tachyarrhythmias was based on heart rate and ECG morphology, such that tachycardias with atrial rates equal to or greater than 240 beats per minute (bpm), with an undulating baseline lacking an isoelectric baseline in at least one lead (saw tooth), were classified as AFL and the others lacking these 2 characteristics as AT. Contemporary electrophysiology studies (EPSs) and improvement in mapping techniques have led to a more precise classification based on pathophysiologic mechanisms.[2]

Regular atrial arrhythmias are now classified as

1. Focal ATs (formerly ATs), which have the following characteristics
   • Origin outside the sinus node and from a discrete portion of the atrium (<2 cm^2)

Disclosures: The authors have nothing to disclose.
Division of Cardiology, University of North Carolina, Chapel Hill, 160 Dental Circle, Burnett-Womack Building, CB #7075, Chapel Hill, NC 27599, USA
* Corresponding author.
E-mail address: Paul_mounsey@med.unc.edu

Heart Failure Clin 9 (2013) 501–514
http://dx.doi.org/10.1016/j.hfc.2013.07.002
1551-7136/13/$ – see front matter © 2013 Elsevier Inc. All rights reserved.

- Centrifugal spread of activation from the discrete portion
- Mechanism automatic, triggered activity, or microreentry
- Propagation occurring over a short duration of the cycle length (**Fig. 1**)
- Rate above 100 bpm but less than 240 bpm
- Warming up and cooling down properties

2. Macroreentrant AT (formerly AFL), with the following characteristics
   - Mechanism is macroreentry involving a large portion of the atrium
   - Propagation occurring around an area of fixed or functional barrier
   - Propagation occurring over most of the duration of the cycle length (**Fig. 2**)

For the remainder of this review, AT refers to focal AT and AFL refers to macroreentrant AT, based on the newer classification. This distinction is not often made in publications. Sometimes the new classifications are implied and knowledge of this by readers is assumed, whereas in other instances, writers use the old classification. Some studies group AT and AFL together as ATs,

distinguishing them from AF. Further complicating the scenario is that a patient may exhibit each of these various tachyarrhythmias at different times. This confusion in terminologies makes the exact prevalence of AT and AFL in the general population, let alone in heart failure patients, uncertain. Although there is a robust amount of literature on AF (often including AFL) in the general population and in heart failure patients, studies on AT and AFL are sparse. Few studies have made efforts to separate these various atrial arrhythmias and, from this limited information, the following is known. The prevalence of AT has been reported to be 0.34% in an asymptomatic population, rising to 0.46% in a population with symptoms,[3] whereas the prevalence of AFL is largely speculative. The incidence of AFL is, however, reported to be approximately 0.07% in the United States, amounting to 200,000 new cases per year, among which 80,000 patients are diagnosed with AFL only (without AF).[4] These numbers are overshadowed by those of AF, which has a prevalence of 2.2 million in the United States (0.7%–1% of the population) and an incidence that stands at 0.1%.[5] Generally, in cardiac disease states, the

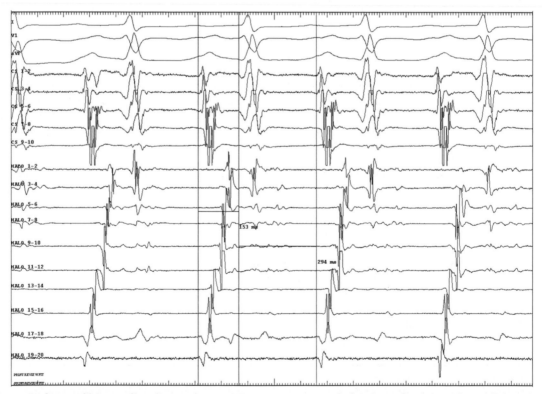

Fig. 1. Surface and intracardiac electrograms at 200 mm/s paper speed, showing a focal AT with a cycle length of 447 ms (153 + 294), which is 134 bpm. Surface leads I, VI, and aVF are shown as well as coronary sinus (CS) leads and Halo catheter leads spanning the crista terminalis in the right atrium. The duration of endocardial activation across large regions of the right atrium (Halo electrodes) and representing the left atrium (CS) is 153 ms, which is only 34% of the entire tachycardia cycle length and is depicted by the first caliper.

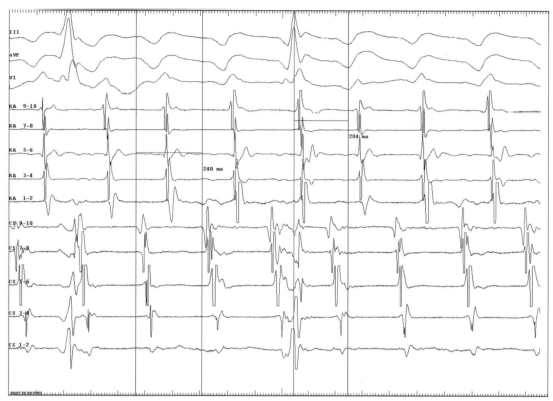

Fig. 2. Surface and intracardiac electrograms at 200 mm/s paper speed, showing macroreentry in the right atrium (typical AFL), with a cycle length of 240 ms (first set of calipers), which is 250 bpm with a 3:1 AV block. Intracardiac leads consist of a 20-pole catheter that has its proximal 10 electrodes (RA 1–2 to RA 9–10) along the right atrium lateral wall and the distal 10 (CS 1–2 to 9–10) in the coronary sinus. Endocardial activation spans a large portion of the entire tachycardia cycle, and its duration depicted by the second caliper is 204 ms, which is 85% of the entire tachycardia cycle length.

prevalence of these arrhythmias increases as corroborated by a study of 917 patients post–acute myocardial infarction, of whom 7% had AF, 3% had AFL, and 3.6% had AT.[6] In heart failure, which may represent a final common pathway for many cardiac conditions, the prevalence of AF is reported to be between 20% and 50% (depending on New York Heart Association class)[7,8] and, although the exact prevalence of AFL and AT are not as well known, their numbers most likely increase as the prevalence of AF increases.

WHY ARE AT AND AFL MORE PREVALENT IN HEART FAILURE PATIENTS?

First, the risk factors for atrial arrhythmias are the same as those for heart failure, so these conditions afflict the same patients. These risk factors include advanced age, hypertension, diabetes, obesity, and cigarette smoking.[4,8,9] In addition, some of the structural changes in the atria of

heart failure patients are shared by those with atrial arrhythmias. Wyndham and colleagues[10] excised tissue samples from the culprit AT focus in a patient, and histology revealed markedly increased levels of mononuclear infiltrates and connective tissue. Josephson and colleagues[11] also demonstrated an increase in wall thickness, endocardial thickness, and inflammatory cells as well as increased mesenchymal cells. In addition, they noted multicomponent atrial electrograms around the foci of atrial tachyarrhythmias depicting slow and asynchronous conduction similar to that seen in diseased ventricles in ventricular tachycardia studies. Similar findings are seen in the atria of patients with heart failure and are attributable to myocardial stretch from pressure and volume changes. In essence, the structural and neuroendocrine alterations in heart failure probably facilitate the development of atrial tachyarrhythmias by complex and interrelated mechanisms (discussed in articles elsewhere in this issue).

WHAT ARE THE EFFECTS OF AT AND AFL ON HEART FAILURE?

Tachyarrhythmias with uncontrolled ventricular response can be the sole cause of heart failure in patients with no other risk factors. The first reported case of suspected tachycardia-mediated cardiomyopathy (TCM) was by Gossage and Hicks in 1913[12] and, since then, animal models of chronic atrial pacing mimicking AT have confirmed the predictable development of reversible heart failure.[13]

Given the aforementioned observations, AT and AFL may, therefore, be either the cause or consequence of heart failure, thereby evoking uncertainty and confusion in the management of new patients with both disorders. This scenario may require aggressive treatment of the arrhythmia and subsequent observation for a few months before it can be determined whether a patient has TCM or heart failure due to another cause with concurrent tachyarrhythmia. Sometimes the left ventricle end diastolic dimension may help distinguish between the two, with left ventricular dimension less than or equal to 6.1 cm being 100% sensitive for TCM and 71.4% specific in a patient presenting with heart failure and an apparently new tachyarrhythmia.[14]

Uncertainty and confusion may also be found in scenarios in which heart failure coexists with AT originating from sites close to the sinoatrial node having a positive P-wave axis on ECG leads II, III, and aVF, giving the initial impression of sinus tachycardia secondary to heart failure.[15] It may take several days to weeks of Holter monitoring of the pattern of tachycardia to make the distinction. Patterns of sudden dips in the heart rate to a new lower baseline alternating with sudden jumps to the higher baseline heart rate may be the first clue that the diagnosis is AT rather than sinus tachycardia, which shows more gradual diurnal fluctuations. EPS may be required in difficult cases.

AT and AFL are common causes of heart failure exacerbation and hospitalization. In patients with preexisting heart failure, they may result in further deterioration in ejection fraction, pushing patients with mild systolic dysfunction to severe dysfunction. This worsening in ejection fraction affects the prognosis and could, for example, be of importance in determining whether a patient requires prophylactic implantable cardioverter defibrillator (ICD) therapy.[8]

Uncontrolled ventricular rates in patients with atrial tachyarrhythmias may increase the likelihood of other morbidities, like myocardial infarction, in patients with ischemic cardiomyopathy or unnecessary ICD firing, with its attendant increased mortality.[16] These arrhythmias have often influenced the choice of ICD type in heart failure patients (single ventricular chamber vs dual, atrial, and ventricular chambers) to facilitate supraventricular tachycardia discrimination.[17,18] In patients with cardiac resynchronization therapy, conducted ventricular beats due to AT and AFL reduce biventricular pacing that may reduce its benefit or cause deterioration in patients with prior response.[19] If the percentage of biventricular pacing suddenly drops in-between evaluations, atrial tachyarrhythmias should be sought and it may be prudent to set up a lower detection or monitor-only zone to pick these up. In addition to these comorbidities, the presence of AT and AF in heart failure patients admitted for myocardial infarction portends an almost 2-fold increase in 30-day mortality, more so if the ejection fraction is between 25% and 35%.[20] Lastly, the onset of AT and AFL may be the first indicator of development of hyperthyroidism, pulmonary embolism, or even progression of the underlying myocardial disease.

In addition to the direct effects of AT and AFL on heart failure, there are several indirect effects. AT and AFL complicate the treatment of heart failure patients by typically making them require higher doses of nodal blocking agents, possibly with associated hypotension, by increasing the need for digoxin, anticoagulation, and antiarrhythmic agents along with their attendant risks.

WHAT IMPACT DOES HEART FAILURE HAVE ON THE MANAGEMENT OF AT AND AFL?

The structural and neurohormonal changes in heart failure facilitate the development of AT and AFL, which in turn leads to further adverse remodeling, which in turn predisposes patients to more atrial tachyarrhythmias, thereby setting up a vicious cycle. By so doing, heart failure encourages the development of new atrial tachyarrhythmias while increasing the burden of preexisting AT and AFL and encouraging recurrence.

The presence of heart failure also influences the treatment strategy of atrial tachyarrhythmias. Restoration of sinus rhythm is highly likely to be attempted given that AT and AFL can precipitate and perpetuate acute decompensation and hospitalizations. In heart failure exacerbations, the authors are inclined to promptly cardiovert patients rather than use nodal blocking agents. Cardioversion is useful in AFL but has limited success in AT. If deciding on a conservative strategy of using AV nodal blocking agents, choices are limited to β-blockers and digoxin. Nondihydropyridine calcium channel blockers, commonly used in the general population, are negatively inotropic and, therefore, contraindicated in most patients with systolic dysfunction. Given the high cathecholaminergic state of heart failure decompensation, digoxin is less desirable given its potential morbidity and mortality[21] and reduced efficacy.[22]

Also, because of the high catecholaminergic state of heart failure, higher than usual doses of β- blockers may be needed—a challenge in a population that may already have low blood pressure from multiple drugs and may not be able to tolerate higher doses of β-blockers or may only be able to tolerate them at the cost of reducing or discontinuing other medications, like angiotensin-converting enzyme inhibitors. Not all acutely decompensated patients, however, may immediately be given β-blockers because of pulmonary edema and the risk of initial worsening.[8] Having considered all these factors, a combination of digoxin and β-blockers is often needed.[23]

Lastly, a conservative approach in treating AT and AFL in heart failure patients is more likely to require antiarrhythmic medication, and there are essentially 2 choices with good safety profile in heart failure: amiodarone[24] and dofetilide.[25] This limitation is because commonly prescribed antiarrhythmic class IC agents[26] and sotalol[27] are absolutely and relatively contraindicated in heart failure, respectively. Dronedarone, another widely used drug in the general population, caused new heart failure and death in patients with chronic atrial arrhythmias or decompensated heart failure, so its use is limited in patients with preexisting heart failure.[28]

Multiple challenges, therefore, exist to a pharmacologic therapy of AT and AFL in heart failure.

CONSIDERATIONS FOR THE ABLATION OF AT AND AFL IN HEART FAILURE PATIENTS

There is a need for definitive therapy for AT and AFL in heart failure patients, particularly given the high efficacy of catheter ablation in the general population, with 85% to 90% success in AT and 90% to 93% in AFL.[29–31] Moreover, approximately 10% of patients with atrial tachyarrhythmias in heart failure, after elimination of the arrhythmia, may be essentially cured of heart failure, leading to a retrospective diagnosis of tachycardia-related cardiomyopathy.[15] In essence, heart failure adds an urgency to the treatment of AT and AFL as well as the need for early consideration of definitive therapy.

A caveat to ablation is that its potential complications may be higher in this population, with more comorbidities, impacts of polypharmacy, propensity for renal insufficiency, drug-drug interactions, and other factors. These factors require meticulous preprocedural planning in patients with heart failure, who may initially be too sick for the procedure. Under these circumstances, cardioversion may be a useful temporizing measure. Besides influencing the timing of procedure, the presence of heart failure has an impact on periablation management. Ablation of complex left-sided AT and AFL may last for several hours, a serious challenge in those with preexisting orthopnea and paroxysmal nocturnal dyspnea. This may require preprocedural aggressive diuresis sometimes at the cost of an acceptable temporary worsening of renal function. When this is inadequate, an early evaluation by anesthesia staff may be helpful in planning the procedure.

Other considerations include the presence of ICD and cardiac resynchronization therapy devices in an increasing proportion of heart failure patients, introducing the risk of lead dislodgement. This may inform the choice of diagnostic catheters and the choice of electroanatomic mapping systems. For example, a bulky catheter, like a Halo catheter, which encircles the tricuspid annulus, may not be elected to be used a patients with multiple leads, or a decision may be made to avoid inserting a diagnostic catheter into the coronary sinus of patients with left ventricular leads. Because coronary sinus activation is often used as an intracardiac timing reference, its unavailability requires an alternative reference site or even technology.

The presence of heart failure may also influence the choice of ablation catheters, especially with regards to open irrigation catheters, which add to the periprocedural fluid input. This additional fluid load should carefully assessed so that intraprocedure or postprocedure additional diuretics may be given as needed.

Once these scenarios and the peculiarities of AT and AFL in heart failure patients have been addressed, there should be few differences between ablation of these arrhythmias in patients with heart failure compared with those without.

ABLATION OF AT

Success in the ablation of AT depends on an understanding of the arrhythmia mechanism. ATs have been localized to several predictable areas of the atria and surrounding structures with the following frequencies (**Table 1**).[32]

Rarely, ATs have also been localized to the noncoronary aortic cusp,[33] superior vena cava (SVC),[34] or the ligament of Marshall.[35] These AT foci are typically 2 cm[2] or less in area, and the aim of catheter ablation is to identify the site of

Table 1
Distribution of the anatomic locations of foci of atrial tachycardias in both atria

Right Atrium	Distribution
Crista terminalis	31%
Tricuspid annulus	22%
Perinodal tissue	11%
Coronary sinus os	8%
Interatrial septum	<1%
Right atrial appendage	<1%
Total	73%

Left Atrium	Distribution
Pulmonary veins	19%
Superior mitral annulus	4%
Coronary sinus body	2%
Interatrial septum	<1%
Left atrial appendage	<1%
Roof	<1%
Total	27%

earliest atrial activation, apply radiofrequency energy, and eliminate them.

Localizing Atrial Tachycardias

The surface P-wave morphology of the AT may be helpful in predicting the site of origin and hence help in planning the procedure using algorithms that have been developed. **Fig. 3** shows an adapted and simplified algorithm that partially summarizes the elegant work of Kalman and colleagues.[32]

There are exceptions to the rule and that most algorithms are developed in patients with clear isoelectric baselines, resulting in undistorted P waves and mostly normal hearts, so extrapolation to patients with structural abnormalities with distortion from chamber enlargement may render ECG prediction less reliable.

Induction and Mapping of ATs

Mapping of a focal AT entails recording electrograms from various parts of the atrial endocardium, with the aim of localizing the earliest point of activation, which is consistent with the point of origin. This point usually precedes the surface P wave by 38 ± 7 ms in duration.[36]

At the time of EPS, if tachycardia is not present, then it may have to be induced by pacing rapidly in the atrium (burst pacing) or programmed extra stimuli. Isoproterenol or other sympathomimetic agents may need to be given in addition to these protocols to induce tachycardia. Antiarrhythmic agents should be discontinued at least 5 half-

lives before EPS when possible and limiting sedation as much as possible may also facilitate tachycardia initiation.

Multielectrode diagnostic catheters are placed in the heart, which can simultaneously record signals from different regions of the heart to give a general idea of the activation sequence. For example, a 20-electrode catheter (Halo) can be wrapped along the lateral wall of the right atrium partly overlapping the crista terminalis. Propagation along this Halo catheter enables determining if the lateral wall is activated before the septum or determining if the activation sequence proceeds from a superior to inferior direction or vice versa. A catheter with between 4 and 10 electrodes is usually placed in the coronary sinus, which interrogates the proximal portion of the os all the way to the area around the mitral annulus on the left side. Coronary sinus propagation enables determining if AT activation is from left atrium to right atrium or vice versa. Once the chamber of origin of the tachycardia is known, a roving catheter can then be used to interrogate the area of interest in detail until the earliest point of activation is found. This area of earliest activation may also demonstrate low and multicomponent voltage indicative of an abnormal focus. Radiofrequency ablation (RFA) is applied at a power of 30 W to 50 W for approximately 30 to 60 seconds. Termination of tachycardia and an inability to reinitiate it approximately 30 minutes after the last RFA application is a good indicator of success.

Other forms of mapping include 3-D electroanatomic mapping (**Fig. 4**), which involves reconstruction of the shell of the atria on which the activation sequence of the tachycardia is superimposed to identify and target the area of earliest activation for RFA.[37]

Finally, if the tachycardia cannot be reproduced in an electrophysiology laboratory in a patient with previously documented AT, the ECG can be used to initially predict the area of origin and then a roving catheter can be moved around the large initial area of interest with intermittent atrial pacing until P-wave morphologies similar to that of the clinical tachycardia (pace mapping) are reproduced. This area is then targeted for ablation.[38]

ABLATION OF ATRIAL FLUTTER

Ablation of macroreentrant atrial tachyarrhythmia differs from AT in that there is no discrete focus to be identified and targeted for RFA but rather a critical isthmus that permits sustenance of the tachycardia, which can be interrupted with a line of RFA lesions. Ablation of AFL is thus targeted to the precise circuit along which the wave front of

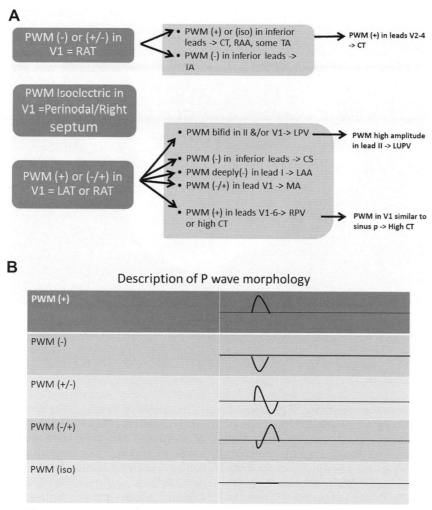

Fig. 3. (*A*) A modified and simplified algorithm showing how ECG P-wave morphology (PWM) can be used to predict the anatomic site of origin of ATs. This partially summarizes the work of Kistler and colleagues.[32] (*B*) A table with visual representation of different P-wave morphologies. CT, Crista terminalis; LAT, left atrial tachycardia; LUPV, left upper pulmonary vein; MA, Mitral annulus; RAA, right atrial appendage; RAT, right atrial tachycardia; RPV, right pulmonary vein.

the tachycardia conducts (**Figs. 5–7**). The boundaries of such circuits are typically formed by regions of functional or anatomic conduction block. Multiple circuits have been described in the right and left atria, with the most common in the right atrium and responsible for the initiation of typical AFL. AFLs are classified into the following[2]:

1. Counterclockwise cavotricuspid isthmus (CTI)–dependent right AFL (typical flutter)
2. Clockwise CTI–dependent right AFL (reverse typical flutter)
3. Lesion macroreentrant AT (scar-related AFL)
4. Left atrial macroreentrant tachycardia (left AFL)

The circuit along which typical flutter travels involves the crista terminalis as it runs along the lateral wall of the right atrium, extending from the

SVC superiorly to the inferior vena cava (IVC) inferiorly. Its continuation inferiorly blends with the anterior lip of the IVC and the eustachian ridge, which extends medially from the IVC toward the interatrial septum, all forming a single continuous unit that in turn forms the posterior limit of what is known as the CTI. The anterior limit of the CTI is the annulus of the tricuspid valve. The wave front of typical flutter ascends in a counterclockwise fashion caudocranially along the interatrial septum to the roof of the right atrium and courses anterior to the crista terminalis to descend along the right atrial lateral wall. Its path is then funneled into the CTI, which is the narrowest portion of the circuit and is also the area of slow conduction that permits the wavelength of the arrhythmia to fit into the fixed circuit and still have an excitable

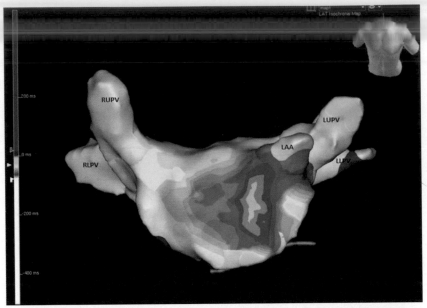

Fig. 4. Electroanatomic map of the left atrium showing the activation pattern of a left AT with a radial spread from the anterior wall of the atrium. Point of earliest activation is the white spot followed by the region in red, then orange, then yellow, and so on. Blue indicates the latest activated regions. LAA, left atrial appendage; LLPV, left lower pulmonary vein; LUPV, left upper pulmonary vein; RLPV, right lower pulmonary vein; RUPV, right upper pulmonary vein.

gap that perpetuates the arrhythmia.[39] In cases of the reverse typical flutter, the wave front moves in a clockwise fashion caudocranially along the lateral wall of the right atrium, crosses the roof, and descends along the interatrial septum from where it is funneled into the CTI. Ablation of typical flutter is essentially ablation along the CTI from its anterior to its posterior limit[40] with the aim of creation of a line of bidirectional block.[41]

Lesion macroreentrant atrial tachyarrhythmias are those with circuits around anatomic scars in the atrium. Commonly these scars are from atriotomies, septal patches for ASD repairs, suture lines, and scar formed by previous ablation. In these scenarios, the goal of EPS is to identify the circuit, delineate the narrowest portion, and then attempt to create a line of RFA lesions along this narrow isthmus in such a way that one connects at both ends to nonconducting structures. For example, a line of RFA lesions may be created from the anatomic line of scar to the SVC, the IVC, or the tricuspid annulus.

Several other described flutters include a lower loop reentry flutter, which rotates around the IVC, traversing the CTI anteriorly and the low posterior right atrium posteriorly. This is a variant of typical flutter and can be ablated along the CTI. An upper loop reentry flutter rotates around the SVC. Mixed variants (double loop or figure of 8) are essentially a combination.[2]

Left-sided AFLs also exist and these are common in patients who have had catheter or surgical AF therapy. These have been arbitrarily classified as peripulmonary vein reentry (roof-dependent) flutters, perimitral annular (mitral isthmus–dependent) flutters, and periseptal flutters (see **Fig. 7**). Ablating these flutters requires mapping and applying RFA lesions along narrowest and/or most accessible portion of the circuit.[42]

ALTERNATIVES TO ABLATION OF AT/AFL: ABLATION OF THE AV NODE

"Ablate and pace" is an old strategy that involved AV nodal ablation with implantation of a dual-chamber permanent pacemaker and was reserved for patients refractory to all medications. It produced excellent relief of symptoms[43] but has been largely overtaken by the advent of catheter ablation. In the current state of electrophysiology, few patients who are intolerant of or allergic to multiple medications and also not amenable to catheter ablation may qualify for it. With increasing knowledge of the deleterious effects of chronic right ventricular pacing, however, particularly in patients with cardiomyopathies,[44] biventricular pacemaker implantation has become the preferred mode because it prevents worsening of heart failure and reduces hospitalization.[45]

A

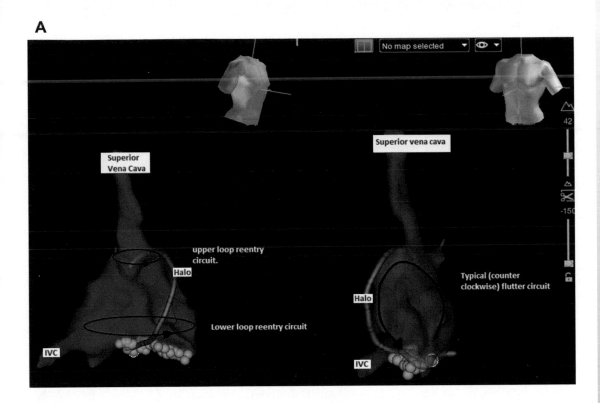

B

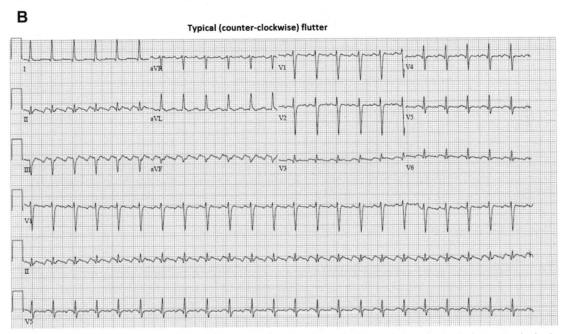

Fig. 5. (*A*) Electroanatomic map of the right atrium showing the activation pattern of a typical counterclockwise flutter circuit, an upper loop reentry, and a lower loop reentry flutter circuit. The reverse typical flutter runs clockwise instead of counterclockwise along the same circuit. The blue spheres represent RFA lesions created along the CTI. Halo, Halo catheter hugging crista terminalis. (*B*) Surface ECG of a patient showing typical counterclockwise (CTI-dependent) flutter.

A

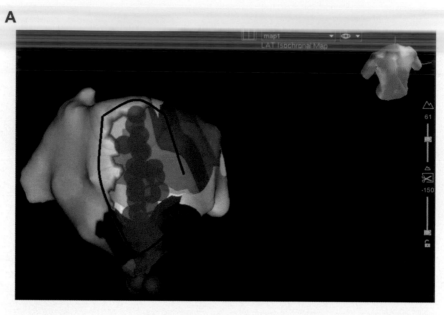

B

Atypical flutter (scar related)

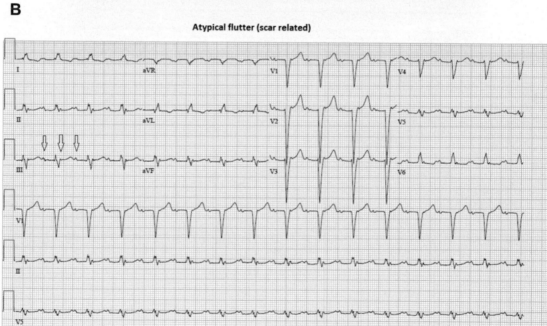

Fig. 6. (*A*) Electroanatomic mapping of the right atrium showing the activation pattern of a scar-related AFL along the lateral wall. Point of earliest activation is the region in red followed by yellow, then green, then blue, and purple. There is a gap of excitable tissue (*gray*) between the head and the tail of the arrow, indicating the head and tail, respectively, of the arrhythmia wave front. The line of red dots represents the area of scar in this instance made by prior RFA lesions. (*B*) A surface ECG of a patient showing atypical flutter secondary to a right atriotomy scar. The arrows point to positive flutter waves in lead III.

WHEN AFL IS REALLY AF

In patients with atypical AFL, in particular arising from the left atrium after a prior AF ablation, mapping not uncommonly reveals a much disorganized rhythm, which is actually AF rather than AFL. Redo AF ablation may be scheduled in such patients with the understanding that the success of catheter ablation in heart failure patients with recurrent persistent AF is at best modest. More extensive ablation is usually

A

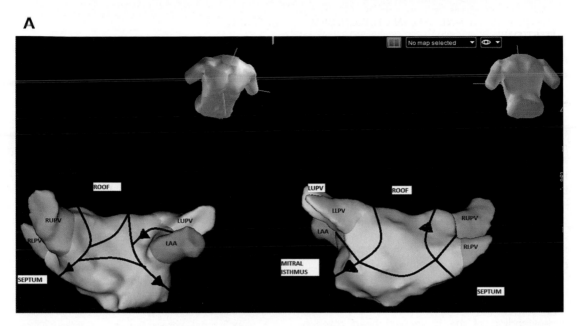

B

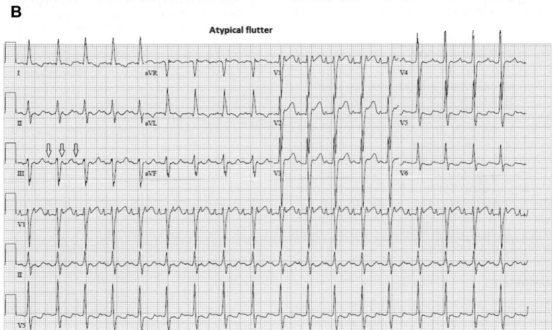

Fig. 7. (*A*) Electroanatomic anatomic map of the anterior and posterior surfaces of the left atrium showing some of the possible multiple paths/circuits of a left AFL. LAA, left atrial appendage; LLPV, left lower pulmonary vein; LUPV, left upper pulmonary vein; RLPV, right lower pulmonary vein; RUPV, right upper pulmonary vein. (*B*) A surface ECG of a patient showing atypical flutter, which in this case was a left AFL. The arrows point to positive flutter waves in lead III.

required in such patients and a hybrid epicardial-endocardial catheter ablation may offer an increased efficacy, particularly when performed simultaneously rather than in a staged fashion. The largest cohort that underwent this strategy to date was reported by Gehi and colleagues.[46] They reported a 66% rate of freedom from arrhythmia 12 months post–single hybrid procedure in spite of an average left atrial size of 5.1 cm. This is a promising result.

ABLATION OF AT AND AFL IN CHALLENGING SITUATIONS

AT and typical AFL have been reported as the most common supraventricular arrhythmias occurring late after cardiac transplantation. Typical AFLs tend to occur in the donor heart whereas the ATs commonly originate from the recipient atria or peri-suture areas. Ablations have been successfully performed by delivering RFA to CTI in cases of AFL and by ablation of atrioatrial electrical connections across anastomotic suture lines or ablation of the foci of origin in either the donor or recipient atria without prohibitive complications.[47] Similarly, AT originating from the anastomotic pulmonary veins of donors propagating across suture lines into the atria of lung transplant recipients have been reported and ablated by pulmonary vein isolation.[48]

Patients with congenital heart diseases and heart failure commonly develop atrial tachyarrhythmias. The challenges in these cases include understanding of the congenital heart disease and its hemodynamic consequences and of the altered anatomy that may render certain areas inaccessible. Ablation in this cohort requires extensive planning and a multidisciplinary approach. Concomitant corrective surgeries and arrhythmia substrate ablation may be useful in this cohort as may be preemptive techniques during surgery, such as extension of surgical cuts to areas of anatomic and physiologic barriers to prevent future arrhythmias. Success of catheter ablation is in the range of 80% to 90%[49] in such patients, with a 10% to 25% risk for recurrence.[50]

Finally, to show the breadth of patient population that may benefit from catheter ablation, AFL ablation has been performed successfully and without complications even in patients on left ventricular assist devices.[51]

SUMMARY

AT and AFL are common tachyarrhythmias in the heart failure population. They commonly lead to, exacerbate, and increase the morbidity and mortality associated with heart failure and, thereby, warrant urgent and early definitive therapy in the form of catheter ablation. Catheter ablation requires careful patient stabilization and extensive preprocedural planning, particularly with regards to anesthesia, strategy, catheter choice, mapping system, and fluid balance, to increase efficacy and limit adverse effects. Heart failure may limit the success of catheter ablation with higher reported recurrence rates[52] and, in selected patients, a hybrid epicardial-endocardial ablation can be considered.

REFERENCES

1. Markides V, Peters NS. Mechanisms underlying the development of atrial arrhythmias in heart failure. Heart Fail Rev 2002;7:243–53.
2. Saoudi N, Cosio F, Waldo A, et al. Classification of atrial flutter and regular atrial tachycardia according to electrophysiologic mechanism and anatomic bases: a statement from a joint expert group from the Working Group of Arrhythmias of the European Society of Cardiology and the North American Society of Pacing and Electrophysiology. J Cardiovasc Electrophysiol 2001;12:852–66.
3. Poutiainen AM, Koistinen MJ, Airaksinen KE, et al. Prevalence and natural course of ectopic atrial tachycardia. Eur Heart J 1999;20:694–700.
4. Granada J, Uribe W, Chyou PH, et al. Incidence and predictors of atrial flutter in the general population. J Am Coll Cardiol 2000;36:2242–6.
5. Fuster V, Rydén LE, Cannom DS, et al, American College of Cardiology, American Heart Association Task Force, European Society of Cardiology Committee for Practice Guidelines, European Heart Rhythm Association, Heart Rhythm Society. ACC/AHA/ESC 2006 guidelines for the management of patients with atrial fibrillation: full text: a report of the American College of Cardiology/American Heart Association Task Force on practice guidelines and the European Society of Cardiology Committee for Practice Guidelines (Writing Committee to Revise the 2001 guidelines for the management of patients with atrial fibrillation) developed in collaboration with the European Heart Rhythm Association and the Heart Rhythm Society. Europace 2006;8:651–745.
6. Liberthson RR, Salisbury KW, Hutter AM, et al. Atrial tachyarrhythmias in acute myocardial infarction. Am J Med 1976;60:956–60.
7. Savelieva I, Camm AJ. Atrial fibrillation and heart failure: natural history and pharmacological treatment. Europace 2003;5:S5–19.
8. Hunt SA, Abraham WT, Chin MH, et al, American College of Cardiology, American Heart Association Task Force on Practice Guidelines, American College of Chest Physicians, International Society for Heart and Lung Transplantation, Heart Rhythm Society. ACC/AHA 2005 Guideline Update for the Diagnosis and Management of Chronic Heart Failure in the Adult: a report of the American College of Cardiology/American Heart Association Task Force on Practice Guidelines (Writing Committee to Update the 2001 Guidelines for the Evaluation and Management of Heart Failure): developed in collaboration with the American College of Chest Physicians and the International Society for Heart and Lung Transplantation: endorsed by the Heart Rhythm Society. Circulation 2005;112:154–235.

9. Kannel WB, Wolf PA, Benjamin EJ, et al. Prevalence, incidence, prognosis, and predisposing conditions for atrial fibrillation: population-based estimates. Am J Cardiol 1998;82:2N–9N.

10. Wyndham CR, Arnsdort MF, Levitsky S. Successful surgical excision of focal paroxysmal atrial tachycardia. Observations in vivo and in vitro. Circulation 1980;62:1365–72.

11. Josephson ME, Spear JF, Harken AH, et al. Surgical excision of automatic atrial tachycardia: anatomic and electrophysiologic correlates. Am Heart J 1982;104:1076–85.

12. Gossage AM, Braxton Hicks JA. On auricular fibrillation. QJM 1913;6:435–40.

13. Whipple GH, Sheffield LT, Woodman EG, et al. Reversible congestive heart failure due to rapid stimulation of the normal heart. Proc New Engl Cardiovasc Soc 1961–1962;20:39–40.

14. Jeong YH, Choi KJ, Song JM, et al. Diagnostic approach and treatment strategy in tachycardia-induced cardiomyopathy. Clin Cardiol 2008;31:72–8.

15. Medi C, Kalman JM, Haqqani H, et al. Tachycardia-mediated cardiomyopathy secondary to focal atrial tachycardia: long-term outcome after catheter ablation. J Am Coll Cardiol 2009;53:1791–7.

16. Poole JE, Johnson GW, Hellkamp AS, et al. Prognostic importance of defibrillator shocks in patients with heart failure. N Engl J Med 2008;359:1009–17.

17. Dorian P, Philippon F, Thibault B, et al. Randomized controlled study of detection enhancements versus rate-only detection to prevent inappropriate therapy in a dual-chamber implantable cardioverter-defibrillator. Heart Rhythm 2004;1:540–7.

18. Friedman PA, McClelland RL, Bamlet WR, et al. Dual-chamber versus single-chamber detection enhancements for implantable defibrillator rhythm diagnosis: the detect supraventricular tachycardia study. Circulation 2006;113:2871–9.

19. Gasparini M, Galimberti P, Ceriotti C. The importance of increased percentage of biventricular pacing to improve clinical outcomes in patients receiving cardiac resynchronization therapy. Curr Opin Cardiol 2013;28:50–4.

20. Pedersen OD, Bagger H, Køber L, et al, TRACE Study Group. Impact of congestive heart failure and left ventricular systolic function on the prognostic significance of atrial fibrillation and atrial flutter following acute myocardial infarction. Int J Cardiol 2005;100:65–71.

21. The effect of digoxin on mortality and morbidity in patients with heart failure. The Digitalis Investigation Group. N Engl J Med 1997;336:525–33.

22. Sarter BH, Marchlinski FE. Redefining the role of digoxin in the treatment of atrial fibrillation. Am J Cardiol 1992;69:71G–81G.

23. Khand AU, Rankin AC, Martin W, et al. Carvedilol alone or in combination with digoxin for the management of atrial fibrillation in patients with heart failure? J Am Coll Cardiol 2003;42:1944–51.

24. Singh S, Fletcher RD, Fisher S, et al. Congestive heart failure: survival trial of antiarrhythmic therapy (CHF STAT). The CHF STAT Investigators. Control Clin Trials 1992;13:339–50.

25. Møller M, Torp-Pedersen CT, Køber L. Dofetilide in patients with congestive heart failure and left ventricular dysfunction: safety aspects and effect on atrial fibrillation. The Danish Investigators of Arrhythmia and Mortality on Dofetilide (DIAMOND) Study Group. Congest Heart Fail 2001;7:146–50.

26. Preliminary report: effect of encainide and flecainide on mortality in a randomized trial of arrhythmia suppression after myocardial infarction. The Cardiac Arrhythmia Suppression Trial (CAST) Investigators. N Engl J Med 1989;10:406–12.

27. Pratt CM, Camm AJ, Cooper W, et al. Mortality in the survival with ORal D-sotalol (SWORD) trial: why did patients die? Am J Cardiol 1998;81:869–76.

28. Connolly SJ, Camm AJ, Halperin JL, et al. Dronedarone in high-risk permanent atrial fibrillation. N Engl J Med 2011;365:268–76.

29. Xia Y, Ju WZ, Chen ML, et al. Catheter ablation of focal atrial tachycardia: the topographic distribution and long-term outcome. Zhonghua Xin Xue Guan Bing Za Zhi 2012;40:231–6 [in Chinese].

30. Pérez FJ, Schubert CM, Parvez B, et al. Long-term outcomes after catheter ablation of cavo-tricuspid isthmus dependent atrial flutter: a meta-analysis. Circ Arrhythm Electrophysiol 2009;2:393–401.

31. Lee G, Sanders P, Kalman JM. Catheter ablation of atrial arrhythmias: state of the art. Lancet 2012;380:1509–19.

32. Kistler PM, Roberts-Thomson KC, Haqqani HM, et al. P-wave morphology in focal atrial tachycardia: development of an algorithm to predict the anatomic site of origin. J Am Coll Cardiol 2006;48:1010–7.

33. Ouyang F, Ma J, Ho SY, et al. Focal atrial tachycardia originating from the non-coronary aortic sinus: electrophysiological characteristics and catheter ablation. J Am Coll Cardiol 2006;48:122–31.

34. Dong J, Schreieck J, Ndrepepa G, et al. Ectopic tachycardia originating from the superior vena cava. J Cardiovasc Electrophysiol 2002;13:620–4.

35. Polymeropoulos KP, Rodriguez LM, Timmermans C, et al. Images in cardiovascular medicine. Radiofrequency ablation of a focal atrial tachycardia originating from the Marshall ligament as a trigger for atrial fibrillation. Circulation 2002;105:2112–3.

36. Chen SA, Chiang CE, Yang CJ, et al. Radiofrequency catheter ablation of sustained intra-atrial reentrant tachycardia in adult patients. Identification of electrophysiological characteristics and endocardial mapping techniques. Circulation 1993;88:578–87.

37. Natale A, Breeding L, Tomassoni G, et al. Ablation of right and left ectopic atrial tachycardias using a three-dimensional non fluoroscopic mapping system. Am J Cardiol 1998;82:989–92.

38. Singh B, Sapra R, Gupta RK, et al. Pace mapping for the localization of focal atrial tachycardia arising near the mitral annulus. Indian Heart J 2004;56:58–60.

39. Feld GK, Fleck RP, Chen PS, et al. Radiofrequency catheter ablation for the treatment of human type 1 atrial flutter. Identification of a critical zone in the reentrant circuit by endocardial mapping techniques. Circulation 1992;86:1233–40.

40. Fischer B, Haissaguerre M, Garrigues S, et al. Radiofrequency catheter ablation of common atrial flutter in 80 patients. J Am Coll Cardiol 1995;25: 1365–72.

41. Moreira JM, Alessi SR, Rezende AG, et al. Catheter ablation of atrial flutter. Electrophysiological characterization of posterior and septal isthmus block. Arq Bras Cardiol 1998;71:37–47 [in Portuguese].

42. Jaïs P, Shah DC, Haïssaguerre M, et al. Mapping and ablation of left atrial flutters. Circulation 2000; 101:2928–34.

43. Kay GN, Ellenbogen KA, Giudici M, et al. Ablate and Pace Trial: a prospective study of catheter ablation of the AV conduction system and permanent pacemaker implantation for treatment of atrial fibrillation. APT Investigators. J Interv Card Electrophysiol 1998;2:121–35.

44. Wilkoff BL, Dual Chamber and VVI Implantable Defibrillator Trial Investigators. The Dual Chamber and VVI Implantable Defibrillator (DAVID) Trial: rationale, design, results, clinical implications and lessons for future trials. Card Electrophysiol Rev 2003;7:468–72.

45. Brignole M, Botto G, Mont L, et al. Cardiac resynchronization therapy in patients undergoing atrioventricular junction ablation for permanent atrial fibrillation: a randomized trial. Eur Heart J 2011;32:2420–9.

46. Gehi AK, Mounsey JP, Pursell I, et al. Hybrid epicardial-endocardial ablation using a pericardioscopic technique for the treatment of atrial fibrillation. Heart Rhythm 2013;10:22–8.

47. Li YG, Grönefeld G, Israel C, et al. Radiofrequency catheter ablation in patients with symptomatic atrial flutter/tachycardia after orthotopic heart transplantation. Chin Med J (Engl) 2006;119:2036–41.

48. Nazmul M, Munger TM, Powell BD. Atrial tachycardia originating from a donor pulmonary vein in a lung transplant recipient. Circulation 2011;124: 1288–9.

49. Lam W, Friedman RA. Electrophysiology issues in adult congenital heart disease. Methodist Debakey Cardiovasc J 2011;7:13–7.

50. Akar JG, Kok LC, Haines DE, et al. Coexistance of type I atrial flutter and intra-atrial re-entrant tachycardia in patients with surgically corrected congenital heart disease. J Am Coll Cardiol 2001; 38:377–84.

51. Maury P, Delmas C, Trouillet C, et al. First experience of percutaneous radio-frequency ablation for atrial flutter and atrial fibrillation in a patient with HeartMate II left ventricular assist device. J Interv Card Electrophysiol 2010;29:63–7.

52. Landolina M, Cantù F, De Ferrari GM, et al. The role of invasive electrophysiology in the management of patients with chronic heart failure. Heart Fail Monit 2002;3:49–59.

Catheter Ablation of Atrial Fibrillation in Heart Failure

Senthil Kirubakaran, MRCP, MD[a],*,
Mark D. O'Neill, DPhil, FRCP, FHRS[b]

KEYWORDS

- Atrial fibrillation • Catheter ablation • Heart failure • Impaired ventricular function

KEY POINTS

- Modest efficacy rates (50%–88%) have been reported for rhythm control of AF with catheter ablation over the short term in patients with heart failure.
- Maintenance of sinus rhythm after ablation is associated with improvements in ventricular systolic function (reverse ventricular remodeling); NHYA functional class; and quality of life.
- Equivalent improvements in ventricular function are seen in patients with paroxysmal and persistent AF.
- Greater improvements in ventricular function are seen in patients with idiopathic cardiomyopathy.
- Reverse ventricular remodeling occurs even in patients with controlled ventricular rates during AF before catheter ablation.
- Efficacy of catheter ablation for AF is less than in patients with normal ventricular function with the requirement for more procedures.
- Some evidence shows catheter ablation of AF to be superior to optimal rate control with greater improvements in exercise tolerance, NYHA functional class, and reverse ventricular remodeling.
- Patient selection for catheter ablation of AF is reasonable in selected patients with heart failure and should be made after considering such factors as the degree and cause of ventricular dysfunction, the underlying atrial substrate, atrial size, and coexisting comorbidities.

INTRODUCTION

Atrial fibrillation (AF) and heart failure (HF) are two epidemics of cardiovascular disease. They often coexist, with their interaction creating a vicious pathophysiologic circle where HF promotes AF and vice versa. This is a considerable therapeutic challenge, with an integrated approach to the management of each condition required to achieve the most favorable outcome for the patient. Although well-established pharmacologic and nonpharmacologic treatments are used for the treatment of HF, the availability of efficacious and safe antiarrhythmic drugs for the treatment of AF in patients with HF is limited. Catheter

ablation is an effective treatment for patients with AF in the absence of significant structural heart disease. This article discusses the role of catheter ablation for the treatment of AF in patients with HF.

TREATMENT OF AF IN HF

The adverse hemodynamic, electrophysiologic, and structural effects of AF in patients with HF and the associated morbidity and increased mortality emphasize the importance of identifying and treating AF in these patients. Analysis of the Cardiac Resynchronisation in Heart Failure trial showed the prevalence of AF in the HF population in those with no prior documented history of AF to

No conflicts of interest.
[a] Cardiothoracic Department, Guy's and St Thomas' NHS Trust, Westminster Bridge Road, London SE1 7EH, UK;
[b] Divisions of Imaging Sciences and Biomedical Engineering and Cardiovascular Medicine, Medical Engineering Centre, 3rd Floor, Lambeth Wing, St. Thomas' Hospital, London SE1 7EH, UK
* Corresponding author.
E-mail address: senthilk1uk@yahoo.co.uk

be 39% (159 of 404 patients), with 22% detected only using device-based diagnostic telemetry.[1] Furthermore, an estimated 5% to 10% of HF hospitalization is caused by the development of new AF or associated rapid ventricular rates.[2–4] This together with the detrimental effects on left ventricular ejection fraction (LVEF) highlights the importance of intensive screening for AF in this population group to initiate strategies to improve treatment with pharmacologic agents or catheter ablation. However, despite these adverse effects, controversy exists as to whether patients with HF respond better to rhythm restoration or ventricular rate control.

The Atrial Fibrillation Investigation of Rhythm Management (AFFIRM) and Rate Control versus Electrical Cardioversion of Persistent Atrial Fibrillation studies showed no difference in the development of HF or hospitalization for HF[5,6] between a rate or rhythm control strategy. Similarly, three other prospective randomized trials (How to Treat Chronic Atrial Fibrillation,[7] Strategies of Treatment of Atrial Fibrillation,[8] and Pharmacologic Intervention in Atrial Fibrillation[9]) showed equivalent outcomes in both arms. However, extrapolation of these results specifically to patients with HF should be done with caution, because the number of patients with HF in these studies was small. The Atrial Fibrillation and Congestive Heart Failure (AF-CHF) was the first randomized prospective trial to assess rhythm and rate control for AF in patients with HF. After a mean follow-up of 3 years, the investigators found no difference in mortality, hospitalization for HF, and stroke between the two groups.

Although these studies have shown equivalent outcomes for rhythm and rate control strategies, the potential benefits of sinus rhythm (SR) might have been offset by the limited efficacy and potentially deleterious effects of antiarrhythmic drugs. Currently, the available pharmacologic agents for rhythm control in patients with HF are amiodarone, sotalol, and dofetilide. The DIAMOND-CHF study showed dofetilide to be an effective class III antiarrhythmic agent in patients with HF.[10] However, despite this finding there was no associated mortality benefit with dofetilide treatment in patients with HF. Amiodarone seems to be the most effective agent; however, its use has been associated with the increased risk of symptomatic bradycardia requiring implantation of a permanent pacemaker[11] and has not been found to reduce mortality in this population group.[12] Upstream therapies with angiotensin receptor blockers and 3-hydroxy-3-methylglutaryl coenzyme A reductase inhibitors seem to have a modest success at reducing AF in patients with HF, because of their possible effects on structural remodeling.[13–17]

Despite the use of these antiarrhythmic drugs, the recurrence rate of AF after successful cardioversion is as high as 44% to 67% after 1 year.[18] Further support for the development of either more efficacious pharmacologic agents or the use of nonpharmacologic treatments came from further analysis of the AFFIRM and AF-CHF trials. The AFFIRM study showed that maintenance of SR was associated with a 47% reduction in the risk of death, whereas the use of antiarrhythmic drugs and the presence of congestive cardiac failure increased the risk of death by 49%, thus reversing the benefit of SR.[19] Post hoc analysis of the AFFIRM and AF-CHF trials demonstrated better survival rates in patients who remained in SR.[19] Further evidence for the maintenance of SR in patients with HF comes from the CAFE II Study comparing rate versus rhythm control with amiodarone and cardioversion in which a greater proportion of rhythm control patients had improved LVEF, quality of life, and natriuretic peptide levels.[20] Restoration and maintenance of SR with pharmacologic agents and electrical cardioversion has also been shown to improve ventricular function in patients with idiopathic cardiomyopathy.[21,22] These findings together with the adverse prognostic effects of AF in patients with HF have been one of the major drivers in developing more efficacious rhythm control approaches to AF in patients with HF to interrupt the vicious circle of AF and HF progression.[23–25]

Stulak and colleagues[26] evaluated whether improved rhythm control for AF in patients undergoing the Cox-Maze procedure improves ventricular function and functional status in a cohort of patients with HF. They reported 97% success rates in treating AF in the 37 patients with ventricular dysfunction. Improved rhythm control was associated with a significant improvement in LVEF (43%–55%; $P<.01$), which correlated with an improvement in functional status. However, the Cox-Maze procedure is an invasive procedure associated with significant complications. This study did, however, strengthen the argument for improved rhythm control strategies in the HF population.

One promising approach is catheter ablation. Over a decade ago, Haissaguerre and colleagues[27] made the pivotal discovery that focal discharges from the pulmonary veins (PVs) initiate AF and ablation of these triggers prevented AF in up to 70% of patients.[28] However, the frequent existence of multiple foci, inconsistencies in PV firing during the procedure, and the high incidence of PV stenosis led to an empiric approach to electrically isolate all the PVs from the left atrium using either a segmental ostial approach[29] or wide anatomic circumferential antral ablation.[30] Numerous studies have since demonstrated the efficacy and safety of PV isolation (PVI) in patients with paroxysmal AF in those who failed antiarrhythmic therapy.[31–36] However, patients with persistent and long-standing persistent AF frequently have significant atrial electrophysiologic and structural changes responsible for arrhythmia maintenance for which PVI alone has been shown to be an ineffective ablation strategy.[37–40] Since then, further approaches with modest success rates have been reported by different groups, including ablation of complex fractionated atrial electrograms (CFAE), which are thought to represent critical sites of slow and discontinuous conduction[38,41]; a stepwise approach including PVI, linear ablation, and CFAE[39,42,43]; ganglionated plexi ablation[44,45]; and ablation of focal rotors[46,47] thought to be responsible for sustaining persistent AF. Although durable PVI remains the building block of an effective catheter ablation procedure for AF, there is consensus that this alone is inadequate for the treatment of patients with nonparoxysmal AF.

CATHETER ABLATION OF AF IN HF SECONDARY TO LV DYSFUNCTION

The efficacy and safety of catheter ablation for AF was then extended to patients with impaired LV function and HF where the prevalence of AF is higher (**Table 1**). In 2004, Chen and colleagues[48] retrospectively reviewed 377 patients who had undergone catheter ablation for AF. A total of 94 of these patients had impaired LV function, defined as an LVEF of less than 40%, of which 56% of patients had persistent AF. Despite the high proportion of patients with persistent AF, only PVI was performed. After a single procedure, the AF recurrence rate was 27%, which was higher compared with those with normal LV function (13%; $P<.05$). A total of 85% of these patients underwent a second procedure to reisolate the PVs. After a mean follow-up of 14 months, 74% of patients had no AF recurrences off antiarrhythmic drugs. More importantly, the improvement in rhythm control was associated with a trend to an increased LVEF of 4.6% along with an improved quality of life. Complication rates did not differ between patients with reduced and normal ventricular function.

A prospective study by Hsu and colleagues[49] published in the same year also evaluated the efficacy and effects of restoration and maintenance of SR by catheter ablation of AF in 58 patients with LV dysfunction. A total of 91% of patients had persistent AF with a mean duration of 80 ± 45 months and mean New York Heart Association (NYHA)

class of 2.3 ± 0.5 and LVEF $35 \pm 7\%$.[49] Contrary to the previous study, left atrial (LA) linear ablation was performed between the two superior PVs (roof line) and from the mitral valve annulus to the left PV (mitral isthmus line) in addition to PVI. A total of 50% of patients required a second procedure because of AF recurrence. After a mean follow-up of 12 ± 7 months, 78% of patients with HF remained in SR compared with 84% in the control group with normal ventricular function ($P = .34$). This was associated with a significant decrease in mean NYHA class by 0.9, improved quality of life as assessed using the Short Form-36 questionnaire, and improved exercise capacity. Maintenance of SR was associated with reverse ventricular remodeling with overall improvements in LVEF of 21% and reductions in LV size, with the greatest improvements seen in the first 3 months after the ablation. Reverse ventricular remodeling occurred irrespective of the cause of LV dysfunction; however, a greater improvement was seen in those with isolated dilated cardiomyopathy compared with those with concurrent structural heart disease (LVEF increase of $24 \pm 10\%$ and $16 \pm 14\%$, respectively; $P<.001$). Consistent improvements in ventricular function were also seen in patients with persistent AF with poor and adequate rate control, with greater improvements in LVEF seen in those with poor rate control (LVEF increase $23 \pm 10\%$ and $17 \pm 15\%$, respectively; $P<.001$). As to be expected, the only variable associated with no improvement of LVEF was AF recurrence; however, among the 12 patients with AF recurrence, four patients still had an improvement in LVEF because of a reduction in AF burden with ablation converting persistent to paroxysmal AF.

This study highlighted an important finding: regardless of the cause of HF or prior rate control, improvements of ventricular function were seen in all groups, with the greatest improvement in those patients with poor ventricular rate control and the absence of coexisting structural heart disease. Of these patients, 92% had significant improvements in LVEF suggesting that most patients with AF and idiopathic cardiomyopathy have some degree of tachycardia-induced cardiomyopathy, further strengthening the argument for recognition of this patient group and consideration for rhythm control with catheter ablation.

Two years later, a similar smaller prospective study by Tondo and colleagues[50] with a different ablation strategy of PVI, mitral, and cavotricuspid isthmus lines confirmed these findings in 40 patients with LV dysfunction and AF. After a mean follow-up of 14 ± 2 months, 87% of patients with impaired LV function were in SR with significant improvements in LVEF of $14 \pm 2\%$, exercise

Table 1
Summary of clinical trials examining the efficacy and safety of catheter ablation for AF in patients with impaired left ventricular function

Groups	Chen et al,[48] 2004		Hsu et al,[49] 2004		Tondo et al,[50] 2006		Gentlesk et al,[51] 2007		Nademanee et al,[57] 2008	Lutomsky et al,[52] 2008	
	Low LVEF	Normal LVEF	Low LVEF	Normal LVEF	Low LVEF	Normal LVEF	Low LVEF	Normal LVEF	Low LVEF	Low LVEF	Normal LVEF
Sample size	94	283	58	58	40	65	67	299	129	18	52
Mean age (y)	57 ± 8	55 ± 11	56 ± 10	56 ± 10	57 ± 10	56 ± 8	54	54	67	56.4 ± 10.6	58.5 ± 8.9
Paroxysmal AF	41%	55%	9%	9%	25%	23%	70%	82%	40%	100%	100%
Ischemic HD	—	—	21%	9%	25%	29%	18%	9%	—	17%	15%
Valvular HD	16%	13%	16%	5%	25%	18%	9%	5%	17%	—	—
Mean AF duration (mo)	72 ± 48	60 ± 24	80 ± 45	79 ± 53	36 ± 12	48 ± 12	67	71	40	—	—
Mean NYHA class	2.72	1.06	2.3 ± 0.5	1.3 ± 0.5	2.8 ± 0.1	—	—	—	—	—	—
Mean LVEF (%)	36 ± 8	54 ± 3	35 ± 7	66 ± 7	33 ± 2	64 ± 6	42 ± 9	61 ± 6	31 ± 7	41 ± 6.5	60 ± 6
Mean LA diameter (mm)	47 ± 8	45 ± 5	50 ± 7	46 ± 6	48 ± 4	44 ± 3	44 ± 7	48 ± 6	—	—	—
Ablation type	PVI ± CTI	PVI ± CTI	PVI ± LINES	PVI ± LINES	PVI ± Mitral ± CTI	PVI ± Mitral + CTI	PVI	PVI	CFAE	PVI	PVI
Complications (%)											
Procedure deaths	0	0	0	0	0	0	—	—	0	0	0
Stroke	2	1	2	2	0	0	—	—	5	0	0
Tamponade	0	0	2	0	0	2	—	—	9	0	0
Periprocedure pulmonary edema	1	0	—	—	—	—	—	—	—	0	0
Procedure duration (min)	—	—	218 ± 65	232 ± 90	225 ± 48	234 ± 50	—	—	—	—	—
Mean follow-up (mo)	14 ± 6	15 ± 8	12 ± 7	12 ± 6	14 ± 2	14 ± 2	20	20	27	6	6
AF recorded after first procedure	27%	13%	—	—	45%	29%	—	—	—	50%	27%
Mean number procedures	1.2	1.1	1.5	1.5	1.3	1.2	1.6 ± 0.8	1.3 ± 0.5	1.7	1	1

Groups	Khan et al,[63] 2008		Choi et al,[64] 2010		De Potter et al,[53] 2010		MacDonald et al,[65] 2011		Jones et al,[67] 2013	
	PVI	AVN/BiV	PVI	Drugs for Rhythm Control	Low LVEF	Normal LVEF	PVI	Rate	PVI	Rate
Sample size	41	40	14	13	36	36	22	19	26	26
Mean age (y)	60	61	56 ± 11	63 ± 14	52	51	62	64	64 ± 10	62 ± 9
Paroxysmal AF	49%	55%	67%	73%	39%	—	0	0	0	0
Ischemic HD	—	—	33%	40%	25%	—	50%	47%	38%	27%
Valvular HD	—	—	—	—	11%	—	—	—	—	—
Mean AF duration (mo)	48	47	44 ± 34	56 ± 46	44	78	44	64	23 ± 22	24 ± 29
Mean NHYA class	—	—	1.7 ± 0.8	2 ± 0.8	—	—	2.9 ± 0.4	2.9 ± 0.4	2.46 ± 0.5	2.5 ± 0.5
Mean LVEF (%)	27 ± 8	29 ± 7	37 ± 6	34 ± 11	41 ± 8	63 ± 5	16 ± 7	20 ± 6	22 ± 8	25 ± 7
Mean LA diameter (mm)	49 ± 5	47 ± 6	45 ± 7	48 ± 9	42 ± 6	42 ± 5	—	—	50 ± 6	46 ± 7
Ablation type	PVI ± LINES ± CFAE	NA	PVI	NA	PVI + LINES	PVI + LINES	PVI ± CFAE ± LINES	NA	PVI + LINES + CFAE	NA
Complications (%)	0	0	0	0	0	0	0	0	0	0
Procedure deaths	0	0	0	0	0	0	0	0	0	0
Arrhythmia free off AAD	74%	87%	84%	—	—	—	—	79%	—	—
Arrhythmia free on AAD	69%	78%	71%	87%	92%	86%	87%	89%	50%	73%
Mean NYHA change	—	-0.9	—	—	—	—	—	—	—	—
Mean LVEF change	4.6% (ns)	+21 ± 13%	—	+14 ± 2%	—	+14%	—	+10%	+9.8%	-1.8%
Mean change in LV size (LVIDs)	—	+8 ± 7 mm	—	—	—	+3 mm	—	—	+2.7 mm (ns)	-0.6 mm (ns)
Mean LA change (mm)	—	—	—	—	—	—	—	—	—	—
Improvement in exercise capacity	—	Yes	Yes	Yes	Yes	Yes	—	—	—	—
Improvement in QOL	Yes	Yes	Yes	Yes	Yes	Yes	—	—	—	—

(continued on next page)

Table 1
(continued)

Groups	Khan et al,[63] 2008		Choi et al,[64] 2010		De Potter et al,[53] 2010		MacDonald et al,[65] 2011		Jones et al,[67] 2011	
	PVI	AVN/BiV	PVI	Drugs for Rhythm Control	Low LVEF	Normal LVEF	PVI	Rate	PVI	Rate
CVA	0	0	0	0	0	1 (TIA)	1	0	0	0
Tamponade	1	0	1	NA	0	0	2	0	1	0
Intraprocedure pulmonary edema	1	0	0	NA	0	0	1	0	1	NA
Procedure duration (min)	—	—	—	NA	—	—	205	NA	333 ± 61	NA
Mean follow-up (mo)	6	6	16 ± 13	16 ± 13	14	17	6	6	12	12
AF recurrence after first procedure	—	100%	27%	60%	50%	55.6%	50%	100%	31%	—
Mean number procedures	1.2	NA	—	NA	1.4	1.4	—	NA	—	NA
Arrhythmia free off AAD	71%	0%	73%	—	—	—	—	—	92%	NA
Arrhythmia free on AAD	88%	0%	—	40%	69.4%	69.4%	50%	0%	—	NA
Mean NYHA change	—	—	−0.4 (P<.01)	−0.2 (P = ns)	—	—	—	—	—	—
Mean LVEF change	+8 ± 8%	−1 ± 4%	+13%	+2% (P = ns)	+8%	—	+4.5 ± 11%	+2.8 ± 6.7%	+10.9 ± 11%	+5.4 ± 3.6%
Mean change in LV sizes	—	—	—	—	—	—	20 ± 50 ml	10 ± 32 ml	—	—
Improvement in exercise capacity	Yes (P<.001 cf AVN and BiVp)	Yes	—	—	—	—	No	No	Yes (Vo₂max)	No
Improvement in QOL	Yes (P<.01 cf AVN and BiVp)	Yes	—	—	—	—	No	No	Yes	No

Abbreviations: AAD, antiarrhythmic drugs; AVN, atrioventricular node; BiVp, biventricular pacing; CTI, cavo-tricuspid isthmus; CVA, (cerebrovascular accident); LA, left atrial; LVID, left ventricular internal dimension; NYHA, New York Heart Association; QOL, quality of life; TIA, transient ischemic attack.

capacity, and quality of life. There were no significant differences in outcomes between the HF and control groups, apart from a higher proportion of patients with HF on antiarrhythmic drugs, 38% compared with 23%, respectively.

Gentlesk and colleagues[51] prospectively evaluated the effect of PVI on LVEF in 67 patients with AF (70% paroxysmal) and decreased LVEF (≤50%). Isolation of the PVs was performed followed by ablation of non-PV triggers, which were identified after administration of isoproterenol and atrial burst pacing. After 20 months of follow-up, AF control defined as freedom from AF or greater than 90% reduction in AF burden determined using transtelephonic monitoring was 86%. This compared favorably with those patients with normal LV function, although more repeat procedures were required (1.6 ± 0.8 vs 1.3 ± 0.6; P<.05). This was associated with a significant improvement in LVEF (from 42 ± 9% to 56 ± 8%; P<.001), with more than 70% of patients returning to normal ventricular function (EF>55%) at 20 months follow-up (Fig. 1). Furthermore, assessments were made of LA function, with a significant increase in LA ejection fraction observed 6 months after catheter ablation and SR maintenance (from 0.32 ± 0.11 to 0.54 ± 0.18; P<.01), which supports the hypothesis that improvement in LVEF might in part be a result of improved atrial transport function.

Similar to Hsu and colleagues,[49] the improvement in ventricular function was not confined to those with poor ventricular rate control, with 88% of the patients having adequate rate control during AF before the ablation, which was defined as heart rates of less than 100 bpm for less than 50% of the time using transtelephonic monitoring for 2 to 3 weeks. These authors concluded that even when AF is not persistent, with well-controlled ventricular rates, reverse ventricular remodeling still occurs and highlighted the presence of an underrecognized group of patients with cardiomyopathy that would benefit by improved rhythm control with catheter ablation.

Similar findings were reported by Lutomsky and colleagues[52] who examined the impact of PVI on cardiac function using cardiac magnetic resonance imaging (CMRI) in patients with paroxysmal AF and impaired LV systolic function. Seventy patients with short periods of AF, defined as less than 24 hours, underwent CMRI before and 6 months after PVI. After a mean follow-up of 152 days, patients with impaired LVEF had lower success rates compared with those with preserved ventricular function (50% vs 73%; P<.05); however, a significant improvement in LVEF was seen (41 ± 6% to 51 ± 12%; P = .004). Interestingly, some patients with previously normal ventricular function who developed AF recurrence after catheter ablation had impaired LV function in follow-up, further supporting the important deleterious impact of AF on ventricular function. The authors concluded that even short periods of paroxysmal AF in patients with HF might have a detrimental effect on LVEF.

The reported success rates for catheter ablation for AF in patients with HF are inferior to patients without structural heart disease, with higher recurrence rates and more redo procedures required. To identify whether this is a consequence of LV dysfunction itself or confounding factors, such as LA size, AF duration, and AF type, a case control matching design study was performed by De Potter and colleagues.[53] In this study 36 patients with depressed LV function (LVEF<50%) and 36 patients with normal LVEF were matched for age, LA size, AF duration, and AF type. Circumferential PV ablation together with a roof, inferior LA, and mitral isthmus lines were performed. A successful outcome was defined as freedom from AF or any episode of AF or atrial flutter episodes of less than 30 seconds. After a mean follow-up of 16 months and a mean of 1.4 procedures, 69.4% had successful outcomes in both groups. There were no differences in outcomes or complication rates between the two groups suggesting that impaired LV systolic function itself is not a predictor of poor success rates or outcomes after catheter ablation. LA size was found to be the only predictor of AF recurrence after ablation: mean LA size was 40.9 ± 5.5 mm in the successful group and 44.7 ± 5.3 mm in the unsuccessful group (P<.01) and reflects more advanced atrial remodeling in the HF population. This has recently been

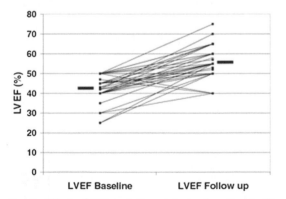

Fig. 1. Effect of PVI on left ventricular function in 67 patients with idiopathic cardiomyopathy. Mean increase in LVEF from 42 ± 9% to 57 ± 7%; P<.001. (*From* Gentlesk PJ, Sauer WH, Gerstenfeld EP, et al. Reversal of left ventricular dysfunction following ablation of atrial fibrillation. J Cardiovasc Electrophysiol 2007;18:12; with permission.)

confirmed in a study assessing the degree of atrial remodeling using CMRI,[54] where patients with LV systolic dysfunction displayed a comparatively greater degree of structural remodeling quantified using late gadolinium MRI than patients with normal LVEF. LA size has been identified as an independent predictor of AF recurrence after catheter ablation in patients with preserved ventricular function with a traditional upper limit of 55 mm being used for exclusion from catheter-based therapies for AF and enrollment for clinical trials.[55,56] As with previous studies in the HF population, reverse ventricular remodeling was evident in those patients who maintained SR after catheter ablation, with an increase in mean LVEF from 42.1% to 56.5% (P<.001) after 6 months. Those patients with idiopathic cardiomyopathy had the largest increase in LVEF.

Following Nadamanee and colleagues initial study describing an alternative approach to AF ablation, in which CFAE were targeted with high procedural success rates, this approach was used in high-risk patients with AF, similar to the cohort studied in the AFFIRM trial.[41,57] The cohort of 771 patients was at least 65 years old or had at least one or more risk factors for a stroke (hypertension, diabetes, structural heart disease, prior stroke or transient ischemic attack, or HF and LVEF ≤40%). A total of 129 patients had impaired LV systolic function with a mean LVEF of 30% in a more elderly population group compared with the previous studies described. A total of 60% of patients had persistent AF and the ablation strategy consisted of electrogram guided (CFAE) ablation alone. After a mean follow-up of 27 months, the AF recurrence rate after multiple procedures was 11%. Similar to previous studies, a significant improvement in LVEF was seen in those who maintained SR from 31 ± 7% to 41 ± 10% (P<.001) compared with those who remained in AF (24 ± 8% to 23.5 ± 9%; P = ns). Multivariate analysis and Cox regression analysis showed SR to be an independent predictor of a favorable prognosis. This was demonstrated in patients with both preserved and impaired LV systolic function (Fig. 2). The authors concluded the improvement in LV function in the HF cohort after maintenance of SR resulted in improved survival.

Rhythm Control with Catheter Ablation Versus Rate Control in Patients with Depressed Ventricular Systolic Function

Although the studies described have clearly shown improvements in ventricular function with catheter ablation of AF, more modest improvements were observed in studies using the "ablate and pace" strategy.[58–61] Greater improvements have been seen in patients who received a biventricular (BiV) pacemaker and AV node (AVN) ablation.[62] Although this approach provides effective rate control with evidence of reverse ventricular remodeling, it does not restore atrioventricular synchrony, and atrial systole has a significant contribution to cardiac output. The Pulmonary Vein Antrum Isolation versus AV Node Ablation with Biventricular Pacing for the Treatment of Atrial Fibrillation in Patients with Congestive Heart Failure (PABA-CHF) randomized multicenter trial was therefore undertaken to compare PVI and AVN ablation with BiV pacing in patients with depressed ventricular function, with an LVEF of less than 40% with NYHA Class II or III symptoms.[63] A total of 81 patients underwent randomization with 41 undergoing PVI with or without linear lines and fractionated electrogram ablation and 40 BiV

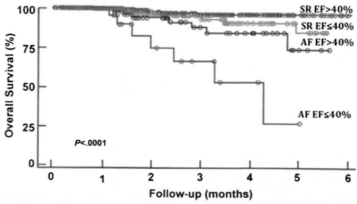

Fig. 2. Kaplan-Meier survival curves for four patient groups after catheter ablation for AF: (1) SR and EF >40%, (2) SR and EF ≤40%, (3) AF and EF >40%, and (4) AF and EF ≤40%. (*From* Nademanee K, Schwab MC, Kosar EM, et al. Clinical outcomes of catheter substrate ablation for high-risk patients with atrial fibrillation. J Am Coll Cardiol 2008;51:847; with permission.)

pacing and AVN ablation. Both groups were matched in terms of LVEF, LA size, type of AF, and age. At 6 months follow-up, all the patients in the AVN ablation and pacing group were in AF, whereas 88% of patients in the PVI group had no AF recurrence with antiarrhythmic drugs. Furthermore, progression of AF (from paroxysmal to persistent to long-standing persistent) did not occur in any of the patients undergoing PVI but occurred in 30% of those who underwent AVN ablation and pacing. Conversely, all the patients in persistent AF before ablation who had AF recurrence were only having paroxysms of AF, compared with 5% in the AVN ablation and BiV pacing group. The change in ventricular function and atrial size during follow up was significantly different between the two groups. At 6 months, the mean LVEF increased by $8 \pm 8\%$ compared with a decrease of $1 \pm 4\%$ in the AVN ablation and pacing group ($P<.001$). Similarly, the LA internal diameter decreased in the PVI group by 0.4 ± 0.3 cm and increased in the AVN ablation and pacing group by 0.1 ± 0.2 cm ($P<.001$). The improved maintenance of SR with PVI, and therefore reverse ventricular remodeling effects, were associated with greater improvements in function capacity measured during a 6-minute walk test and quality of life compared with AVN ablation and pacing and adds further support for the important contribution of atrial systole to cardiac output in patients with depressed ventricular function. Further analysis showed that greater improvements in LVEF, functional capacity, and quality of life were seen in patients with persistent AF undergoing PVI compared with the paroxysmal patients with AF. Complication rates were similar in both groups. In the PVI group, one patient had pericardial tamponade and two had PV stenosis and pulmonary edema. In the BiV pacing group, one patient had lead dislodgement and one had a pneumothorax. The authors concluded that rhythm control with catheter ablation and PVI provided superior morphologic and functional improvements compared with the best rate control strategy with AVN ablation and BiV pacing. The finding of greater benefit in patients with persistent AF compared with paroxysmal AF contradicts current beliefs that patients with persistent AF have advanced disease, particularly impaired ventricular function, which precludes them from catheter ablation. In light of these trials, one might argue that patients with persistent AF and HF have more to gain from catheter ablation because of the greater improvements in ventricular function, functional class, and quality of life.

Following these studies demonstrating the benefits of catheter ablation for AF in patients with HF,

three studies were reported comparing conventional rate or rhythm control with pharmacologic agents and catheter ablation. Choi and colleagues[64] performed a retrospective case control trial to evaluate cardiac function and outcomes in patients with LV dysfunction treated with either catheter ablation or conventional medication with rate and rhythm control strategies. Two groups consisting of 14 patients in the catheter ablation group and 13 in the medication group were evenly matched in terms of age, NYHA class, LVEF, AF duration, AF type, and LA size. After a mean follow-up of 16 ± 13 months, 73% of patients treated with catheter ablation remained in SR, which was associated with a significant improvement in LVEF from 37% to 51% and improvements in NYHA functional class. Conversely, only 40% of control subjects remained in SR, and showed no change in LVEF or NHYA functional class on follow-up echocardiography.

After this, another study was conducted to compare a rhythm control strategy by catheter ablation against rate control using pharmacologic agents in patients with more severe impairment of LV function and persistent AF.[65] Twenty patients were randomized to catheter ablation and 18 to medical rate control. At the end of the 6-month follow-up period, SR was maintained in 50% of patients in the ablation group and 0% in the rate control group. Comparison between the two strategies revealed no significant difference in change in LVEF or LV dimensions, 6-minute walk test, or quality of life when measured using the Kansas City Cardiomyopathy Questionnaire and Minnesota Living with Heart Failure Questionnaire. These results are contrary to the previous beneficial results reported in patients undergoing catheter ablation. The authors commented that maintenance of SR in their study was lower than previous studies (50% compared with 78%–96%), which was because the study group recruited, which was older, had more severe systolic dysfunction and longer AF durations. These clinical characteristics are associated with atrial dilatation and fibrosis and decreased procedural success.[66] In view of these findings they performed a post hoc analysis to identify whether patients in SR demonstrated any improvements in cardiac structure or function. They identified significant improvements in LVEF, which occurred within 1 week of SR; however, this was not associated with any improvement in exercise capacity or quality of life. They speculated that the improvement in LV function observed might have been as a consequence of measuring LVEF in SR rather than AF, because there were no other observed improvements in functional exercise capacity or N-terminal prohormone of brain natriuretic peptide (NT-proBNP) and the improvement in LVEF was observed. Further effort at ablation when significant reverse ventricular remodeling is unlikely to occur.

More recently, Jones and colleagues[67] conducted a single-center prospective randomized control trial comparing catheter ablation with rate control for persistent AF. Fifty-two patients met the inclusion criteria of LVEF less than or equal to 35% assessed using radionucleotide ventriculography, NYHA Class II to IV, and on optimal HF medical therapy. Appropriate rate control, defined as a mean resting heart rate less than or equal to 80 bpm and after a 6-minute walk test of less than or equal to 110 bpm was achieved in 96% of patients in the rate control group at 3 months. A stepwise catheter ablation strategy was used that included PVI; linear lesions (roof, mitral, and cavotricuspid isthmus); and CFAE ablation. The 1-year arrhythmia-free survival was 72% after a single ablation procedure and after multiple procedures it was 92%. There was one serious procedural complication requiring emergency pericardiocentesis and sternotomy to repair a perforation at the atrioventricular groove. Other complications included one groin hematoma, one chest infection 2 weeks postablation, and one patient with postprocedural pulmonary edema. In keeping with previous studies, catheter ablation and maintenance of SR was associated with reverse structural and functional remodeling with a significant decrease in LA and RA area and an increase in LVEF at 12 months. When compared with stringent rate control, the primary end point of peak Vo_2 had increased significantly in the ablation group and decreased in the rate control group (difference + 3.07 ml/kg/min; 95% confidence interval, 0.56–5.59; P = .018). For the secondary end points, ablation also improved quality-of-life scores assessed using the Minnesota questionnaire (P = .019) and decreased brain natriuretic peptide (BNP) (P = .045), and showed nonsignificant trends toward improved 6-minute walk test (P = .095) and EF (P = .055). This study reported high success rates after catheter ablation that may reflect the younger cohort of patients enrolled with a high proportion of nonischemic cardiomyopathy. Although these are promising results, ablation procedures were extensive with mean procedure times of 333 ± 61 minutes and ablation times of 80 ± 19 minutes. Nevertheless, this study demonstrates that maintenance of SR after catheter ablation in patients with HF in the short term is associated with greater improvements in symptoms, neurohormonal status, and objective physiologic exercise capacity compared with rate control for persistent AF.

Meta-analysis

The results of these clinical trials represent a heterogenous group of patients with different ages, AF types and durations, ablation strategy, and follow-up, and therefore outcomes of AF ablation in patients with HF are difficult to analyze. Two meta-analyses were performed to assess the role of catheter ablation for AF in patients with HF. The first performed by Wilton and colleagues[68] compared the safety and efficacy of AF ablation in patients with and without LV dysfunction. They reported that those with ventricular dysfunction were 1.5 times more likely to have AF recurrences after a single ablation procedure compared with those with preserved ventricular function. However, after repeat procedures, similar success rates were reported in both groups without increased risk or complication rates. It is not surprising that repeat procedures are required in those with ventricular dysfunction because of the more complex atrial substrate and larger atrial size. Reassuringly, this does not seem to be associated with increased risk; however, the previously mentioned studies are small with incomplete reporting in some of the studies. The consistent finding of improved LVEF after catheter ablation and maintenance of SR in the studies was highlighted by this meta-analysis and is an important finding. After catheter ablation, patients with LV dysfunction experienced an absolute improvement in LVEF of 11% (95% confidence interval, 7%–14%) (**Fig. 3**).

A second meta-analysis reviewed nine studies (of which six were common to both meta-analyses) with 354 patients, of which four were cohort studies, three case controlled, and two randomized controlled studies.[69] Study patients were mainly male with a mean age of 49 to 62 years with moderately impaired LV systolic function with LVEF range from 35% to 43%. Similar to the previous meta-analysis, LVEF improved after ablation by a mean difference of 11.1% (**Fig. 4**) with the presence of coronary artery disease being inversely related to LVEF improvement (P<.0001). This meta-analysis found no association between the degree of LVEF improvement and the proportion of patients with persistent or paroxysmal AF.

Complication rates were reported in seven out of the nine studies and out of the 268 patients who underwent AF ablation, 18 developed complications (6.7%), which included four strokes (1.5%), five pericardial effusions/tamponade (1.9%), two episodes of periprocedural pulmonary edema (0.8%), two cases of pulmonary stenosis (0.8%), three with minor groin bleeding (1.2%), and one patient required readmission 1 week after

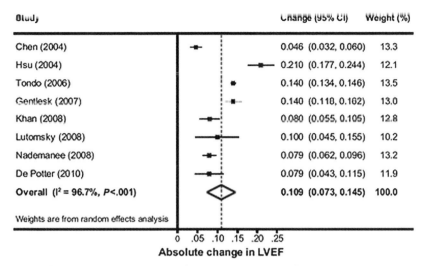

Fig. 3. Meta-analysis of absolute change in LVEF after catheter ablation for AF in patients with impaired ventricular systolic function. (*From* Wilton SB, Fundytus A, Ghali WA, et al. Meta-analysis of the effectiveness and safety of catheter ablation of atrial fibrillation in patients with versus without left ventricular systolic dysfunction. Am J Cardiol 2010;106:1289; with permission.)

discharge with HF. Quality of life was not assessed in this meta-analysis because of the heterogeneity in the measures used in the studies.

The evidence suggests that improved rhythm control with catheter ablation in patients with HF is feasible and moderately efficacious in the short term (between 60% and 88%) and is associated with reverse atrial and ventricular remodeling[70] and improved ventricular systolic function, which improves exercise capacity and quality of life. The improvement in ventricular function might in part be related to improved ventricular rate control and rhythm regularization. There is some evidence that regularization of ventricular rhythm

independent of rate can improve hemodynamics. In two studies, after AVN ablation, regular right ventricular pacing at equivalent ventricular rates to that observed during AF was associated with improved cardiac outputs, decreased filling pressures, and improved LVEF.[71,72] The mechanism for reversal of arrhythmia-induced cardiomyopathy may be similar to that observed after suppression[73] and ablation[74] of frequent ventricular ectopy. However, rate or rhythm regularization alone cannot explain all the observed results. For example, the PABA-CHF trial comparing AVN ablation and BiV pacing with PVI demonstrated no improvements in LVEF in those treated with BiV pacing. In addition,

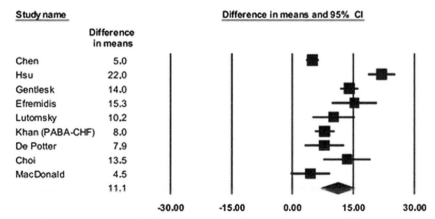

Fig. 4. Change in left ventricular systolic function after catheter ablation for AF. The *diamond* represents the mean difference in LVEF, and width is 95% confidence interval. (*From* Dagres N, Varounis C, Gaspar T, et al. Catheter ablation for atrial fibrillation in patients with left ventricular systolic dysfunction. A systematic review and meta-analysis. J Card Fail 2011;17:967; with permission.)

consistent improvements in LV function were seen in patients with adequate ventricular rate control or short (<24 hours) episodes of AF.[49,51,52,67] Another possible explanation for the improvement in LV function might be related to technical issues with quantification of LVEF in SR and AF and the use of nonmasked operators. Calculation of LVEF during AF is associated with an underestimation of LVEF because of beat-beat variability.[75] For example, the PABA-CHF study comparing catheter ablation and CRT with AVN ablation was comparing LVEF postintervention in SR and AF, with 12% of patients in AF after catheter ablation compared with 100% after Cardiac Resynchronisation Therapy (CRT) and AVN ablation, which might have influenced the improvements in LVEF observed. However, two studies did perform baseline and follow-up LVEF measurements during SR and found equivalent increases in LVEF after catheter ablation comparable with the other studies.[51,52] Another explanation for an improvement in LVEF could be improved atrial transport function associated with SR, which was suggested by the improvement in LA function after catheter ablation in two studies.[51,76]

Another important consideration when interpreting changes in LVEF is the imaging modality used. Most of the studies used transthoracic echocardiography, which measures LVEF during one cardiac cycle. However, nuclear imaging is a more reliable modality for LVEF assessment in AF because its value is calculated by measuring a composite beat created during 20 minutes of recorded heartbeats.

Catheter Ablation for AF and Effects on Diastolic Function

Isolated diastolic HF or HF with preserved LV dysfunction accounts for 30% to 50% of patients with HF and is associated with AF particularly in the elderly.[77–83] A substudy of the CHARISMA trial also identified the association of diastolic dysfunction with new-onset AF and vascular events after myocardial infarction.[78] The severity and degree of diastolic dysfunction seem to be associated with risk for the development of AF.[82] A study by Jais and colleagues[81] highlighted the significant differences in measures of diastolic function in patients labeled as "lone AF" compared with age-matched control subjects.

Frequently the onset of AF in these patients is associated with significant hemodynamic effects caused by the presence of impaired LV relaxation and reduced LV filling further exposed by the loss of atrial contractility. The mechanism for the increase in incidence of AF in patients with diastolic

HF is incompletely understood, but in part is related to the common etiologies, the presence of raised ventricular filling pressures and associated atrial stretch, dilatation, and contractile dysfunction. An increasing LA pressure and volume is positively correlated with the degree and severity of diastolic dysfunction.[84,85] This increase in LA pressure and size creates a favorable substrate for the maintenance of AF by increasing dispersion of refractoriness and alterations in anisotropic and conduction properties.

There is now favorable evidence on the efficacy of catheter ablation for AF in patients with LV systolic dysfunction; however, studies with isolated diastolic dysfunction are limited. The first prospective trial was in 2005 by Reant and colleagues[86] who evaluated 48 patients with paroxysmal and persistent AF and diastolic dysfunction. Compared with healthy control subjects in SR, LA dimensions were greater and measures of diastolic function using echocardiography and tissue Doppler were reduced. After catheter ablation that involved PVI and linear lesions and a mean follow-up of 11 months, reverse morphologic LA remodeling and improvements in LV diastolic function were observed. This study suggested that in part impaired diastolic function caused by AF and maintenance of SR with catheter ablation could potentially reverse this process. In 2011, Cha and colleagues[87] evaluated and compared the long-term efficacy of catheter ablation for AF in patients with normal LV function and abnormal diastolic and systolic function. One year after ablation, elimination rates for AF off antiarrhythmic drugs were 84% in those with normal LV function and 62% and 75% with abnormal LV systolic function and diastolic function, respectively. However, after a 5-year follow-up period the success rates in patients were poor, with only 33% of patients free from AF in the systolic dysfunction group and 40% in the diastolic dysfunction group (**Fig. 5**).

Similar to previous studies, those patients with LV systolic dysfunction had a significant increase in LVEF from 35% to 56% with AF recurrence being a predictor of reverse LV remodeling. However, fewer patients had improvements in diastolic function, with only 30% demonstrating an improvement compared with 49% in those with systolic dysfunction. The authors concluded that AF ablation in patients with diastolic dysfunction is relatively efficacious after 1 year; however, in the long term arrhythmia recurrence was high. They acknowledged in this study that patients with diastolic dysfunction were older with a high proportion of comorbidities, such as hypertension, and suggested that during longer follow-up, progression of diastolic dysfunction and redevelopment

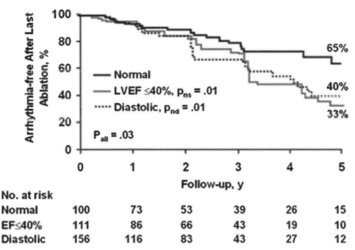

Fig. 5. Long-term freedom from AF recurrence after ablation in patients with left ventricular systolic and diastolic dysfunction. (*From* Cha YM, Wokhlu A, Asirvatham SJ, et al. Success of ablation for atrial fibrillation in isolated left ventricular diastolic dysfunction: a comparison to systolic dysfunction and normal ventricular function. Circ Arrhythm Electrophysiol 2011;4:728; with permission.)

of the vulnerable substrate may predispose to AF recurrence. One year later, Hu and colleagues[88] assessed the relationship between diastolic dysfunction, LA substrate quantified by measuring atrial voltages, and efficacy of catheter ablation in patients with paroxysmal AF. As in the previous study, patients with diastolic dysfunction were older. Patients with diastolic dysfunction had significantly lower atrial voltages compared with those with normal ventricular function after adjusting for age and hypertension. After catheter ablation, AF recurrence in those with diastolic dysfunction was higher at 30% compared with 10% in the normal LV function group. Further analysis also showed that low atrial voltages were predictors of AF recurrence after ablation.

Thus, the presence of atrial structural remodeling, in particular atrial fibrosis, is associated with poorer outcomes after catheter ablation because of a favorable substrate for the maintenance of reentry circuits and sites for non-PV ectopy and could explain the higher recurrence rates of AF in patients with diastolic dysfunction.[89,90]

PATIENT SELECTION FOR CATHETER ABLATION FOR AF IN PATIENTS WITH HF

Although the current studies suggest modest efficacy rates with catheter ablation of AF in patients with HF, these are largely based on cohort studies in experienced high-volume centers with significant heterogeneity in patient selection and outcome measures. The studied population in most studies was selected and not representative of the average patient with HF with concomitant AF

(eg, patients were frequently younger and with a relatively high LVEF). Therefore, generalized recommendations on catheter ablation for all patients with AF in the HF population cannot be made; however, based on the current available evidence, highly selective patients should be considered on an individual basis. The studies do, however, highlight several important factors, which are relevant when selecting patients for catheter ablation.

As with patients with normal ventricular function, LA dilatation is an important predictor of AF recurrence in the HF population secondary to more advanced structural remodeling and atrial fibrosis. In the general population LA diameters of greater than 55 mm have more recently been excluded from catheter ablation and in the HF population LA diameters greater than 45 mm in two studies have been associated with AF recurrence and poorer outcomes.

Baseline LVEF is also an important factor and as alluded to previously many studies demonstrating reasonable outcomes at 1 year recruited patients with an average LVEF between 35% and 45%. MacDonald and colleagues[65] who recruited patients with a lower LVEF reported poorer outcomes with catheter ablation compared with previous studies and therefore highlighted the importance of LVEF for patient selection.

Although shorter AF durations have been reported as a predictor of success after catheter ablation for persistent AF in patients with preserved LVEF, the AF durations in the current studies have been variable, between 36 and 80 months, with similar efficacy rates. Contrary to studies on catheter ablation in patients with preserved LV systolic function, patients with persistent AF seemed to derive significant benefit from catheter ablation and one might argue have more to gain, because these patients are more likely to have an associated tachycardia-induced cardiomyopathy, which potentially could be reversed by catheter ablation and maintenance of SR.

Finally, the cause of ventricular dysfunction has been shown to be a predictor of success, with patients diagnosed with idiopathic cardiomyopathy having greater success rates and reverse remodeling after catheter ablation, which is likely related to a higher proportion of patients with a tachycardia-induced cardiomyopathy in this group.

Patients with HF and AF are a challenging group. It is important to recognize that AF is one aspect of the management of the patient with HF. Patients should be treated with optimal HF medical therapy before considering catheter ablation analogous to patient selection for CRT. When deciding on a nonpharmacologic strategy for the treatment of AF in these patients one must formulate an estimate for the likelihood of maintaining SR incorporating the previously mentioned factors and coexisting comorbidities. Additional information on the underlying atrial substrate from advanced imaging modalities may be useful to further assess the likelihood of success after catheter ablation. For example, Akkaya and colleagues[54] recently showed a greater improvement in LVEF after catheter ablation in patients with HF in those with less atrial remodeling assessed using late gadolinium CMRI.

Catheter ablation in the HF population is associated with longer procedure and higher fluoroscopy times, more repeat procedures, and complication rates reported by some studies as high as 13%. Although the studies have reported modest success rates, the follow-up of these patients is limited and between 6 and 20 months. In keeping with previous studies on catheter ablation of AF[91] the success rates are likely to diminish during longer follow-up. Therefore, thorough discussions with the patient at the outset about short-term success rates, requirement for multiple procedures, complication rates, and unproved long-term success rates are important before deciding on catheter ablation for AF in patients with HF.

SUMMARY

Current evidence is supportive for a beneficial role in maintenance of SR in patients with HF with AF by catheter ablation. Catheter ablation for AF seems to be superior to rate control and pharmacologic rhythm control. The benefit is not restricted to type of AF (paroxysmal or persistent); however, greater benefit is seen in patients with idiopathic dilated cardiomyopathy where AF is a significant contributor to depressed ventricular function and symptoms. The studies have demonstrated improved rhythm control with better quality of life and reverse ventricular and atrial remodeling. Given the increased morbidity and mortality associated with AF in the presence of HF, one would expect improved ventricular function after catheter ablation to be associated with improvements in these parameters. However, no large-scale trials have been reported demonstrating a mortality benefit with catheter ablation in this patient cohort, because none of the studies were robust or powered sufficiently to assess mortality differences. Larger trials are required, such as the ongoing CASTLE-AF and RAFT-AF trials, to evaluate whether catheter ablation of AF in patients with HF is associated with improved mortality compared with conventional treatment. This has been recognized in the 2012 Consensus Statement on catheter ablation of AF, which states that "catheter ablation of AF is reasonable in highly selected patients with HF."[92]

REFERENCES

1. Hoppe UC, Casares JM, Eiskjaer H, et al. Effect of cardiac resynchronization on the incidence of atrial fibrillation in patients with severe heart failure. Circulation 2006;114:18–25.
2. Michalsen A, Konig G, Thimme W. Preventable causative factors leading to hospital admission with decompensated heart failure. Heart 1998;80:437–41.
3. Tsuyuki RT, McKelvie RS, Arnold JM, et al. Acute precipitants of congestive heart failure exacerbations. Arch Intern Med 2001;161:2337–42.
4. Chin MH, Goldman L. Factors contributing to the hospitalization of patients with congestive heart failure. Am J Public Health 1997;87:643–8.
5. Wyse DG, Waldo AL, DiMarco JP, et al, The Atrial Fibrillation Follow-up Investigation of Rhythm Management (AFFIRM) Investigators. A comparison of rate control and rhythm control in patients with atrial fibrillation. N Engl J Med 2002;347:1825–33.
6. Blackshear JL, Safford RE. AFFIRM and RACE trials: implications for the management of atrial fibrillation. Card Electrophysiol Rev 2003;7:366–9.
7. Opolski G, Torbicki A, Kosior DA, et al. Rate control vs rhythm control in patients with nonvalvular persistent atrial fibrillation: the results of the Polish How to Treat Chronic Atrial Fibrillation (HOT CAFE) Study. Chest 2004;126:476–86.

8. Carlsson J, Miketic S, Windeler J, et al. Random-ized trial of rate-control versus rhythm-control in persistent atrial fibrillation: the Strategies of Treat-ment of Atrial Fibrillation (STAF) study. J Am Coll Cardiol 2003;41:1690–6.

9. Hohnloser SH, Kuck KH, Lilienthal J. Rhythm or rate control in atrial fibrillation–Pharmacological Intervention in Atrial Fibrillation (PIAF)· a rando-mised trial. Lancet 2000;356:1789–94.

10. Moller M, Torp-Pedersen CT, Kober L. Dofetilide in patients with congestive heart failure and left ven-tricular dysfunction: safety aspects and effect on atrial fibrillation. The Danish Investigators of Arrhythmia and Mortality on Dofetilide (DIAMOND) Study Group. Congest Heart Fail 2001;7:146–50.

11. Weinfeld MS, Drazner MH, Stevenson WG, et al. Early outcome of initiating amiodarone for atrial fibrillation in advanced heart failure. J Heart Lung Transplant 2000;19:638–43.

12. Roy D, Talajic M, Nattel S, et al. Rhythm control versus rate control for atrial fibrillation and heart failure. N Engl J Med 2008;358:2667–77.

13. Pedersen OD, Bagger H, Kober L, et al. Trandolap-ril reduces the incidence of atrial fibrillation after acute myocardial infarction in patients with left ven-tricular dysfunction. Circulation 1999;100:376–80.

14. Swedberg KP, Coen-Solal A. Prevention of atrial fibrillation in symptomatic chronic heart failure by candesartan: results of the CHARM study. J Am Coll Cardiol 2004;43(Suppl A):222A.

15. Wachtell K, Lehto M, Gerdts E, et al. Angiotensin II receptor blockade reduces new-onset atrial fibrilla-tion and subsequent stroke compared to atenolol: the Losartan Intervention For End Point Reduction in Hypertension (LIFE) study. J Am Coll Cardiol 2005;45:712–9.

16. Young-Xu Y, Jabbour S, Goldberg R, et al. Useful-ness of statin drugs in protecting against atrial fibrillation in patients with coronary artery disease. Am J Cardiol 2003;92:1379–83.

17. Shiroshita-Takeshita A, Brundel BJ, Burstein B, et al. Effects of simvastatin on the development of the atrial fibrillation substrate in dogs with conges-tive heart failure. Cardiovasc Res 2007;74:75–84.

18. Lafuente-Lafuente C, Mouly S, Longas-Tejero MA, et al. Antiarrhythmic drugs for maintaining sinus rhythm after cardioversion of atrial fibrillation: a sys-tematic review of randomized controlled trials. Arch Intern Med 2006;166:719–28.

19. Corley SD, Epstein AE, DiMarco JP, et al. Rela-tionships between sinus rhythm, treatment, and survival in the Atrial Fibrillation Follow-Up Investiga-tion of Rhythm Management (AFFIRM) Study. Cir-culation 2004;109:1509–13.

20. Shelton RJ, Clark AL, Goode K, et al. A randomised, controlled study of rate versus rhythm control in patients with chronic atrial fibrillation and heart failure: (CAFE-II Study). Heart 2009;95:924–30.

21. Peters KG, Kienzle MG. Severe cardiomyopathy due to chronic rapidly conducted atrial fibrillation: complete recovery after restoration of sinus rhythm. Am J Med 1988;85:242–4.

22. Van Gelder IC, Crijns HJ, Blanksma PK, et al. Time course of hemodynamic changes and Improve-ment of exercise tolerance after cardioversion of chronic atrial fibrillation unassociated with cardiac valve disease. Am J Cardiol 1993;72:560–6.

23. Benjamin EJ, Levy D, Vaziri SM, et al. Independent risk factors for atrial fibrillation in a population-based cohort: the Framingham Heart Study. JAMA 1994;271:840–4.

24. Poole-Wilson PA, Swedberg K, Cleland JG, et al. Comparison of carvedilol and metoprolol on clinical outcomes in patients with chronic heart failure in the Carvedilol Or Metoprolol European Trial (COMET): randomised controlled trial. Lancet 2003;36:7–13.

25. Middlekauff HR, Stevenson WG, Stevenson LW. Prognostic significance of atrial fibrillation in advanced heart failure. A study of 390 patients. Circulation 1991;84:40–8.

26. Stulak JM, Dearani JA, Daly RC, et al. Left ventric-ular dysfunction in atrial fibrillation: restoration of sinus rhythm by the Cox-maze procedure signifi-cantly improves systolic function and functional status. Ann Thorac Surg 2006;82:494–500 [discus-sion: 500–1].

27. Haissaguerre M, Jaise P, Sha D, et al. Spontaneous initiation of atrial fibrillation by ectopic beats origi-nating in the pulmonary veins. N Engl J Med 1998;339:659–66.

28. Haissaguerre M, Jais P, Shah DC, et al. Electro-physiological end point for catheter ablation of atrial fibrillation initiated from multiple pulmonary venous foci. Circulation 2000;101:1409–17.

29. Oral H, Scharf C, Chugh A, et al. Catheter ablation for paroxysmal atrial fibrillation: segmental pulmo-nary vein ostial ablation versus left atrial ablation. Circulation 2003;108:2355–60.

30. Pappone C, Oreto G, Rosanio S, et al. Atrial electro-anatomic remodeling after circumferential radiofre-quency pulmonary vein ablation: efficacy of an anatomic approach in a large cohort of patients with atrial fibrillation. Circulation 2001;104:2539–44.

31. Wilber DJ, Pappone C, Neuzil P, et al. Comparison of antiarrhythmic drug therapy and radiofrequency catheter ablation in patients with paroxysmal atrial fibrillation: a randomized controlled trial. JAMA 2010;303:333–40.

32. Wazni OM, Marrouche NF, Martin DO, et al. Radio-frequency ablation vs antiarrhythmic drugs as first-line treatment of symptomatic atrial fibrillation: a randomized trial. JAMA 2005;293:2634–40.

33. Pappone C, Rosanio S, Augello G, et al. Mortality, morbidity, and quality of life after circumferential pulmonary vein ablation for atrial fibrillation: outcomes from a controlled nonrandomized long-term study. J Am Coll Cardiol 2003;42:185–97.

34. Ouyang F, Bansch D, Ernst S, et al. Complete isolation of left atrium surrounding the pulmonary veins: new insights from the double-Lasso technique in paroxysmal atrial fibrillation. Circulation 2004;110:2090–6.

35. Haissaguerre M, Shah DC, Jais P, et al. Mapping-guided ablation of pulmonary veins to cure atrial fibrillation. Am J Cardiol 2000;86:9K–19K.

36. Nair GM, Nery PB, Diwakaramenon S, et al. A systematic review of randomized trials comparing radiofrequency ablation with antiarrhythmic medications in patients with atrial fibrillation. J Cardiovasc Electrophysiol 2009;20:138–44.

37. Elayi CS, Di Biase L, Barrett C, et al. Atrial fibrillation termination as a procedural endpoint during ablation in long-standing persistent atrial fibrillation. Heart Rhythm 2010;7:1216–23.

38. Elayi CS, Verma A, Di Biase L, et al. Ablation for longstanding permanent atrial fibrillation: results from a randomized study comparing three different strategies. Heart Rhythm 2008;5:1658–64.

39. Haissaguerre M, Hocini M, Sanders P, et al. Catheter ablation of long-lasting persistent atrial fibrillation: clinical outcome and mechanisms of subsequent arrhythmias. J Cardiovasc Electrophysiol 2005;16:1138–47.

40. Oral H, Knight BP, Tada H, et al. Pulmonary vein isolation for paroxysmal and persistent atrial fibrillation. Circulation 2002;105:1077–81.

41. Nademanee K, McKenzie J, Kosar E, et al. A new approach for catheter ablation of atrial fibrillation: mapping of the electrophysiologic substrate. J Am Coll Cardiol 2004;43:2044–53.

42. Haissaguerre M, Sanders P, Hocini M, et al. Catheter ablation of long-lasting persistent atrial fibrillation: critical structures for termination. J Cardiovasc Electrophysiol 2005;16:1125–37.

43. O'Neill MD, Wright M, Knecht S, et al. Long-term follow-up of persistent atrial fibrillation ablation using termination as a procedural endpoint. Eur Heart J 2009;30:1105–12.

44. Nakagawa H, Scherlag BJ, Patterson E, et al. Pathophysiologic basis of autonomic ganglionated plexus ablation in patients with atrial fibrillation. Heart Rhythm 2009;6:S26–34.

45. Lu Z, Scherlag BJ, Lin J, et al. Autonomic mechanism for initiation of rapid firing from atria and pulmonary veins: evidence by ablation of ganglionated plexi. Cardiovasc Res 2009;84:245–52.

46. Narayan SM, Krummen DE, Shivkumar K, et al. Treatment of atrial fibrillation by the ablation of localized sources: CONFIRM (Conventional Ablation for Atrial Fibrillation With or Without Focal Impulse and Rotor Modulation) trial. J Am Coll Cardiol 2012;60:628–36.

47. Narayan SM, Patel J, Mulpuru S, et al. Focal impulse and rotor modulation ablation of sustaining rotors abruptly terminates persistent atrial fibrillation to sinus rhythm with elimination on follow-up: a video case study. Heart Rhythm 2012;9:1436–9.

48. Chen MS, Marrouche NF, Khaykin Y, et al. Pulmonary vein isolation for the treatment of atrial fibrillation in patients with impaired systolic function. J Am Coll Cardiol 2004;43:1004–9.

49. Hsu LF, Jais P, Sanders P, et al. Catheter ablation for atrial fibrillation in congestive heart failure. N Engl J Med 2004;351:2373–83.

50. Tondo C, Mantica M, Russo G, et al. Pulmonary vein vestibule ablation for the control of atrial fibrillation in patients with impaired left ventricular function. Pacing Clin Electrophysiol 2006;29:962–70.

51. Gentlesk PJ, Sauer WH, Gerstenfeld EP, et al. Reversal of left ventricular dysfunction following ablation of atrial fibrillation. J Cardiovasc Electrophysiol 2007;18:9–14.

52. Lutomsky BA, Rostock T, Koops A, et al. Catheter ablation of paroxysmal atrial fibrillation improves cardiac function: a prospective study on the impact of atrial fibrillation ablation on left ventricular function assessed by magnetic resonance imaging. Europace 2008;10:593–9.

53. De Potter T, Berruezo A, Mont L, et al. Left ventricular systolic dysfunction by itself does not influence outcome of atrial fibrillation ablation. Europace 2010;12:24–9.

54. Akkaya M, Higuchi K, Koopmann M, et al. Higher degree of left atrial structural remodeling in patients with atrial fibrillation and left ventricular systolic dysfunction. J Cardiovasc Electrophysiol 2013;24(5):485–91.

55. Berruezo A, Tamborero D, Mont L, et al. Pre-procedural predictors of atrial fibrillation recurrence after circumferential pulmonary vein ablation. Eur Heart J 2007;28:836–41.

56. McCready JW, Smedley T, Lambiase PD, et al. Predictors of recurrence following radiofrequency ablation for persistent atrial fibrillation. Europace 2011;13:355–61.

57. Nademanee K, Schwab MC, Kosar EM, et al. Clinical outcomes of catheter substrate ablation for high-risk patients with atrial fibrillation. J Am Coll Cardiol 2008;51:843–9.

58. Wood MA, Brown-Mahoney C, Kay GN, et al. Clinical outcomes after ablation and pacing therapy for atrial fibrillation: a meta-analysis. Circulation 2000;101:1138–44.

59. Kay GN, Ellenbogen KA, Giudici M, et al. The Ablate and Pace trial: a prospective study of catheter ablation of the AV conduction system and

permanent pacemaker implantation for treatment of atrial fibrillation. APT Investigators. J Interv Card Electrophysiol 1998;2:121–35.

60. Ozcan C, Jahangir A, Friedman PA, et al. Long-term survival after ablation of the atrioventricular node and implantation of a permanent pacemaker in patients with atrial fibrillation. N Engl J Med 2001; 344:1043–51.

61. Brignole M, Menozzi C, Gianfranchi L, et al. Assessment of atrioventricular junction ablation and VVIR pacemaker versus pharmacological treatment in patients with heart failure and chronic atrial fibrillation: a randomized, controlled study. Circulation 1998;98:953–60.

62. Doshi RN, Daoud EG, Fellows C, et al. Left ventricular-based cardiac stimulation post AV nodal ablation evaluation (the PAVE study). J Cardiovasc Electrophysiol 2005;16:1160–5.

63. Khan MN, Jais P, Cummings J, et al. Pulmonary-vein isolation for atrial fibrillation in patients with heart failure. N Engl J Med 2008;359:1778–85.

64. Choi AD, Hematpour K, Kukin M, et al. Ablation vs medical therapy in the setting of symptomatic atrial fibrillation and left ventricular dysfunction. Congest Heart Fail 2010;16:10–4.

65. MacDonald MR, Connelly DT, Hawkins NM, et al. Radiofrequency ablation for persistent atrial fibrillation in patients with advanced heart failure and severe left ventricular systolic dysfunction: a randomised controlled trial. Heart 2011;97:740–7.

66. Oakes RS, Badger TJ, Kholmovski EG, et al. Detection and quantification of left atrial structural remodeling with delayed-enhancement magnetic resonance imaging in patients with atrial fibrillation. Circulation 2009;119:1758–67.

67. Jones DG, Haldar SK, Hussain W, et al. A randomized trial to assess catheter ablation versus rate control in the management of persistent atrial fibrillation in heart failure (ARC-HF). J Am Coll Cardiol 2013;61:1894–903.

68. Wilton SB, Fundytus A, Ghali WA, et al. Meta-analysis of the effectiveness and safety of catheter ablation of atrial fibrillation in patients with versus without left ventricular systolic dysfunction. Am J Cardiol 2010;106:1284–91.

69. Dagres N, Varounis C, Gaspar T, et al. Catheter ablation for atrial fibrillation in patients with left ventricular systolic dysfunction. A systematic review and meta-analysis. J Card Fail 2011;17:964–70.

70. Efremidis M, Sideris A, Xydonas S, et al. Ablation of atrial fibrillation in patients with heart failure: reversal of atrial and ventricular remodelling. Hellenic J Cardiol 2008;49:19–25.

71. Clark DM, Plumb VJ, Epstein AE, et al. Hemodynamic effects of an irregular sequence of ventricular cycle lengths during atrial fibrillation. J Am Coll Cardiol 1997;30:1039–45.

72. Verma A, Newman D, Geist M, et al. Effects of rhythm regularization and rate control in improving left ventricular function in atrial fibrillation patients undergoing atrioventricular nodal ablation. Can J Cardiol 2001;17:437–45.

73. Duffee DF, Shen WK, Smith HC. Suppression of frequent premature ventricular contractions and improvement of left ventricular function in patients with presumed idiopathic dilated cardiomyopathy. Mayo Clin Proc 1998;73:430–3.

74. Yarlagadda RK, Iwai S, Stein KM, et al. Reversal of cardiomyopathy in patients with repetitive monomorphic ventricular ectopy originating from the right ventricular outflow tract. Circulation 2005; 112:1092–7.

75. Schneider J, Berger HJ, Sands MJ, et al. Beat-to-beat left ventricular performance in atrial fibrillation: radionuclide assessment with the computerized nuclear probe. Am J Cardiol 1983;51:1189–95.

76. Lemola K, Desjardins B, Sneider M, et al. Effect of left atrial circumferential ablation for atrial fibrillation on left atrial transport function. Heart Rhythm 2005; 2:923–8.

77. Kosiuk J, Van Belle Y, Bode K, et al. Left ventricular diastolic dysfunction in atrial fibrillation: predictors and relation with symptom severity. J Cardiovasc Electrophysiol 2012;23:1073–7.

78. Jons C, Joergensen RM, Hassager C, et al. Diastolic dysfunction predicts new-onset atrial fibrillation and cardiovascular events in patients with acute myocardial infarction and depressed left ventricular systolic function: a CARISMA substudy. Eur J Echocardiogr 2010;11:602–7.

79. Elesber AA, Redfield MM. Approach to patients with heart failure and normal ejection fraction. Mayo Clin Proc 2001;76:1047–52.

80. Moon J, Rim SJ, Cho IJ, et al. Left ventricular hypertrophy determines the severity of diastolic dysfunction in patients with nonvalvular atrial fibrillation and preserved left ventricular systolic function. Clin Exp Hypertens 2010;32:540–6.

81. Jais P, Peng JT, Shah DC, et al. Left ventricular diastolic dysfunction in patients with so-called lone atrial fibrillation. J Cardiovasc Electrophysiol 2000;11:623–5.

82. Tsang TS, Barnes ME, Gersh BJ, et al. Risks for atrial fibrillation and congestive heart failure in patients >/=65 years of age with abnormal left ventricular diastolic relaxation. Am J Cardiol 2004;93: 54–8.

83. Tsang TS, Gersh BJ, Appleton CP, et al. Left ventricular diastolic dysfunction as a predictor of the first diagnosed nonvalvular atrial fibrillation in 840 elderly men and women. J Am Coll Cardiol 2002; 40:1636–44.

84. Tsang TS, Barnes ME, Gersh BJ, et al. Left atrial volume as a morphophysiologic expression of left

ventricular diastolic dysfunction and relation to cardiovascular risk burden. Am J Cardiol 2002;90: 1284–9.

85 Pritchett AM, Mahoney DW, Jacobsen SJ, et al. Diastolic dysfunction and left atrial volume: a population-based study. J Am Coll Cardiol 2005; 45:87–92.

86. Reant P, Lafitte S, Jais P, et al. Reverse remodeling of the left cardiac chambers after catheter ablation after 1 year in a series of patients with isolated atrial fibrillation. Circulation 2005;112: 2896–903.

87. Cha YM, Wokhlu A, Asirvatham SJ, et al. Success of ablation for atrial fibrillation in isolated left ventricular diastolic dysfunction: a comparison to systolic dysfunction and normal ventricular function. Circ Arrhythm Electrophysiol 2011;4:724–32.

88. Hu YF, Hsu TL, Yu WC, et al. The impact of diastolic dysfunction on the atrial substrate properties and outcome of catheter ablation in patients with paroxysmal atrial fibrillation. Circ J 2010;74(10):2074–8.

89. Akoum N, Daccarett M, McGann C, et al. Atrial fibrosis helps select the appropriate patient and strategy in catheter ablation of atrial fibrillation: a DE-MRI guided approach. J Cardiovasc Electrophysiol 2011;22:16–22.

90. Verma A, Wazni OM, Marrouche NF, et al. Pre-existent left atrial scarring in patients undergoing pulmonary vein antrum isolation: an independent predictor of procedural failure. J Am Coll Cardiol 2005;45:285–92.

91. Tilz RR, Rillig A, Thum AM, et al. Catheter ablation of long-standing persistent atrial fibrillation: 5-year outcomes of the Hamburg Sequential Ablation Strategy. J Am Coll Cardiol 2012;60:1921–9.

92. Calkins H, Kuck KH, Cappato R, et al. 2012 HRS/EHRA/ECAS Expert Consensus Statement on Catheter and Surgical Ablation of Atrial Fibrillation: recommendations for patient selection, procedural techniques, patient management and follow-up, definitions, endpoints, and research trial design. Europace 2012;14:528–606.

Surgical Treatment of Atrial Fibrillation in the Heart Failure Population

Stephen R. Large, MA, MS, FRCS, FRCP, MBA*,
Samer A.M. Nashef, MB ChB, FRCS, PhD

KEYWORDS

• Atrial fibrillation • Heart failure • Maze procedure • Surgery • Treatment

KEY POINTS

- Surgery to correct a structural heart valve problem can restore sinus rhythm in approximately one-fifth of patients with atrial fibrillation (AF), and the addition of a maze procedure will increase this proportion.
- Evidence shows that the maze procedure may restore atrial function in some patients and may have beneficial effects on functional symptoms and prognosis.
- The addition of a maze procedure for patients with AF undergoing valve or coronary surgery adds little risk and may be beneficial.
- The role of the maze procedure as an isolated treatment for lone AF in the context of heart failure with no structurally correctable cause is unknown.
- Future progress will determine the appropriate indications for treatment and the risks and benefits of any intervention.

INTRODUCTION

Atrial fibrillation (AF) is common, affecting approximately 2% of the population, with this proportion increasing with age.[1] It brings with it an irregular pulse, a loss of coordinated atrial contraction, a 5-fold increase in the risk of stroke, a doubling of mortality, worsening quality of life, and a progression from occasional (paroxysmal) to continuous (persistent) AF. Structural changes are seen in atria with AF (myocyte hypertrophy, fibrosis, inflammation, and apoptosis)[2] and, with a poorly controlled ventricular rate, changes typical of dilated cardiomyopathy are seen. AF is a strong and independent risk factor for the development of heart failure, and both conditions frequently coexist, partly because of overlapping risk factors.[3] In addition to this association, AF reduces cardiac function by reducing ventricular filling

through both loss of atrial contraction and reduced diastolic interval time. This impairment of cardiac pumping action adds fatigue, dizziness, and breathlessness to palpitations in the panoply of symptoms attributable to AF.

Heart failure is also common, and its prevalence also increases with age. It affects at least 10% of the population older than 70 years and has been defined by the European Society of Cardiology as "an abnormality of cardiac structure or function leading to failure of the heart to deliver oxygen at a rate commensurate with the requirements of the metabolizing tissues, despite normal filling pressures (or only at the expense of increased filling pressures)".[3] Its natural history is progressive and the outcome is not good, with survival worsening with increasing severity of heart failure, so much so that patients with drug-resistant advanced heart failure (New York Heart

Disclosures: The authors have nothing to disclose.
Papworth Hospital, Cambridge CB23 3RE, UK
* Corresponding author.
E-mail address: srl24@cam.ac.uk

heartfailure.theclinics.com

Association class IV) can expect a survival rate of only 8% at 2 years.[4] Two mechanisms are thought to account for this: further events leading to myocyte death, such as recurrent myocardial infarction, and myocardial injury, resulting in activation of the renin-angiotensin-aldosterone and sympathetic nervous systems. These systemic responses themselves lead to further myocardial injury, producing a pathophysiologic vicious cycle, resulting in many of the clinical features of the heart failure syndrome, including myocardial electrical instability.[5]

The symptoms and signs of heart failure have some similarity to those of AF. The 2 conditions coexist at a prevalence between 10% and 50% (Fig. 1).[6,7] The probability exists that when combined with AF, the prognosis of heart failure worsens. Certainly the likelihood of stroke increases by a further 3.5-fold when AF and heart failure combine.

MANAGEMENT OF AF IN HEART FAILURE

The management of patients with AF with and without coexisting heart failure follows a series of steps:

1. Identification of correctable predisposing causes
2. Identification of features that favor a rhythm control or a rate control strategy
3. Assessment of thromboembolism risk and implementation of prophylaxis

The treatment of AF per se requires the identification of treatable causes (hyperthyroidism, electrolyte disorders, uncontrolled hypertension, mitral valve disease, ischemic heart disease) and precipitating factors (recent surgery, chest infection, exacerbation of chronic pulmonary disease, acute myocardial ischemia, acute alcohol excess). Treatment directed at the predisposing cause has a variable likelihood of success in correcting AF. Surgery has a role to play in this regard, especially with cardiac structural and ischemic presentations, and is addressed in the following section.

If AF cannot be corrected through treating an underlying cause, pharmacologic management of rate, rhythm, and thromboembolic risk is required. Counterintuitively, the pharmacologic pursuit of sinus rhythm in patients with AF does not seem to improve long-term survival, perhaps even being associated with slightly worse prognosis than merely controlling heart rate. Six trials have failed to show any improvement in prognosis with rhythm control.[8–13] The unadjusted hazard ratio for the rhythm-control group, compared with the rate-control group, was 1.06 (95% confidence interval [CI], 0.86–1.30). Most of those in the rhythm-management group were on amiodarone. Perhaps the complexities of drug therapy and the circumstances that led to AF and heart failure are too much to expect stable sinus rhythm to be consistently and safely achieved. If AF is permanent, the risk of stroke can be quantified using a scoring system that guides appropriate anticoagulation.[14] The main hazard of long-term

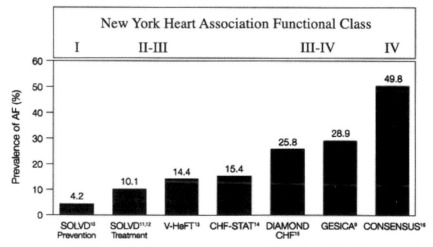

Fig. 1. Prevalence of atrial fibrillation (AF) in several major heart failure trials. CHF-STAT, Congestive Heart Failure Survival Trial of Antiarrhythmic Therapy; CONSENSUS, Cooperative North Scandinavian Enalapril Survival Study; DIAMOND CHF, Danish Investigations of Arrhythmia and Mortality on Dofetilide Congestive Heart Failure study; GESICA, Grupo de Estudio de la Sobrevida en la Insuficiencia Cardiaca en Argentina; SOLVD, Studies of Left Ventricular Dysfunction; V-HeFT, Vasodilator in Heart Failure Trial. (*From* Maisel WH, Stevenson LW. Atrial fibrillation in heart failure: epidemiology, pathophysiology, and rationale for therapy. Am J Cardiol 2003;91(6):2; with permission.)

antiooagulant therapy is bleeding. The risk of anticoagulant-related bleeding can also be quantified using a similar clinical tool, HAS-BLED (H, hypertension; A, abnormal liver or renal function; S, stroke history; B, bleeding predisposition; L, labile INR [international normalised ratio]; E, elderly [age 65 years and older]; D, drugs or alcohol usage),[15] which identifies patients at higher risk. It is possible, of course, that the "holy grail" of sinus rhythm in patients presenting with AF and heart failure can be achieved with a surgical approach.

SURGICAL TREATMENT IN HEART FAILURE AND AF

Heart failure from a variety of causes can be treated well with surgery. Correction of structural abnormalities of the heart, such as replacing a stenotic or regurgitant aortic valve or correcting mitral regurgitation through valve repair or replacement, often abolishes all of the symptoms and signs of heart failure, and can be associated with a markedly improved prognosis. Even coronary artery bypass grafting may improve some of the symptoms of heart failure in selected patients with hibernating, viable myocardium. The effects of correction of a structural valve defect on coexisting AF are less certain. In mitral regurgitation complicated by AF, correcting the valve lesion will restore sinus rhythm in 21% of patients.[16] The rate of sinus rhythm restoration correlated inversely with left ventricular end-systolic diameter. This effect is not commonly seen in patients with AF who have revascularization for myocardial ischemia.

A direct surgical approach to AF is a recent development. Because of an incomplete understanding of its pathophysiology, AF was not regarded as a surgical condition until recently.

Several major breakthroughs have occurred in understanding of the mechanisms of AF. The first is the observation by Haïssaguerre and colleagues[17] that AF often originates in the vicinity of the pulmonary veins. Surgery that is specifically directed at AF began in the 1980s when Williams and colleagues[18] described left atrial isolation. This procedure electrically isolated the fibrillating left atrium from the rest of the heart. Guiraudon and colleagues[19] developed a "corridor" procedure, effectively isolating both atria but leaving intact the connection between the sinoatrial and atrioventricular nodes. Of course, a feature of both the left atrial isolation and the corridor procedure is that the left atrium continues to fibrillate.

In 1987, James Cox[20] proposed the construction of an electrical "maze" throughout the left and right atria. The principle behind this operation is that through electrically isolating the pulmonary veins from the atrial body, and partitioning atrial tissues into a maze in which the "paths" are narrow enough to block the large (≈ 5 cm: **Fig. 2**) macro-reentry circuits, AF can be surgically abolished and sinus rhythm restored.

CURRENT SURGICAL APPROACHES IN AF

The lines of electrical isolation in the maze procedure have been extensively studied since the technique was introduced in 1987. Several modifications to the maze lesion set have been proposed and accepted. One set of lesions in common use

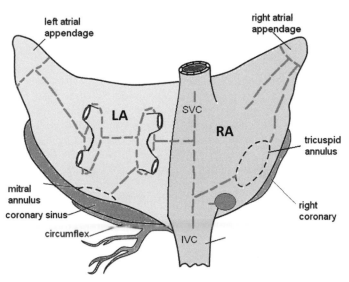

Fig. 2. A maze procedure lesion set: the posterior aspect of the atria is shown. The bold broken lines show the lesion set. IVC, inferior vena cava; LA, left atrium; RA, right atrium; SVC, superior vena cava.

nowadays is illustrated in **Fig. 2**. The maze procedure was originally performed by cutting and suturing atrial tissue along prescribed lines (the "cut-and-sew" maze). Despite reports of a high rate of restoration of electrical sinus rhythm, the cut-and-sew maze procedure never achieved widespread use, possibly because it is a major cardiac operation that requires full median sternotomy and cardiopulmonary bypass, and the extensive suture lines are time-consuming with a predictably substantial bleeding risk. Attention was therefore focused on replacing surgical cuts with electrical isolation achieved through other means, such as radiofrequency, cryotherapy, and even electrocautery. A multitude of devices were developed and marketed to this end, and the number of modified maze procedures performed worldwide increased sharply.

The complete maze procedure, whether achieved using the cut-and-sew method or with the aid of an energy device, still requires median sternotomy and cardiopulmonary bypass to allow access to the mitral and tricuspid annuli, which mark the end point of some of the maze isolation lines. In an attempt to reduce the magnitude of the operation, alternative and less-invasive approaches have been described.

Pulmonary vein isolation instead of the full maze procedure has been proposed based on Haïssaguerre's finding that the pulmonary vein region is responsible for most AF triggers. This procedure is less complex than a full maze, and can be achieved using a port-access approach, which avoids median sternotomy and cardiopulmonary bypass. Some have combined this approach with left atrial appendage exclusion with a view to reducing further the risk of thromboembolism, and with vagal denervation, in an attempt to increase effectiveness. These less-invasive techniques have been reported to achieve sinus rhythm restoration rates of between 52% and 80% at 1 year,[21,22] markedly inferior to those reported for the full maze. To address this gap, a hybrid approach[23] was proposed in which some lesions are created using a port-access surgical approach and others percutaneously in an attempt to achieve as complete a lesion set as possible while avoiding median sternotomy and cardiopulmonary bypass.

The maze procedure, with its many guises and methods of delivery, can now be considered to be firmly established as part of the modern cardiac surgeon's armamentarium. However, no consensus exists on the optimal surgical approach to AF. A full surgical maze procedure undoubtedly has the highest level of effectiveness, but in the context of heart failure, such an invasive procedure should be approached with caution in view of the limited cardiac functional reserve. If surgical treatment is being contemplated for AF in heart failure, the decision must take account of both the effectiveness of the proposed approach and its attendant risk.

Before addressing the role of the maze procedure as a treatment for AF in the setting of heart failure, the state of the evidence must be appreciated for its effectiveness in AF generally. In isolated symptomatic longstanding AF, wherein the predominant symptoms are fatigue and troublesome palpitations, no doubt exists that the maze procedure is effective in reducing symptoms and, probably, thromboembolic risk.[24] The restoration of sinus rhythm varies between 50% and more than 95%, and the success rate depends on several factors. The highest success rates are achieved in AF of relatively recent onset in otherwise normal atria without excessive enlargement, in the absence of other cardiac lesions, in paroxysmal rather than persistent AF, and are enhanced by the completeness of the lesion set created by the maze procedure. However, even in chronic longstanding AF, the maze procedure has a higher success rate of restoring sinus rhythm than percutaneous, open, or port-access pulmonary vein isolation.[25]

A recent review of Cox's own experience[20] with this procedure in lone AF reported an attendant mortality of 1.4% and a freedom from AF of 93% at 1 year and 84% at 10 years. The incidence of stroke was 0.5% at 10 years, with all patients in stable sinus rhythm free of oral anticoagulants.

The incidence of stroke was similarly low after a successful surgical maze procedure in 433 patients. This finding was independent of the CHADS$_2$ (C, congestive heart failure; H, hypertension; A, age 75 years and older; D, diabetes mellitus; S$_2$, prior stroke [or transient ischemic attack or thromboembolism]) score and warfarin use, but was associated with diabetes and previous neurologic events.[26] Ad and colleagues[27] recently investigated the potential benefit from Cox maze surgery in patients with impaired ventricular function (left ventricular ejection fraction $\leq$40%). The sample was small (n = 42) with a mean age of 61.1 $\pm$ 12.9 years, and additive European System for Cardiac Operative Risk Evaluation (EuroSCORE) of 7.5 $\pm$ 3.1. One operative death (2.3%) and no strokes or transient ischemic attacks were reported at follow-up. Ejection fraction improved from 30% $\pm$ 5.0% to 45% $\pm$ 13.0% at a mean of 1.5 $\pm$ 11.3 months after surgery. The return to sinus rhythm at the time of follow-up echocardiography was 86% (35 of 40 patients). The physical functioning and health-related quality of life scores improved (27.0 ± 12.3 to 10.0 ± 0.1, $P = .02$) at 12 months with a significant reduction in symptom severity. The Kaplan-Meier major event-free survival rate at 24 months was 87% (CI, 80.4–91.6; the events considered were redo valve replacement, ventricular assist device implantation, or death).

Therefore, reasonable evidence exists that a maze procedure is effective in restoring sinus rhythm and may allow the withdrawal of anticoagulation in patients in whom this restoration is achieved, and that this can be performed without an attendant increase in the rate of thromboembolic events, but none of this evidence is from randomized controlled trials. Reasons exist to be circumspect in considering this evidence. Patients who are offered major cardiac surgery for AF are almost certainly fitter than the general population with AF. The clinical outcomes achieved in this selected group may not be replicated in typical patients with AF and heart failure, who tend to be older, with structural or myocardial abnormalities. These patients would be symptomatic for a multitude of reasons,[12] perhaps with the heart failure playing a greater role in symptomatology than the AF itself.

Two questions must be answered. The first is whether surgical correction of AF can be justified as a concomitant procedure in patients with AF undergoing major cardiac surgery, such as valve and coronary operations. This question will be answered by the results of further prospective studies, such as the adjunct maze study (the Amaze Trial) to determine whether a maze procedure has added value beyond the production of a regular R-R interval. The second is whether surgical correction of AF as a lone procedure is associated with survival and event-free benefits in patients with heart failure. The answer to this question is unknown, even in patients without heart failure. Much of the anticipated benefits will derive from the restoration of atrial function, which should intuitively be associated with a reduced risk of stroke. Several studies have indicated that some restoration of atrial function can occur[24,28] after surgical maze procedures, but more information is needed to determine whether these benefits justify the risk of a major cardiac intervention in elderly patients in heart failure.

Finally, heart failure and AF may represent a "chicken-and-egg" scenario. Many conditions associated with heart failure are also associated with AF, with documented mechanisms for the effect of mitral lesions and myocardial ischemia on atrial function. However, AF may also cause heart failure, such as through tachycardia-induced cardiomyopathy and, in some patients, atrioventricular valve annular dilatation as a result of the AF and its attendant volume loading and increased atrial and ventricular diastolic pressure. If such a pathophysiologic mechanism is responsible for heart failure, then an argument can be made to manage the AF surgically as a method of heart failure treatment, but much more evidence is needed.

Surgical correction of AF in a well-defined group of patients seems to produce a robust, drug-free cardioversion to sinus rhythm. Evidence shows that this is reasonably safe and effective surgery. Data on maze surgery in the setting of heart failure are limited, but those that are available seem to indicate favorable outcomes, which would mean that the failure of pharmacologic rhythm control in AF may simply reflect the shortcomings and adverse effects of the currently available drugs for rhythm control.

SUMMARY

Surgery to correct a structural heart valve problem can restore sinus rhythm in approximately one-fifth of patients with AF. The addition of a maze procedure will substantially increase this proportion. In patients with troublesome palpitations, the maze procedure can be performed safely and is symptomatically effective. From the viewpoint of effective cardiac function, evidence indicates that the maze procedure may restore some atrial function in some patients, and may be proven in the future to have beneficial effects on functional symptoms and perhaps even prognosis, but the risk/benefit equation remains to be determined. In patients with AF who are undergoing valve or coronary surgery, the addition of a maze procedure adds little risk and may be of benefit, and it is reasonable to assume that this will also apply to the heart failure subset. The role of the maze procedure as an isolated treatment for lone AF in the context of heart failure with no structurally correctable cause is unknown. Future progress in this field will determine the appropriate indications for treatment and the risks and benefits of any intervention, and is likely to require a multidisciplinary approach involving both electrophysiologists and cardiac surgeons.

REFERENCES

1. Kirchhof P, Auricchio A, Bax J, et al. Outcome parameters for trials in atrial fibrillation: executive summary. Recommendations from a consensus conference organized by the German Atrial Fibrillation Competence NETwork (AFNET) and the European Heart Rhythm Association (EHRA). Eur Heart J 2007;28: 2803–17.

2. Frustaci A, Chimenti C, Bellocci F, et al. Histological substrate of atrial biopsies in patients with lone atrial fibrillation. Circulation 1997;96:1180–4.

3. Dickstein K, Cohen-Solal A, Filippatos G, et al, ESC Committee for Practice Guidelines (CPG). ESC Guidelines for the diagnosis and treatment of acute and chronic heart failure 2008: the Task Force for the diagnosis and treatment of acute and chronic heart failure 2008 of the European Society of Cardiology. Developed in collaboration with the Heart Failure Association of the ESC (HFA) and endorsed by the European Society of Intensive Care Medicine (ESICM). Eur Heart J 2008;29:2388–442.

4. Rose E, Gelijns A, Moskowitz A, et al, Randomized Evaluation of Mechanical Assistance for the Treatment of Congestive Heart Failure (REMATCH) Study Group. Long-term use of a left ventricular assist device for end-stage heart failure. N Engl J Med 2001; 345:1435–43.

5. Hohnloser SH, Kuck KH, Lilienthal J. Rhythm or rate control in atrial fibrillation—Pharmacological Intervention in Atrial Fibrillation (PIAF): a randomised trial. Lancet 2000;356:1789–94.

6. McMurray J, Adamopoulos S, Anker S, et al. ESC guidelines for the diagnosis and treatment of acute and chronic heart failure 2012. The Task Force for the Diagnosis and Treatment of Acute and Chronic Heart Failure 2012 of the European Society of Cardiology. Developed in collaboration with the Heart Failure Association (HFA) of the ESC. Eur Heart J 2012; 33:1787–847.

7. Maisel WH, Stevenson LW. Atrial fibrillation in heart failure: epidemiology, pathophysiology, and rationale for therapy. Am J Cardiol 2003;91(6):2–8.

8. Wyse DG, Waldo AL, DiMarco JP, AFFIRM Investigators. A comparison of rate control and rhythm control in patients with atrial fibrillation. N Engl J Med 2002; 347:1825–33.

9. Van Gelder IC, Hagens VE, Bosker HA, et al. A comparison of rate control and rhythm control in patients with recurrent persistent atrial fibrillation. N Engl J Med 2002;347:1834–40.

10. Carlsson J, Miketic S, Windeler J, et al, STAF Investigators. Randomized trial of rate-control versus rhythm control in persistent atrial fibrillation. J Am Coll Cardiol 2003;41:1690–6.

11. Opolski G, Torbicki A, Kosior DA, et al. Rate control vs rhythm control in patients with nonvalvular persistent atrial fibrillation: the results of the Polish How to Treat Chronic Atrial Fibrillation (HOT CAFE) study. Chest 2004;126:476–86.

12. Roy D, Talajic M, Nattel S, et al, Atrial Fibrillation and Congestive Heart Failure Investigators. Rhythm control versus rate control for atrial fibrillation and heart failure. N Engl J Med 2008;358:2667–77.

13. Ogawa S, Yamashita T, Yamazaki T, et al. Optimal treatment strategy for patients with paroxysmal atrial fibrillation: J-RHYTHM study. Circ J 2009;73: 242–0.

14. Lip G, Nieuwlaat R, Pisters R, et al. Refining clinical risk stratification for predicting stroke and thromboembolism in atrial fibrillation using a novel risk factor-based approach the euro heart survey on atrial fibrillation. Chest 2010;137(2):263–72.

15. Pisters R, Lane DA, Nieuwlaat R, et al. A novel user-friendly score (HAS-BLED) to assess 1-year risk of major bleeding in patients with atrial fibrillation: the Euro Heart Survey. Chest 2010;138(5): 1093–100.

16. Large SR, Hosseinpour AR, Wisbey C, et al. Spontaneous cardioversion and mitral valve repair: a role for surgical cardioversion (Cox-maze)? Eur J Cardiothorac Surg 1997;11(1):76–80.

17. Haïssaguerre M, Jaïs P, Shah DC, et al. Spontaneous initiation of atrial fibrillation by ectopic beats originating in the pulmonary veins. N Engl J Med 1998;339(10):659–66.

18. Williams J, Ungerleider R, Lofland G, et al. Left atrial isolation: new treatment for supra-ventricular arrhythmias. J Thorac Cardiovasc Surg 1980;80(3): 373–80.

19. Leitch J, Klein G, Yee R, et al. Sinus node—atrio ventricular node isolation: long term results of the Corridor operation for atrial fibrillation. J Am Coll Cardiol 1991;17(4):970–5.

20. Weimar T, Schena S, Bailey M, et al. The Cox-maze procedure for lone atrial fibrillation a single-center experience over 2 decades. Circ Arrhythm Electrophysiol 2012;5:8–14.

21. Bagge L, Blomstrom P, Nilsson L, et al. Epicardial off-pump pulmonary vein isolation and vagal denervation improve long-term outcome and quality of life in patients with atrial fibrillation. J Thorac Cardiovasc Surg 2009;137:1265–71.

22. Wang JG, Li Y, Shi JH, et al. Treatment of long-lasting persistent atrial fibrillation using minimally invasive surgery combined with irbesartan. Ann Thorac Surg 2011;91:1183–9.

23. Muneretto C, Bisleri G, Bontempi L, et al. Successful treatment of lone persistent atrial fibrillation by means of a hybrid thoracoscopic-transcatheter approach. Innovations (Phila) 2012;7:254–8.

24. Cox J, Ad N, Palazo T, et al. Impact of the maze procedure on stroke rate in patients with atrial fibrillation. J Thorac Cardiovasc Surg 1999;118(5): 833–40.

25. Edgerton J, Edgerton Z, Weaver T, et al. Minimally invasive pulmonary vein isolation and partial autonomic denervation for surgical treatment of atrial fibrillation. Ann Thorac Surg 2008;86(1):35–8.

26. Pet M, Robertson JO, Bailey M, et al. The impact of CHADS(2) score on late stroke after the Cox maze procedure. J Thorac Cardiovasc Surg 2013;146(1): 85–9.

27. Ad N, Henry L, Hunt S. The impact of surgical ablation in patients with low ejection fraction, heart failure, and atrial fibrillation. Eur J Cardiothorac Surg
2011;40(1):70–6.

28. Aikawa M, Watanabe H, Shimokawa T, et al. Preop-
erative left atrial emptying fraction is a powerful predictor of successful maze procedure. Circ J 2009;
73(2):269–73.

Index

Note: Page numbers of article titles are in **boldface** type.

Heart Failure Clin 9 (2013) 541–544
http://dx.doi.org/10.1016/S1551-7136(13)00074-3

heartfailure.theclinics.com

United States Postal Service

Statement of Ownership, Management, and Circulation
(All Periodicals Publications Except Requestor Publications)

1. Publication Title	2. Publication Number	3. Filing Date
Heart Failure Clinics	0 2 5 - 0 5 5	9/14/13

4. Issue Frequency	5. Number of Issues Published Annually	6. Annual Subscription Price
Jan, Apr, July, Oct	4	$224.00

7. Complete Mailing Address of Known Office of Publication (Not printer) (Street, city, county, state, and ZIP+4®)

Elsevier Inc.
360 Park Avenue South
New York, NY 10010-1710

Contact Person
Stephen R. Bushing

Telephone (Include area code)
215-239-3688

8. Complete Mailing Address of Headquarters or General Business Office of Publisher (Not printer)

Elsevier Inc., 360 Park Avenue South, New York, NY 10010-1710

9. Full Names and Complete Mailing Addresses of Publisher, Editor, and Managing Editor (Do not leave blank)

Publisher (Name and complete mailing address)

Linda Belfus, Elsevier, Inc., 1600 John F. Kennedy Blvd. Suite 1800, Philadelphia, PA 19103-2899

Editor (Name and complete mailing address)

Barbara Cohen-Kligerman, Elsevier, Inc., 1600 John F. Kennedy Blvd. Suite 1800, Philadelphia, PA 19103-2899

Managing Editor (Name and complete mailing address)

Adrianne Brigido, Elsevier, Inc., 1600 John F. Kennedy Blvd. Suite 1800, Philadelphia, PA 19103-2899

10. Owner (Do not leave blank. If the publication is owned by a corporation, give the name and address of the corporation immediately followed by the names and addresses of all stockholders owning or holding 1 percent or more of the total amount of stock. If not owned by a corporation, give the names and addresses of the individual owners. If owned by a partnership or other unincorporated firm, give its name and address as well as those of each individual owner. If the publication is published by a nonprofit organization, give its name and address.)

Full Name	Complete Mailing Address
Wholly owned subsidiary of	1600 John F. Kennedy Blvd., Ste. 1800
Reed/Elsevier, US holdings	Philadelphia, PA 19103-2899

11. Known Bondholders, Mortgagees, and Other Security Holders Owning or Holding 1 Percent or More of Total Amount of Bonds, Mortgages, or Other Securities. If none, check box. ☐ None

Full Name	Complete Mailing Address
N/A	

12. Tax Status (For completion by nonprofit organizations authorized to mail at nonprofit rates) (Check one)
The purpose, function, and nonprofit status of this organization and the exempt status for federal income tax purposes:
☐ Has Not Changed During Preceding 12 Months
☐ Has Changed During Preceding 12 Months (Publisher must submit explanation of change with this statement)

PS Form 3526, September 2007 (Page 1 of 3 (Instructions Page 3)) PSN 7530-01-000-9931 PRIVACY NOTICE: See our Privacy policy in www.usps.com

---

13. Publication Title	14. Issue Date for Circulation Data Below
Heart Failure Clinics	July 2013

15. Extent and Nature of Circulation		Average No. Copies Each Issue During Preceding 12 Months	No. Copies of Single Issue Published Nearest to Filing Date
a. Total Number of Copies (Net press run)		203	176
b. Paid Circulation (By Mail and Outside the Mail)	(1) Mailed Outside-County Paid Subscriptions Stated on PS Form 3541. (Include paid distribution above nominal rate, advertiser's proof copies, and exchange copies)	60	56
	(2) Mailed In-County Paid Subscriptions Stated on PS Form 3541 (Include paid distribution above nominal rate, advertiser's proof copies, and exchange copies)		
	(3) Paid Distribution Outside the Mails Including Sales Through Dealers and Carriers, Street Vendors, Counter Sales, and Other Paid Distribution Outside USPS®	12	10
	(4) Paid Distribution by Other Classes Mailed Through the USPS (e.g. First-Class Mail®)		
c. Total Paid Distribution (Sum of 15b (1), (2), (3), and (4))	►	72	65
d. Free or Nominal Rate Distribution (By Mail and Outside the Mail)	(1) Free or Nominal Rate Outside-County Copies Included on PS Form 3541	61	63
	(2) Free or Nominal Rate In-County Copies Included on PS Form 3541		
	(3) Free or Nominal Rate Copies Mailed at Other Classes Through the USPS (e.g. First-Class Mail)		
	(4) Free or Nominal Rate Distribution Outside the Mail (Carriers or other means)		
e. Total Free or Nominal Rate Distribution (Sum of 15d (1), (2), (3) and (4))	►	61	60
f. Total Distribution (Sum of 15c and 15e)	►	133	126
g. Copies not Distributed (See instructions to publishers #4 (page #3))	►	70	50
h. Total (Sum of 15f and g)	►	203	176
i. Percent Paid (15c divided by 15f times 100)		54.14%	52.8%

16. Publication of Statement of Ownership

☐ If the publication is a general publication, publication of this statement is required. Will be printed
in the October 2013 issue of this publication.

☐ Publication not required.

17. Signature and Title of Editor, Publisher, Business Manager, or Owner

Stephen R. Bushing – Inventory /Distribution Coordinator

Date
September 14, 20_3

I certify that all information furnished on this form is true and complete. I understand that anyone who furnishes false or misleading information on this form or who omits material or information requested on the form may be subject to criminal sanctions (including fines and imprisonment) and/or civil sanctions (including civil penalties).

PS Form 3526, September 2007 (Page 2 of 3)

Moving?

Make sure your subscription moves with you!

To notify us of your new address, find your **Clinics Account Number** (located on your mailing label above your name), and contact customer service at:

Email: journalscustomerservice-usa@elsevier.com

800-654-2452 (subscribers in the U.S. & Canada)
314-447-8871 (subscribers outside of the U.S. & Canada)

Fax number: 314-447-8029

Elsevier Health Sciences Division
Subscription Customer Service
3251 Riverport Lane
Maryland Heights, MO 63043

ELSEVIER

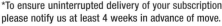